Sympathy
& Science

Sympathy & Science

Women Physicians in American Medicine

REGINA MORANTZ-SANCHEZ

With a New Preface by the Author

The University of North Carolina Press

Chapel Hill & London

Originally published by Oxford University Press in 1985.
Published by the University of North Carolina Press in 2000.

The paper in this book meets the guidelines for permanence
and durability of the Committee on Production Guidelines for
Book Longevity of the Council on Library Resources.

Library of Congress Cataloging-in-Publication Data
Morantz-Sanchez, Regina.
Sympathy and science: women physicians in American medicine /
Regina Morantz-Sanchez.
p.   cm.
Originally published: New York: Oxford University Press, 1985.
Includes bibliographical references and index.
ISBN 0-8078-4890-5 (pbk.: alk. paper)
1. Women physicians—United States—History.   2. Physicians—
United States—History.   3. Medicine—United States—History.
4. Social medicine—United States—History.   I. Title.
R692.M64   2000
610'.82'0973—dc21   00-027309

The author is grateful to the following journals for permission to
quote from her previously published articles: "Making Women
Modern: Middle-Class Women and Health Reform in 19th Century
America," *Journal of Social History* 10 (June 1977); "Professionalism,
Feminism, and Gender Roles: A Comparative Study of Nineteenth-
Century Medical Therapeutics," *Journal of American History* 67
(December 1980); "Feminism, Professionalism and Germs: A Study
of the Thought of Elizabeth Blackwell and Mary Putnam Jacobi,"
American Quarterly 34 (Winter 1982).

04 03 02 01 00   5 4 3 2 1

For
Maxwell M. Markell
zichrono l'vrachah
and
Adam Max Sanchez
l'Torah, u-l'chupah, u-l'maasim tovim

Contents

Preface

When *Sympathy and Science* was first published in 1985, women physicians comprised a mere 14 percent of the profession, although their numbers had been steadily rising since the 1970s. Today, predictions based on medical school enrollments suggest that this figure will reach 40 percent in the first third of the twenty-first century. The presence of women has also increased, although unevenly, in all specialties. It is no longer a shock to encounter a female surgeon, and the field of obstetrics and gynecology, once a male preserve because it was a surgical subspecialty, now attracts large numbers of female medical students. The rhetoric, ideas, and political activism of a resurgent feminist movement helped catalyze these changes, which have resolutely remapped the public landscape in the last thirty years. In addition, new federal and state antidiscrimination legislation and favorable court decisions responsive to decisive social and economic shifts have permanently altered women's opportunities and aspirations in the professions, the world of work, and family life.

It has been more than three decades as well since new scholarship on women began to reconstruct the past in intriguing and innovative ways. Researchers commenced by exploring a broad range of topics, including women's suffrage, changes in women's role in the family, birth control and sexuality, women and abolitionism, colonial witch trials, nineteenth-century female moral reform, and women and work. This literature had become increasingly sophisticated by 1985, making that year an opportune time to publish the first comprehensive study of the history of women in the medical profession in the United States.[1] I was drawn to this topic because it touched on so many questions already being raised regarding the relationship of women to public and private life. At the time, American history was in the midst of a conceptual expansion that resulted in a radical explosion of fields of inquiry and innovative research methodologies. This emergence of what was called "the new social history" enabled investigators for the first time to examine medicine as an artifact of culture. The result was an influx into the history of medicine of young historians who were not physicians and whose view of history was shaped by the Thompsonian social-historical tradition. They linked medical subjects to histories written "from the bottom up."[2]

I was one of those historians, though my interest in women physicians had a personal dimension as well. I understood that entering the academy would place me among the ranks of female professionals. I felt linked in some way with another set of female professionals, women physicians, whom I pictured as struggling to make it in a man's world while attempting to meet the family obligations and role expectations American society imposed on all women. On some level, I believed that I could better comprehend my own private challenges by uncovering their long and complicated history. I was not disappointed.

My aspirations in writing *Sympathy and Science* were relatively straightforward. I wished to combine the best historical scholarship on women with the exciting new work being done in the social history of medicine, producing a volume that would appeal to experts in both fields. In addition, I wanted to offer a narrative spanning all of our nation's history, one that would lay out a useful conceptual framework regarding women and the professions. Finally, I hoped to write a readable account that could appeal to both scholars and the larger public. Judging from the responses of colleagues, physicians, and general readers who have written and spoken to me enthusiastically over the years, I managed in some measure to meet these goals.

Sympathy and Science remains to date the most comprehensive analytical treatment of American women physicians over the last 300 years. Indeed, a range of subsequent scholarship has both expanded its insights and underscored its usefulness as a basic text. The narrative traces the history of women in the medical profession from the colonial period to the present. It recounts the participation of colonial women in healing as nurses, midwives, and practitioners of folk medicine, charts the successful struggles of women in the nineteenth century to enter medical schools and found their own institutions and organizations, and follows women doctors into the latter half of the twentieth century, when their dilemma has been primarily to sustain a significant and rewarding role as full-fledged medical professionals without sacrificing the other privileges and opportunities of womanhood. I argue that the entrance of women into the profession was a consequence of significant alterations in the social and economic realm in the late eighteenth and early nineteenth centuries, resulting in a transformation of family life and the social meaning of gender roles. Some women utilized these changes to insert themselves into public life, choosing a variety of venues. Nineteenth-century middle-class preoccupations with health and fitness created one possible outlet for many women activists, who used their expanded role as mothers to participate in a health reform movement that eventually led them to the conviction that women would make excellent doctors.

Though I carefully chronicle the strong public and professional opposition these women encountered, the book is primarily concerned with what women physicians, who by the turn of the twentieth century numbered almost 5 percent of the profession, managed to accomplish. I examine the hospitals and medical schools they founded. Equally important was their development of a female professional ethos. Their worldview was initially fashioned out of the assumptions of female moral superiority prevalent in the nineteenth century. This notion gave them needed self-confidence and helped many women doctors critique the gradual emergence of impersonal, dehumanized standards of scientific medicine and medical careerism. But it also threatened at times to marginalize them from mainstream professional developments. Indeed, by the last third of the nineteenth century and well into the twentieth, especially as women physicians struggled for an equal place in the profession, they found it more and more self-defeating to retain a perspective on medicine that emphasized their dissimilarities from male colleagues. Some female physicians indicted their sisters for perpetuating a false and outmoded notion of female difference that held them all back. Yet the story of their role in twentieth-century medicine, I argue, is still in large part that of continued wrestling with both the philosophical and cultural (as well as the mundane and practical) implications of what it means to be both a woman *and* a doctor.

Ironically, although historians of women in the 1970s were the first to grapple with the subject of women's health and treatment in the past, U.S. scholars were slow to incorporate insights from the new social history of medicine into mainstream approaches to teaching and scholarship on women.[3] Recent work in the history of the body stimulated by Foucault and feminist theory has, however, dramatically altered this situation. New scholarship committed to refined understandings of the links between power, domination, and resistance in the past has highlighted medicine as an auspicious site for studying complex negotiations between individuals, the professions, bureaucracies, and the state.[4] Also significant in changing contemporary historical scholarship on women is the expansion of research guided by recent theoretical conceptions of gender. In light of these new perspectives, the present seems an appropriate moment to reexamine *Sympathy and Science*. How many of the ideas in the book are still useful, and how have they been modified or enhanced by new scholarly work?

Colonial Beginnings and Separate Spheres

In the chapters that deal with the colonial period and the nineteenth century, *Sympathy and Science* contends that white women's status eventually improved by the second half of the nineteenth century, allowing them to contemplate entering the medical profession for the first time. When originally published, the evidence in *Sympathy and Science* buttressed the work of scholars who were calling into question prevailing assumptions about the existence of a colonial Golden Age—one in which women enjoyed myriad economic opportunities and were not yet subject to the constraints imposed by the rigid sex roles that emerged early in the nineteenth century.[5] The relative openness of social relations in the seventeenth-century colonies, I maintained, did not provide women access to the medical profession. Women did, however, wield authority in the healing arts, most often as midwives, and childbirth was primarily a female-controlled event.

Subsequent scholarship has generally confirmed this view by elaborating on the complexity and unevenness of colonial women's evolving position. For example, Laurel Ulrich's *A Midwife's Tale* treats us to a vivid rendering of the life and female social context of Martha Ballard, a highly respected and very successful midwife, but her story reaffirms my contention that neither medicine's professional impotence in the colonies nor colonial tolerance of occasional gender flexibility enabled women to become licensed doctors.[6] Subsequent research on the seventeenth and eighteenth centuries reinforces a multifaceted and occasionally contradictory portrait of female power and agency, while work on the revolutionary period has verified earlier suspicions that, for women, the end result of republican ideology was a strengthening of the separation of public and private life that led to their banishment from much scientific and intellectual endeavor. We understand even more clearly now why, as I argued fifteen years ago, colonial and revolutionary society was not ready to train women formally in medicine.[7] Still, notwithstanding a recent emphasis on the ways republicanism could confine as well as liberate, Linda Kerber's identification of the emancipatory elements of the ideology of Republican Motherhood and Nancy Isenberg's exploration of the emergence of early women's rights discourse have been helpful in enabling us to understand how some women negotiated more assertive identities in the nineteenth century.[8]

When *Sympathy and Science* was conceived in the mid-1970s, the dominant scholarly paradigm informing scholarship on the nineteenth century was the notion of separate spheres, which focused on white, middle-class, primarily northern women. As then understood, definitions of the concept were not only narrow, but race and class-biased. Historians explored white middle-class women's troubled relationship to emerging concepts of public and private and their struggles to balance newly defined obligations in the domestic sphere with expanded educational opportunities and specifically female forms of public activity. In the beginning, much of the work concentrated on the *prescribed* aspect of these emergent roles, with less attention to how cultural ideologies actually structured women's daily lives.[9]

By the early 1980s, however, historians had begun to expand their understandings of separate spheres, and *Sympathy and Science* was very much a part of this effort. Some scholars argued that women's responsibilities in the bourgeois family eventually catapulted them into new avenues of endeavor, encompassing what has been termed "quasi-political" activity.[10] Others emphasized women's increasing participation in a vibrant consumer economy, underscoring my contention that women were conscientious consumers of health care.[11] Indeed, much of the continued contribution of *Sympathy and Science* lies in its detailed examination of how emerging economic and ideological complexities eventually led some women to pursue a medical education. My work on women physicians describes the ease and frequency with which many white middle-class women moved back and forth between family responsibilities and new forms of participation in the public sphere.[12] It shows how, by midcentury, some of them had already chosen to immerse themselves quite emphatically in both the family and the professionalizing world of science and medicine. Indeed, although many found this effort full of tension and contradiction—and justified their radical choices by utilizing a form of Victorian separate-spheres ideology—they fully believed that women physicians would build a bridge between those two spheres. A favorite story encapsulating their sometimes paradoxical solutions to difficult problems is that of Elizabeth Blackwell's fierce battle to defy middle-class convention by entering medical school, followed by her refusal, after the successful completion of her course at Geneva Medical College two years later, to march in the graduation parade because to do so would be unladylike. How women such as Blackwell managed the personal and professional conflicts that arose out of their efforts is a major theme of the book.

Exploring Diversity

While researching women physicians' lives, I was particularly struck by the multiplicity of their individual choices, within the constraints of prevailing gender and class regimes, a fact that helped to further revise separate-spheres theory. Although the large majority of female doctors practiced primarily among women and children, they lived in both cities and rural towns. Many were suffragists, while others were not; some involved themselves in female reform movements, including the women's medical movement, but others avoided such activities. Some saw themselves as responsible for humanizing the profession; others merely hoped to make a decent living at work more interesting than teaching. Some were highly oriented to professional and scientific change, though a majority were content with general practice. Many believed that women should be trained in medicine to perform a unique role in the delivery of specialized care to women and children, while others hoped to be nothing more or less than family practition- ers and were eager to integrate themselves totally into an increasingly masculinizing professional culture. In other words, women physicians were never a monolithic group, neither in their attitudes toward their place in the profession nor in their assumptions about politics, patient care, or the management of their own private lives.

In order to help illustrate the boundaries at the wide edges of this register of opinion and choice, I compared the differences in the careers and ideas of the two towering leaders of the nineteenth-century wom- en's medical movement, Mary Putnam Jacobi and Elizabeth Black- well. In choosing these two, I sought to explore the range of opinions women doctors could harbor on the important role of the woman phy- sician and her relationship to developments in late nineteenth-century scientific medicine. I argued that Blackwell focused primarily on women's differences from men, while Jacobi spoke much more often of men's and women's shared characteristics.

Meanwhile, as scholars continued to revise and expand the para- digm of separate spheres to better explain women's efforts at shaping their public and familial responsibilities in the nineteenth century, they highlighted what they described as tensions around separatism and in- tegration, and sameness versus difference. I have already noted that nineteenth-women reformers and the institutions they created were often predicated on ideals of female difference and moral superiority.

Indeed, Virginia Drachman argues in her study of the New England Hospital for Women and Children that separatism was a dominant or preferred strategy among the early generation of women doctors, who deliberately stayed within their own institutions.[13] My research on women's medical schools did not support this conclusion, although I readily acknowledge that many women hoped fervently, along with Elizabeth Blackwell, that female students would occupy positions in medicine that "men cannot fully occupy" and exercise an influence that "men cannot wield at all."[14] Moreover, I have argued that some of the disagreements between Blackwell and Jacobi over women's role as doctors could be linked to their differing responses to advances in scientific medicine, and that developments in medicine influenced their thinking as powerfully as did Victorian ideologies about women. I was very clear in my discussion of these two pioneers that they represented a wide spectrum of attitudes and lifestyles. The chapter on Jacobi and Blackwell is richly augmented by two additional chapters of collective biography specifically intended to avert tendencies to interpret women doctors' lives in simplistic dualisms. Rereading those chapters now confirms my view that they still destabilize tendencies to think about women physicians in terms of either/or.[15]

The efforts of *Sympathy and Science* to paint a rich and varied portrait of individual lives and accomplishments did not obviate my historian's desire to understand what those lives had in common as well as how they differed from one another. Did enough women physicians practice an alternative kind of medicine or develop a particular professional style to allow us to conclude that women doctors diverged from their male colleagues in certain particulars? If they did not, does their story still deserve to be separated out from more general histories of the medical profession? What generalizations about women physicians could be made without violating my commitment to the diversity of their lives?

Sympathy and Science makes several inferences, having entered the emerging debates about "gender" just as it became useful to use the term.[16] In discussions of women's health and treatment, I separate notions of gender from an examination of women's behavior. For example, most women physicians believed that they treated patients differently from men. My research confirmed this divergence, but not always in the ways women doctors or other historians would have liked to think. A comparative chapter on obstetrical treatment at two Boston hospitals—one run by men, the other by women—demonstrates, for example, that women doctors did live up to their self image as more empathetic attendants, suggesting that notions of gender affected their delivery of patient care. Women doctors interacted more often with patients in modest ways, prescribing supportive teas and mild drugs more frequently than their male colleagues. They exhibited a greater concern with patients' social situations and took more steps to transition postpartum women into stable environments when they left the hospital. Yet in regard to significantly more controversial therapeutic interventions like the use of forceps, I found male and female doctors' rates of usage to be similar.[17]

On the other hand, female doctors did produce an alternative discourse of women's health and disease that countered, quite emphatically at times, dominant notions of female frailty. Gradually women physicians helped wean Victorian culture away from exaggerated assumptions about the negative role the female reproductive system played in dictating women's health and disease. Women doctors also paid a good deal more attention than male doctors to preventive medicine, a fact in keeping with their argument that they had special contributions to make to the profession. They prided themselves on their interest in what I called "social medicine," and linked it with the public image of the woman doctor, actively involving themselves in a network of public health institutions in the Progressive Era and beyond.

When *Sympathy and Science* was published, historians had not yet invented the term "maternalist state" to refer to late nineteenth- and early twentieth-century governmental changes brought about in response to women's new public activism on behalf of mothers and children. But abundant research in this area in the last decade has both highlighted the importance of the activity I chronicled and located it squarely within new scholarly understandings of maternalist politics. It is clear from *Sympathy and Science* that women physicians, through their work in the Children's Bureau, schools, and other public and private institutions, participated enthusiastically in shaping public health policy, including defining the boundaries of acceptable female adolescent behavior and helping to develop the ambiguous and ambivalent policies of protective constraint that historians like Linda Gordon, Mary Odem, Regina Kunzel, and others have recently explored.[18] Though I also briefly described their participation in the birth control movement, eugenics, and the establishment of sex clinics, additional scholarly work is still needed in this area. Also welcome would be a more thorough examination of women doctors' role in the political debates surrounding the welfare state in general and health care in particular.[19]

Women and Professionalization

In discussing the relationship of women to professionalization at the end of the nineteenth century and the beginning of the twentieth, *Sympathy and Science* highlights the tensions between prevailing concepts of femininity and the evolving professional ethos of scientific medicine. Though women did not choose to become doctors as often as they became teachers in the nineteenth century, medicine was their second most popular occupational preference. Hence, their response to changing developments in the field is an important piece of women physicians' story. I argue that professionalization both encumbered and empowered them in complex ways. It empowered them by establishing an allegedly gender-free standard in which competence was measured by the successful completion of the requirements for a degree. As medical schools gradually opened their doors to women, the number of women doctors grew. But the professionalization process also hindered their progress, because embedded in that increasingly standardized life path was the foundational assumption that aspirants would invariably be men. Medical education and medical lifestyles were tailored to the male life cycle.

In addition, the definition of a medical professional became increasingly intertwined with more modern notions of scientific practice that validated a specific kind of inquiry—controlled laboratory experiments, counting and measuring results, the establishment of protocols of publication and replication. These novel methods of producing knowledge increasingly pushed definitions of the professional physician toward privileging those individuals who could best understand and be identified with experimental protocols and new technologies derived from the laboratory. These forms of knowledge were gendered male, while intuition and empathy were feminized. This development narrowed understandings of professionalism to such an extent that even the traditional bedside skills of male clinicians were often devalued. Medical practitioners such as midwives, whose expertise was grounded in artisanal knowledge and caregiving, lost out when the communities they served embraced doctors, who could more readily be identified with new models of disinterested science.[20]

I suggest that women physicians responded to these conditions by developing a theory of *female* professionalism that helped them stake out a continued place for themselves. They hoped to counteract the masculinized notion of the skilled professional that gained heightened legitimacy with the ascendancy of modern science. Such efforts most often drew them toward "feminine" areas of endeavor: social hygiene and public health work, child-saving, gynecology, pediatrics, obstetrics.

The version of professionalism espoused by some women physicians, I suggest in *Sympathy and Science*, served to critique the narrow careerism and biomedical materialism that they found characteristic of their male colleagues, while also conflating traditional ideas about female self-sacrifice with aspects of an older nineteenth-century ideal—shared by both sexes earlier in the century—of the good practitioner. In subsequent publications I elaborated considerably on these themes.[21] Other historians have taken them up as well. Robyn Muncy, for example, has utilized the idea of female professionalism to characterize the social strategies and political policies of many women activists in the Progressive Era.[22] The fate of this style of female activism in the twentieth century, when "sameness" feminism clashed with and gradually supplanted nineteenth-century notions of female difference, is an integral part of my narrative, especially in the last chapters of the book.[23] Not surprisingly, contemporary scholars, women physicians, and other female professionals still grapple with these issues today.

Recent Scholarship

For lack of solid evidence, *Sympathy and Science* did not take up the question of African American women physicians. My research turned up occasional brief references to a handful of black women pioneers, but the important contextual work on African American women was just beginning when the book was published.[24] Indeed, it was about this time that feminist historians began to move away from a monolithic focus on white women as emblematic of all women's experience and sought, in particular, to regain the history of black women.[25] Estimates suggest that about 115 African American women were trained in medicine by the turn of the century, compared to roughly 7,000 white women, several hundred black male doctors, and approximately 132,000 white men.[26]

Unfortunately, there is still no book-length monograph on the subject of black women physicians, in large part because evidence from before the twentieth century remains difficult to find.[27] In 1985, Darlene Clark Hine began the task of historical reconstruction with an important article, and two years later Gloria Melnick Moldow published an account of the careers of both white and black female physicians in Gilded Age Washington, D.C. The presence in the nation's capital of Howard University, which offered a coeducational medical course to

both blacks and whites, allowed Moldow to provide something no
other historian of women physicians or of black women has offered to
date: an account of the social origins, professional training, and subsequent practice patterns of the city's black women doctors, placed in
the context of evolving professional developments.[28]

In the last fifteen years, black women's history has flourished, with
several new works offering an evocative portrait of the complicated
lives of African American women in the postemancipation period.[29]
These studies have detailed, more than ever before, their problems and
possibilities. Some have suggested that African American women
struggled with "too heavy a load" as they worked to "uplift the race."
Always, they fought a battle on two fronts: *for* better economic and
social conditions for all blacks and *against* the oppression of black
women, not only in the larger culture, but also at home.[30]

Equally valuable are studies of individual black women activists,
white women's reform politics, black women in the nursing profession and other medical institutions, and southern women.[31] This scholarship has deepened our understanding of the rigid constraints white
women's institutional racism placed on black women's access to professional and political development.[32] For example, though Stephanie
Shaw's study of black women professionals does not deal directly
with physicians, read in conjunction with this research on racism, it
offers a stark contrast to my portrait of the daily lives of white women
physicians. The struggle of the black community in the face of late
nineteenth-century Jim Crow restrictions pervasively structured the
education of black girls to communal responsibility, and Hine, Shaw,
and others emphasize the power of this socialization. But the forced
economic marginality of blacks, both North and South, coupled with
educational and occupational discrimination, weakened the ability of
black communities to adequately finance their own training institutions. These conditions help to explain why few black women—or
black men, for that matter—became doctors. As *Sympathy and Science* notes, by the turn of the century medical education became increasingly more expensive, and the percentage of white women physicians became static, just as black women began entering a variety of
professional occupations, including nursing.[33]

Historians have found that, in spite of the patriarchal attitudes of
many black men, black women both enjoyed and encouraged greater
gender role flexibility within their own communities than did white
women. Shaw's work and other studies demonstrate that black women
diverged from white women with respect to work/family patterns in
intriguing ways. Future histories of black and white women physi-

cians may uncover some striking differences. Equally noteworthy is the fact that historians have recently moved beyond attempts to supplement white models only by contrasting them with studies of black women. Many have begun to embrace a multicultural framework that emphasizes ethnic and racial diversity of all kinds, including a reevaluation of international boundaries.[34]

Beyond these new areas of interest, most of the scholarly work published after *Sympathy and Science* has not challenged its conceptual framework, but rather developed, underscored, and amplified its themes.[35] For example, information on sectarian women, though still inadequately mined by scholars, has offered interesting contrasts between these women and regular female practitioners in terms of alternative theories of treatment, attitudes toward the emerging professional ethos, and physician-patient relations, which, among some sectarians, may have been more democratic.[36] Scholars have also begun to look more carefully at the relationship of women physicians to the new medical science that emerged at the end of the nineteenth century. Arleen Tuchman is substantially revising present interpretations of the career of Marie Zakrzewska, the founder of the New England Hospital for Women and Children. By highlighting Zakrzewska's political and scientific background in her native Germany, Tuchman has been able to paint a more nuanced portrait of this enigmatic woman, hitherto imperfectly understood by scholars, while amplifying my discussions of the ties between women physicians and nineteenth-century science.[37]

Another topic explored in *Sympathy and Science* that has benefited from recent feminist theoretical approaches is medical constructions of the female body and the related question of gender and medical treatment. While I have devoted considerable attention to both of these themes in my more recent work, other scholars have also paved the way for increasingly sophisticated approaches to questions we historians grappled with almost two decades ago. We now understand more clearly that the body has a history, and that medical and lay perceptions of anatomy, physical structure, and function are embedded in situated cultural milieus that are not universal, but change through time.[38] These insights have considerably enhanced our perceptions of doctors' encounters with patients, another topic that has recently received increased attention.[39]

In several articles and a newly published book, Ellen More revisits *Sympathy and Science*'s conclusions surrounding the complicated question of women physicians' transition to the twentieth century. Focusing on the notion of striking a "balance," she has expanded my depiction of the various strategies that modern women physicians—required to function in an entirely different medical world from that of their nineteenth-century sisters—adopted to reconcile the dilemmas of equality and difference, not only as full-fledged professionals, but as wives, mothers, and daughters.[40] Recently published biographies and autobiographies have also proved invaluable for exploring these themes.[41] Equally welcome is the first detailed scholarly history of the Woman's Medical College of Pennsylvania, the institution that figured so centrally in my own narrative account of women physicians' complicated struggle for access to equal medical education and expanding professional opportunities.[42]

Comparative perspectives, exemplified by Thomas Bonner's ambitious and insightful study of women's medical education in Europe and the United States, have been especially important in understanding the complexities of American women's access to training.[43] Bonner has demonstrated that, however severe the struggle for women who sought medical education in the United States, barriers lasted longer in Europe. In America, the absence of government regulation enabled women to found their own medical schools by midcentury or to attend the various sectarian schools that welcomed them. Primarily controlled by the state, however, most European universities did not allow women to take the medical degree until the end of the 1860s or the early 1870s. Thus, American women physicians outnumbered their European sisters by significant numbers in the nineteenth century. Many American women eventually sought further training in Europe, rightly convinced of the inferiority of the American system and suspicious of separate women's schools. Ironically, though Europe was late to admit women to the degree, once the decision was taken by state initiative, the policy was protected by law. In contrast, the tradition of private sponsorship of medical education in America enabled U.S. medical schools to discriminate against women well into the twentieth century. While the number of women physicians steadily rose in Europe after 1900, reaching close to 20 percent in Germany by the early 1930s, in the United States the ratio of women doctors stagnated at around 5 percent until the 1960s. In Great Britain before World War II, the figure was double what it was in the United States, with an increase in female physicians since 1900 of 237 percent. As Bonner notes, though Europe and America similarly questioned women's suitability for medicine, the relationship of the state to medical practice eventually determined women's success. In Europe, state control "held private prejudices in check" and "women benefited." In the United States, where "institutions and licensing were more privatized, women often lost out in a complex but discernible way."[44]

New Directions for Future Scholarship

Despite the high quality of new scholarship on women physicians, there is much left to be done. Though work in the last decade and a half has created a textured and sophisticated analysis of black women in various aspects of history that can serve as an excellent backdrop for further studies of black women in the medical profession, we still eagerly await a book-length study. We need to know more as well about the experiences of women of color in medical education and practice. Equally lacking is a better understanding of women's role in sectarian medicine in the early years of the of the twentieth century.[45] Though I have recently elaborated in *Conduct Unbecoming a Woman: Medicine on Trial in Turn-of-the-Century Brooklyn* on the relationship between women physicians and the dominant paradigms of twentieth-century scientific medicine, the topic remains a rich area for further investigation, and the insights of feminist theorists and historians of science on the relationship between science and culture need further amplification.[46]

Women's historians have lately exhibited a great deal of interest in exploring the more recent past, especially women's politics in the twentieth century. They have begun to trace the maternalist impulse through the period of the New Deal and beyond. This work has special relevance to the history of women physicians because of their enthusiastic participation in social medicine. It can help illuminate their differences from their male colleagues and sharpen our grasp of the interface between health concerns and social policy.[47] Missing from our view of twentieth-century developments is a longitudinal understanding of the relationship of women physicians to feminism or of the role the revived feminist movement of the 1960s played in stimulating contemporary women's interest in the professions. How has feminism helped women doctors manage their ambivalent relationship to the dominant American professional ethos or to "nonfeminine" specialties, like surgery?[48]

Contemporary feminism has also focused intensely on issues of women's health. What has been the role of women physicians in this effort, and how have they benefited from it? And what of the relationship between women doctors and patients—female as well as male? Finally, though *Sympathy and Science* linked the history of women physicians to other fascinating topics in recent American history—the emergence of the welfare state and the ascendancy of managed care in the second half of the twentieth century (which provides women doctors with the work hours best suited to marriage and family), women and work, medical research (particularly on women's health), gender relations, sexuality, marriage and family life—many of these subjects remain underexplored.

Optimists are buoyed by the likelihood that women physicians will achieve approximate parity with men in the twenty-first century. They celebrate as well the fact that women now comprise roughly 24 percent of the full-time faculty at U.S. medical schools. Gains have been dramatic and relatively swift. But, according to a study by the Association of American Medical Colleges, the extraordinary advances of the last thirty years are beginning to reach a plateau.[49] What this means for the future of women in medicine remains to be seen. At the very least, it suggests that though overt discriminatory practices have surely diminished, they are still present in muted form. Research on women and the professions suggests that work/family conflicts remain as frustrating as ever.[50] Moreover, it is worth contemplating that women have been invited into the profession at precisely the moment when perhaps the majority of their colleagues deplore the ascendancy of managed care and think that medicine is being degraded and deprofessionalized by the increasing primacy of cost/benefit analyses in determining the outcome of crucial decisions about treatment.

Two recently published autobiographies, both by women surgeons, suggest that in spite of extraordinary advances in the last three decades, women physicians will face the new century still grappling with many of the issues their predecessors could not resolve.[51] Lori Arviso Alford made an extraordinary journey from life on a Navaho reservation to a career as a successful general surgeon and dean at Dartmouth Medical School. Reminding us of women physicians at the dawn of the twentieth century, her account articulates her ongoing struggle to balance the holistic approach to healing characteristic of her Native American heritage with the reductionist, organ-specific focus of Western medical care in general and her chosen specialty in particular. It contributes as well an interesting and important multicultural perspective. Meanwhile, in *Walking Out on the Boys*, the neurosurgeon Frances Conley chronicles how her efforts to be a success in her chosen specialty were thwarted by blatant incidents of gender discrimination, one of which occurred when she was at the pinnacle of her career, after having done "everything right," including forgoing the possibility of children and more conventional forms of familial connection and self-development that might have encumbered her pursuit of professional advancement.

Both these books tell stories that carry extraordinary narrative power when read in the light of women physicians' history. It is my hope that *Sympathy and Science* will continue to provide context for a new generation of historians, physicians, and individuals who believe in the contemporary value of retrieving the past.

Notes

I would like to thank Anne Lombard, Sue Juster, Anna Smith, Steve Peitzman, Michele Mitchell, Charlotte Borst, and, especially, Louise Newman and Barbara Bair for conversations, suggestions, and comments.

1. Two scholarly books on the history of women physicians in the United States preceded the publication of *Sympathy and Science*. Mary Roth Walsh's *"Doctors Wanted: No Women Need Apply": Sexual Barriers in the Medical Profession, 1835–1975* (New Haven: Yale University Press, 1977), charted persistent discrimination against women physicians, dealing less directly with their lives and accomplishments. Virginia Drachman's *Hospital With a Heart: Women Doctors and the Paradox of Separatism at the New England Hospital, 1862–1969* (Ithaca: Cornell University Press, 1984), focused on the history of one important New England training institution.

2. For an example of the new social history of medicine, see David Rosner and Susan Reverby, eds., *Health Care in America: Essays in Social History* (Philadelphia: Temple University Press, 1979), especially the introduction, "Beyond the Great Doctors."

3. My informal impression is that this happened more readily in Great Britain in the 1970s and 1980s.

4. This scholarly literature is now extensive, but three anthologies might serve as introductions: Mary Jacobus, Evelyn Fox Keller, and Sally Shuttleworth, eds., *Body/Politics: Women and the Discourses of Science* (New York: Routledge, 1990); Irene Diamond and Lee Quinby, eds., *Feminism and Foucault: Reflections on Resistance* (Boston: Northeastern University Press, 1988); and Alison M. Jaggar and Susan R. Bordo, eds., *Gender/Body/Knowledge: Feminist Reconstructions of Being and Knowing* (New Brunswick, N.J.: Rutgers University Press, 1989). Also essential reading are Thomas Laqueur, *Making Sex: Body and Gender from the Greeks to Freud* (Cambridge: Harvard University Press, 1990); Barbara Duden, *The Woman Beneath the Skin: A Doctor's Patients in Eighteenth-Century Germany* (Cambridge: Harvard University Press, 1991); and Nancy M. Theriot, *Mothers and Daughters in Nineteenth-Century America: The Biosocial Construction of Femininity* (Lexington: University Press of Kentucky, 1996).

5. The argument is best made in Gerda Lerner's classic article "The Lady and the Mill Girl: Changes in the Status of Women in the Age of Jackson," *American Studies* 10 (Spring 1969): 5–15.

6. Laurel Ulrich, *A Midwife's Tale: The Life of Martha Ballard, Based on Her Diary, 1785–1812* (New York: Alfred A. Knopf, 1990).

7. See especially Kathleen M. Brown, *Good Wives, Nasty Wenches, and Anxious Patriarchs: Gender, Race, and Power in Colonial Virginia* (Chapel Hill: University of North Carolina Press, 1996); Cornelia Dayton, *Women Before the Bar: Gender, Law and Society in Connecticut, 1639–1789* (Chapel Hill: Uni-

versity of North Carolina Press, 1995); Susan Juster, *Disorderly Women: Sexual Politics and Evangelicalism in Revolutionary New England* (Ithaca: Cornell University Press, 1994); and Linda Kerber, *Toward an Intellectual History of Women* (Chapel Hill: University of North Carolina Press, 1997), and *No Constitutional Right to Be Ladies: Women and the Obligations of Citizenship* (New York: Hill & Wang, 1998). See also Joan Landes, *Women and the Public Sphere in the Age of the French Revolution* (Ithaca: Cornell University Press, 1988), and Londa Scheibinger, *"The Mind Has No Sex?": Women in the Origins of Modern Science* (Cambridge: Harvard University Press, 1989).

8. In the end, Kerber comes down on the side of the constraints of republicanism, but she also suggests ways in which women's role as mothers could eventually link them with the state, while admitting that this link was always problematic. Linda Kerber, *Women of the Republic: Intellect and Ideology in Revolutionary America* (Chapel Hill: University of North Carolina Press, 1980), and *No Constitutional Right to Be Ladies*. Nancy Isenberg, *Sex and Citizenship in Antebellum America* (Chapel Hill: University of North Carolina Press, 1998).

9. Barbara Welter's influential article "The Cult of True Womanhood," *American Quarterly* 18 (Summer 1966): 151–74, was a major influence on and exemplar of this early stage of thinking on separate spheres. For my own early discomfort with this approach, which tended to see women primarily as victims, see Regina Morantz, "The Lady and Her Physician," in *Clio's Consciousness Raised: New Perspectives on the History of Women*, ed. Lois Banner and Mary Hartman (New York: Harper Torchbooks, 1973), 38–53.

10. Paula Baker, "The Domestication of Politics: Women and American Political Society, 1780–1920," *American Historical Review* 89 (June 1984): 620–647. Baker's article was stimulated by an abundant literature produced between the mid-1970s and the mid-1980s exploring, delineating, and analyzing this reformist activity.

11. On consumption, see, for example, Elaine Abelson, *When Ladies Go A'Thieving: Middle-Class Shoplifters in the Victorian Department Store* (New York: Oxford University Press, 1989). For more on women as patient consumers, see Regina Morantz-Sanchez, *Conduct Unbecoming a Woman: Medicine on Trial in Turn-of-the-Century Brooklyn* (New York: Oxford University Press, 1999), chap. 6.

12. For a theoretical development of this argument and a discussion of the history of this paradigm, see Linda Kerber, "Separate Spheres, Female Worlds, Woman's Place: The Rhetoric of Women's History," *Journal of American History* 75 (June 1988): 9–39.

13. See below, chap. 4 for their suspicion of separatism.

14. See below, p. 196.

15. A few recent scholars have read into this discussion a kind of binarism that was emphatically absent from the original argument. Ellen More, for example, in an otherwise exemplary new study of women doctors, suggests that I "explored the tension between two typologies of female professionalism: separatist perfectionism and collegial assimilation" (More, *Restoring the Balance: Women Physicians and the Profession of Medicine, 1850–1995* [Cambridge: Harvard University Press, 1999], 9).

16. Joan Scott's *Gender and the Politics of History* (New York: Columbia University Press) was published in 1988. For a still-useful discussion of the dif-

ferences in approach between gender history and women's history, see Louise
Newman, "Critical Theory and the History of Women: What's at Stake in Deconstructing Women's History," *Journal of Women's History* 3 (Winter 1991):
58–68.
17. Below, chap. 8. Contemporary studies note that women physicians probably
spend slightly more time with patients and establish less hierarchical relationships with them while taking a history. Joan M. Altekruse and Susanne W.
McDermott, "Contemporary Concerns of Women in Medicine," in *Feminism
within the Science and Health Professions: Overcoming Resistance*, ed. Sue V.
Rosser (Oxford: Pergamon Press, 1987), 65–88; Steven C. Martin, Robert
Arnold, and Ruth Parker, "Gender and Medical Socialization," *Journal of
Health and Social Behavior* 15 (1988): 161–205; K. D. Bertakis et al., "The
Influence of Gender on Physicians' Practice Style," *Medical Care* 13 (1995):
407–16; and Ludwien Meeuwesen, Cas Schaap, and Cees van der Staak, "Ver-
bal Analysis of Doctor-Patient Communication," *Social Science and Medicine*
32 (1991): 1143–50.
18. On maternalism, see Sonya Michel and Seth Koven, "Womanly Duties: Maternalist Politics and the Origins of Welfare States in France, Germany, Great
Britain, and the United States, 1880–1920," *American Historical Review* 95
(October 1990): 1076–1109. The literature is now voluminous and these are
only representative examples. See Linda Gordon, *Heroes of Their Own Lives:
The Politics and History of Family Violence, Boston, 1880–1960* (New York:
Viking Press, 1988); Regina Kunzel, *Fallen Women, Problem Girls: Unmarried Mothers and the Professionalization of Social Work, 1890–1945* (New
Haven: Yale University Press, 1994); Mary Odem, *Delinquent Daughters:
Protecting and Policing Adolescent Female Sexuality in the United States,
1885–1920* (Chapel Hill: University of North Carolina Press, 1995).
19. There is nothing available that is as detailed on women physicians' participation as, for example, Atina Grossmann's compelling monograph on sex reform in Germany in this period. See *Reforming Sex: The German Movement
for Birth Control and Abortion Reform, 1920–1950* (New York: Oxford University Press, 1995).
20. For the link between the marginalization of midwives and the rise of professional science, see Charlotte G. Borst, *Catching Babies: The Professionalization of Childbirth, 1870-1920* (Cambridge: Harvard University Press, 1995).
See also Regina Morantz-Sanchez, "Feminist Theory and Historical Practice:
ReReading Elizabeth Blackwell," *History and Theory* 31 (December 1992):
51–69. For a very interesting perspective on the complexity of the professionalization process, especially in terms of how its meritocratic values facilitated
women's opportunities even as the masculinization of subject matter and personal lifestyles held their progress in check, see Kirsten Swinth's acute analysis of women in art, *Painting and Professionals: Women Artists and the Development of American Art* (Chapel Hill: University of North Carolina Press:
forthcoming).
21. Morantz-Sanchez, "Feminist Theory and Historical Practice"; "The Gender-
ing of Empathic Expertise: How Women Doctors Became More Empathic
Than Men," in *The Empathic Practitioner: Empathy, Gender, and the Therapeutic Relationship*, ed. Ellen More and Maureen Mulligan (New Brunswick,

N.J.: Rutgers University Press, 1994), 40–58; and *Conduct Unbecoming a Woman*, especially chap. 9.

22. Robyn Muncy, *Creating a Female Dominion in American Reform, 1890–1935* (New York: Oxford University Press, 1991). Although not about women physicians, recent work on women and professionalization has complicated the narrative by carefully delineating class differences between female professionals and clients in ways suggested, but not always fleshed out, in *Sympathy and Science*. These works give us a clearer picture of the professional struggles twentieth-century women physicians coped with, especially those that required them to combat their own marginalization even as they worked to maintain a place in the field for the woman physician. See Patricia Hill, *The World Their Household: The American Woman's Foreign Mission Movement and Cultural Transformation, 1870–1920* (Ann Arbor: University of Michigan Press, 1985), and Linda Gordon, *Heroes of Their Own Lives* (New York: Viking, 1988). More recently, see Odem, *Delinquent Daughters*; Kunzel, *Fallen Women, Problem Girls*; and Elizabeth Lunbeck, *The Psychiatric Persuasion: Knowledge, Gender and Power in Modern America* (Princeton: Princeton University Press, 1994).

23. See Joan C. Williams, "Sameness Feminism and the Work/Family Conflict," *New York Law School Law Review* 34 (March 1990): 347–60.

24. See Dorothy Sterling, ed., *We Are Your Sisters: Black Women in the Nineteenth Century* (New York: W. W. Norton, 1984), 440–50; Margaret Jerrido, "Black Women Physicians: A Triple Burden," *Medical College of Pennsylvania Alumnae Bulletin* 30 (Summer 1979): 44–45.

25. See, for example, Bonnie Thornton Dill, "Race, Class, Gender: Prospects for an All-Inclusive Sisterhood," *Feminist Studies* 9 (Spring 1983): 131–50; Nancy Hewitt, "Beyond the Search for Sisterhood: American Women's History in the 1980's," *Social History* 10 (October 1985): 299–321; Evelyn Brooks Higginbotham, "Beyond the Sound of Silence: Afro-American Women's History," *Gender and History* 1 (Spring 1989): 50–67, and "African American History and the Metalanguage of Race," *Signs* 17 (Winter 1992): 251–74; and Antonia Castañeda, "Women of Color and the Rewriting of Western History: The Discourse, Politics, and Decolonization of History," *Pacific Historical Review* (Winter 1992): 501–33.

26. H. Scott Turner, "History of Women in Medicine," *Los Angeles Journal of Eclectic Medicine* 2 (1905): 125; Darlene Clark Hine, "Physicians, Nineteenth Century," in Darlene Clark Hine, Elsa Barkley Brown, and Rosalyn Terborg-Penn, eds., *Black Women in America: An Historical Encyclopedia* (Bloomington: Indiana University Press, 1993), 2:923–26. See also Todd Savitt, "Entering a White Profession: Black Physicians in the New South," *Bulletin of the History of Medicine* 61 (Winter 1987): 507–40, and "'A Journal of Our Own': The *Medical and Surgical Observer* at the Beginnings of an African-American Medical Profession in Late 19th-Century America," Parts I and II, *Journal of the National Medical Association* 88 (1996): 52–60, 115–22.

27. See Darlene Clark Hine, "Co-Laborers in the Work of the Lord: Nineteenth-Century Black Women Physicians," in *"Send Us a Lady Physician": Women Doctors in America, 1835–1920*, ed. Ruth J. Abram (New York: W. W. Nor-

ton, 1985), 107–20. This lack does not exist for the twentieth century. To my knowledge, more work on black women physicians is presently being done by Hine and Vanessa Northington Gamble, M.D., Ph.D., professor of the history of medicine at the University of Wisconsin. As scholarly supervisor of The Oral History Project on Women and Medicine sponsored by the Archives on Women in Medicine of the Medical College of Pennsylvania, 1975–79, I, along with another interviewer, completed lengthy oral autobiographies of four black women physicians of different ages and specialties. One, the story of Vanessa Northington Gamble, was published in Regina Morantz, Cynthia Pomerleau, and Carol Fenichel, eds., *In Her Own Words: Oral Histories of Women Physicians* (Westport, Conn.: Greenwood Press, 1982). Full transcripts of interviews with Gamble (March 15, 1978), a medical student at the time, Dr. Dorothy Brown (February 27, 1978), Dr. Victoria Nichols (March 24, 1978), and Dr. Jeanne Spurlock (June 2, 1978) are on deposit at the Archives on Women in Medicine, Medical College of Pennsylvania, Philadelphia. Radcliffe Women's Archives also commissioned several oral autobiographies of this kind, and the transcript of my interview with Dr. Eleanor Makel (January 21, 1983) is located at the Schlesinger Library. Fortunately, there are also a number of biographies and autobiographies available for the twentieth century. See, for example, Sara Lawrence Lightfoot, *Balm in Gilead: Journal of a Healer*, Radcliffe Biography Series (New York: Addison Wesley, 1988).

28. Hine, "Co-Laborers in the Work of the Lord." Gloria Melnick Moldow, *Women Doctors in Gilded Age Washington: Race, Gender, and Professionalization* (Urbana: University of Illinois Press, 1987).

29. See, for example, Evelyn Brooks Higginbotham, *Righteous Discontent: The Women's Movement in the Black Baptist Church, 1880–1920* (Cambridge: Harvard University Press, 1999); Deborah Gray White, *Too Heavy a Load: Black Women in Defense of Themselves, 1894–1994* (New York: W. W. Norton, 1999); Tera Hunter, *To 'Joy My Freedom: Southern Black Women's Lives and Labors after the Civil War* (Cambridge: Harvard University Press, 1997); Darlene Clark Hine, *Black Women in White: Racial Conflict and Cooperation in the Nursing Profession, 1890–1950* (Bloomington: Indiana University Press, 1989); Nell Painter, *Standing at Armageddon: The United States, 1877–1919* (New York: W. W. Norton, 1987); Rosalyn Terborg-Penn, *African American Women in the Struggle for the Vote, 1850–1920* (Bloomington: University of Indiana Press, 1998); Glenda Gilmore, *Gender and Jim Crow: Women and the Politics of White Supremacy in North Carolina, 1896–1920* (Chapel Hill: University of North Carolina Press, 1996); Stephanie Shaw, *What a Woman Ought to Be and Do: Professional Women Workers During the Jim Crow Era* (Chicago: University of Chicago Press, 1996); and Susan L. Smith, *Sick and Tired of Being Sick and Tired: Black Women and the National Negro Health Movement, 1915–1950* (Philadelphia: University of Pennsylvania Press, 1995).

30. For an excellent discussion of the larger context of race uplift ideology see Kevin Gaines, *Uplifting the Race: Black Leadership, Politics, and Culture in the Twentieth Century* (Chapel Hill: University of North Carolina Press, 1996). For an excellent analysis of recent historiography on African American gender and sexual relations, see Michele Mitchell, "Silences Broken, Silences

Kept: Gender and Sexuality in African-American History," *Gender and History* 11 (November 1999): 433–44.

31. See, for example, Gail Bederman, *Manliness and Civilization: A Cultural History of Gender and Race in the United States, 1880–1917* (Chicago: University of Chicago Press, 1995); Louise Newman, *White Women's Rights: The Racial Origins of Feminism in the United States* (New York: Oxford University Press, 1999); Hine, *Black Women in White*; Vanessa Northington Gamble, *Making a Place for Ourselves: The Black Hospital Movement, 1920–1945* (New York: Oxford University Press, 1995); Jacquelyn Dowd Hall, *Revolt against Chivalry: Jessie Daniel Ames and the Women's Campaign against Lynching* (New York: Columbia University Press, 1979).

32. Interestingly, the Woman's Medical College of Pennsylvania, partly because it was a Quaker-founded school, had an exemplary record on admitting black women and other racial minorities. See Steve Peitzman, *"A New and Untried Course": Woman's Medical College and Medical College of Pennsylvania, 1850–1998* (New Brunswick, N.J.: Rutgers University Press, 2000).

33. See Shaw, *What a Woman Ought to Be and Do*, and Hine, *Black Women in White*. See also Natalie J. Sokoloff, *Black and White Women in the Professions: Occupational Segregation by Race and Gender, 1960–1980* (New York: Routledge, 1992).

34. See Castañeda, "Women of Color," and several of the essays in Chandra Mohanty, Ann Russo, and Lourdes Torres, eds., *Third World Women and the Politics of Feminism* (Bloomington: Indiana University Press, 1991). See also Barbara Bair and Susan E. Cayleff, eds., *Wings of Gauze: Women of Color and the Experience of Health and Illness* (Detroit: Wayne State University Press, 1993). For sketches of black women physicians in the twentieth century, see More, *Restoring the Balance*.

35. See, for example, Gail L. McDaniel, "Women, Medicine, and Science: Kansas Female Physicians, 1880–1910," *Kansas History* 21 (Fall 1998): 102–17.

36. See Jane Donegan, *"Hydropathic Highway to Health": Women and Water Cure in Antebellum America* (Westport, Conn.: Greenwood Press, 1986); Susan Cayleff, *Wash and Be Healed: The Water-Cure Movement and Women's Health* (Philadelphia: Temple University Press, 1987). See also Naomi Rogers, "Women and Sectarian Medicine," in *Women, Health, and Medicine in America: A Historical Handbook*, ed. Rima Apple (New York: Garland Publishing, Inc., 1990), and Clark Davis, "Called by God, Led by Men: Women Face the Masculinization of American Medicine at the College of Medical Evangelists, 1909–1922," *Bulletin of the History of Medicine* (Fall 1993): 119–48.

37. See Arleen Tuchman, "'Only in a Republic Can it Be Proved That Science Has No Sex': Marie Elizabeth Zakrzewska and the Multiple Meanings of Science in the Nineteenth-Century United States," *Journal of Women's History* 11 (Spring 1999): 121–42. Tuchman is writing a biography of Zakrzewska. Also interesting in this regard is Susan Wells, *Out of the Deadhouse: Nineteenth-Century Women Physicians and Their Writing of Medicine* (Madison: University of Wisconsin Press, 2000).

38. The work of Foucault has been essential here. Studies that have been particularly helpful to me include the following: Duden, *The Woman Beneath the Skin*; Theriot, *Mothers and Daughters in Nineteenth-Century America*;

Laqueur, *Making Sex*; Joan Brumberg, *Fasting Girls: The Emergence of Anorexia Nervosa as a Modern Disease* (Cambridge: Harvard University Press, 1988); and several of Sander Gilman's monographs, including *Disease and Representation: Images of Illness from Madness to AIDS* (Ithaca: Cornell University Press, 1988). Wonderfully provocative is Rachel P. Maines, *The Technology of the Orgasm: "Hysteria," the Vibrator, and Women's Sexual Satisfaction* (Baltimore: Johns Hopkins University Press, 1999). See also Morantz-Sanchez, *Conduct Unbecoming a Woman*, chap. 5.

39. See Alexandra Dundas Todd, *Intimate Adversaries: Cultural Conflict between Doctors and Women Patients* (Philadelphia: University of Pennsylvania Press, 1989); Wendy Mitchinson, *The Nature of Their Bodies: Women and Their Doctors in Victorian Canada* (Toronto: University of Toronto Press, 1991); Patricia A. Vertinsky, *The Eternally Wounded Woman: Women, Doctors, and Exercise in the Late Nineteenth Century* (New York: St. Martin's Press, 1990); Nancy Theriot, "Women's Voices in Nineteenth-Century Medical Discourse: A Step Toward Deconstructing Science," *Signs* 19 (Autumn 1993): 1–31; Morantz-Sanchez, *Conduct Unbecoming a Woman*, chap. 6. See also my "Comment: Negotiating Power at the Bedside: Nineteenth-Century Patients and Their Gynecologists," forthcoming in *Feminist Studies*.

40. See Ellen More, "The Blackwell Medical Society and the Professionalization of Women Physicians," *Bulletin of the History of Medicine* 61 (Winter 1987): 603–28; and "'A Certain Restless Ambition': Women Physicians and World War I," *American Quarterly* 41 (December 1989): 636–60; and *Restoring the Balance*, where she offers a number of important biographical sketches.

41. See, for example, Joycelyn Elders, M.D., *From Sharecropper's Daughter to Surgeon General of the United States of America* (New York: Morrow, 1996); Mary Canaga Rowland, *As Long as Life: The Memoirs of a Frontier Woman Doctor* (Seattle: Storm Peak Press, 1994); *Doc Susie* (Carpenteria, Calif.: Manifest Publications, 1991); Eva Salber, *The Mind Is Not the Heart: Recollections of a Woman Physician* (Durham: Duke University Press, 1989); Beulah Parker, *The Evolution of a Psychiatrist* (New Haven: Yale University Press, 1987); Ellen Lerner Rothman, *White Coat: Becoming a Doctor at Harvard Medical School* (New York: William Morrow, 1999); Perri Klass, *A Not Entirely Benign Procedure* (New York: G. Putnam & Sons, 1987); Morantz, Pomerleau, and Fenichel, *In Her Own Words*; Frances K. Conley, M.D., *Walking Out on the Boys* (New York: Farrar, Straus and Giroux, 1998).

42. Peitzman, *"A New and Untried Course."*

43. Thomas Bonner, *To the Ends of the Earth: Women's Search for Education in Medicine* (Cambridge: Harvard University Press, 1992). See also Shirley Roberts, *Sophia Jex-Blake: A Woman Pioneer in Nineteenth-Century Medical Reform* (New York: Routledge, 1993), and, for the Australian case, Rosemary Pringle, *Sex and Medicine: Gender, Power and Authority in the Medical Profession* (Cambridge, England: Cambridge University Press, 1998).

44. Bonner, *To the Ends of the Earth*, 166, 164.

45. For needed avenues of research, see Naomi Rogers's excellent historiographical essay, "Women in Sectarian Medicine."

46. This literature is now very rich. A good place to start would be Evelyn Fox Keller, *Reflections on Gender and Science* (New Haven: Yale University Press, 1985); Ruth Bleier, *Science and Gender: A Critique of Biology and Its*

Theories on Women (Elmsford, N.J.: Pergamon Press, 1984); Ruth Bleier, ed., *Feminist Approaches to Science* (Elmsford, N.J.: Pergamon Press, 1986); Ludmilla Jordanova, *Sexual Visions: Images of Gender in Science and Medicine between the Eighteenth and Twentieth Centuries* (Madison: University of Wisconsin Press, 1989); Sandra Harding and Jean F. O'Barr, *Sex and Scientific Inquiry* (Chicago: University of Chicago Press, 1987); and Donna Harraway, *Simians, Cyborgs, and Women* (New York: Routledge, 1991). See also anthropologist Joan Cassell's *The Woman in the Surgeon's Body* (Cambridge: Harvard University Press, 1998).

47. See, for example, Ellen Leopold, *A Darker Ribbon: Breast Cancer, Women, and Their Doctors in the Twentieth Century* (Boston: Beacon Press, 1999).

48. See Cassell, *The Woman in the Surgeon's Body*.

49. See Janet Bickel et al., *Women in U.S. Academic Medicine Statistics, 1998* (Washington, D.C.: American Association of Medical Colleges, 1998), especially 1–2. See the Winter 2000 issue of the *Journal of the American Women's Medical Association* (vol. 55) for an update on a wide range of issues related to the current status of women physicians.

50. See Cassell, *The Woman in the Surgeon's Body*. Especially instructive in this regard for all professionals is Constance Coiner and Diana Hume George, eds., *The Family Track* (Urbana: University of Illinois Press, 1998).

51. Lori Arviso Alford, M.D., *The Scalpel and the Silver Bear: The First Navaho Woman Surgeon Combines Western Medicine and Traditional Healing* (New York: Bantam Books, 1999); Conley, *Walking Out on the Boys*. For a perspective on Conley's early career as a surgeon, see my interview with her, June 20, 1977, Archives on Women in Medicine, Medical College of Pennsylvania.

Acknowledgments

The longer it takes to finish a book, the more debts an author accumulates. My list is extensive. First, several people gave me significant encouragement at the early stages of this study. Gerda Lerner, William Chafe, John Blake, James Cassedy, Judith Walzer Leavitt, James W. Reed, Nancy P. Weiss, Ronald Walters, Carl Degler, Guenter Risse, Ronald Numbers, Kirk Jeffrey, Joyce Antler, Ellen Chesler, Martin Pernick, Eric Foner, Patricia Spain Ward, and Lois Banner all expressed enthusiasm in this project at a time when I myself hardly believed that it would ever come to fruition.

During the course of the research, I received courteous and efficient help from the staffs of a number of libraries, including the Special Collections at Columbia, Stanford and Cornell Universities, the Stanford Medical School Library, the Huntington Library, the Social Welfare Archives, University of Minnesota, the Michigan Historical Collections, the Deering Library, Northwestern University, the Rudolph Matas Library, Tulane University, the American Philosophical Society Library, the Schlesinger Library at Radcliffe College, the Massachusetts Historical Society, and the University of Kansas Medical Library. Michael W. Sedlak of Northwestern University Library tendered meticulous research assistance, and Eric Case of the University of Kansas Medical Library handled efficiently more interlibrary loans than he bargained for.

Dorothy Hanks's cheerful assistance during the two years I worked in the reading room of the National Library of Medicine and the good-natured flexibility of Richard Wolfe, director of the Countway Library, in providing me with manuscript material at a particularly crucial period in my research are still remembered with appreciation. Eleanor Lewis at the Sophia Smith Collection went out of her way several times to furnish me with needed documents, and each effort was accompanied by enthusiasm for this work. Alice McCone and Beatrice McLeod generously shared with me the diaries and letters of their great aunts, Drs. Harriet Belcher and Anna M. Fullerton, respectively. Claire Schultz and Carol Fenichel, then with the Florence A. Moore Library of the Medical College of Pennsylvania, also furnished indispensable assistance. But it is to Sandra Chaff, director, Margaret Jerrido, assistant archivist, and later Jill Gates Smith at the Archives and Special Collections on Women in Medicine of the same institution that I owe my greatest debt of gratitude. Their wholehearted faith in this project has never failed. Not only have they been careful to direct me to archival material that I otherwise might have missed during my visits to Philadelphia, but they have also researched new collections for me long distance, in order to keep me updated. They have never turned down a request for aid; I fear I will not be able to properly repay them for their help.

I am grateful to a number of institutions for the financial assistance that made my research possible. Early stages of this project were supported by a two-year grant from the National Library of Medicine, a grant-in-aid from the National Council of Learned Societies, a summer stipend and a Senior Fellowship from the National Endowment for the Humanities, and two summer Faculty Research Grants from the University of Kansas. I spent 1982–83 as a fellow of the Charles Warren Center of Harvard University. The last stages of this book were completed there under most pleasant circumstances, featuring outstanding secretarial support from Pat Denault and Peggy Burtlet.

My colleagues at the University of Kansas, both those in history and in women's studies, have been especially encouraging. Additionally, the secretarial staff of my own department provided me with prompt, cheerful and efficient aid. Janet Crow's agreeable manner does not detract in any way from her ability to expedite requests with brisk competence. Sandee Kennedy, my typist, has been a patient and extraordinarily skillful assistant. Her unsolicited expressions of enthusiasm for the book have buoyed my spirits at times when the completion of this project appeared to be elusive.

Sue Zschoche furnished research assistance of superior quality. Her intelligence and skill in understanding my goals and in sifting through large amounts of material saved me time and energy. She is a fine historian in her own right, and our conversations about her findings were always very helpful to me. Her assistance with the statistical portions of this work was essential, as was her friendship in these past several years.

Phil Paludan, David Katzman, Bill Chafe, John Clark, Janet Sharistanian, Allan Brandt, Joan Brumberg, Barbara Rosenkrantz, Michael Fellman, Joyce Antler, Constance McGovern, George Sanchez, Rita Napier, Edna Manzer and Barbara Sicherman all read portions of the manuscript and offered helpful suggestions.

Rosalind Rosenberg, Ellen Chesler, Gloria Melnick Moldow, Judith Walzer Leavitt, James W. Reed, Anita Clair Fellman, Ann Schofield, and Clifford Griffin read through the entire manuscript at least once, and some of them more than once. Each of them is responsible for improvements in thought and word. Their confidence in me and in this project has been unflagging. I will always be in their debt. My respect and gratitude goes also to Sheldon Meyer of Oxford University Press for his friendship, patience and enthusiasm for this project; and to Pam Nicely, my skillful copyeditor, special thanks for making its final production stages a wholly pleasant experience.

I am grateful to my many friends who gave me moral and emotional support. Henry Balser, Ari Averett, Mark Fitzerman, Alice Blue, Will Docter, Stan Stern, Ann Schofield, Bea Chorover, Jo Jeanne Calloway, Lee Denner, Steve Shaw, Esther Gross, Sue Ellmaker, Rita Napier, Joan Meisel, and Bill and Lorna Chafe were always there when I needed them. Rosalind Rosenberg never once stopped believing in this undertaking and offered encouragement all along the way. Jim Reed was always willing to give advice and several times dropped what he was currently doing to read a chapter and offer suggestions.

My mother, Rosalind Markell, and Jane Merriweather, Susan English Bower and especially Kerry Trotter kept my young daughters, Alison and Jessica, busy and satisfied when I had to work. As the years passed and Alison and Jessica grew old enough to take care of themselves, they became a support network of last resort. They believed in this book and respected my right to seé it to its finish, even when it meant giving up time with their mother. In the last stages of completion, they even babysat for their new brother, Adam Max. Their love has been more to me than they will ever know.

My father died before this book was completed. But his stubborn insistence that I could accomplish anything that I set my mind to do was a lesson that sustained me long after I could no longer hear him tell me so in person.

George Sanchez came into my life after I had spent more years than I want to admit working on this project. Yet his contribution to it has been immeasurable. We both know how important he was to its completion.

Sympathy
& Science

Introduction

In 1916, when Pauline Stitt was seven years old, her mother gave her a set of Louisa May Alcott's books for Christmas. She started out reading *Little Women* and before long went on to *Little Men*. Halfway through the book she discovered Nan, the girl who planned to be a doctor. "I rushed to my mother," Stitt recalled, "and demanded, 'Mama, you know this girl Nan? She is going to be a doctor. Well, Mama, are girls ever doctors?' " "Yes, certainly," Stitt's mother answered. "Oh, for goodness sake," responded the daughter. "Well, then, that's what I'm going to be. . . . I didn't know before that girls could be doctors." Seventeen years later Pauline Stitt received her medical degree from the University of Michigan.[1]

This is a book about women physicians. It traces their history in the medical profession in the United States. Beginning with a discussion of the colonial period, when women were not members of the profession but participated in healing as nurses, midwives, and practitioners of folk medicine, the narrative moves to an examination of the antebellum health reform movement and its role in making public the idea that health is a female responsibility. Finally, the book describes the entrance of women into the profession and tells the story of their long struggle to become respected professionals in the eyes of male colleagues and the public at large. Because of the book's scope and a disconcerting lack of source material, black women physicians and sectarian women have been largely passed over in this account. Each group deserves further scrutiny, and it is my hope that this study will inspire others to pursue topics which I have been forced by time and circumstance to omit.

The entrance of women into the medical profession in the nineteenth century was integrally connected to the rise of feminism.

Throughout this book, feminism will be defined as broadly as possible. It will signify a movement that at its core intended to connect women in some integral way with public life. Feminism generated an extensive spectrum of public activity for women and a wide range of ideological explanations to justify that public activity. Feminists disagreed about many things. They differed, for example, over whether the best means to accomplish their goals would be to press for women's suffrage. Some argued that the suffrage was a sine qua non of women's full participation in the community. Others believed that women's work would best be confined to those concerns which were most obviously "feminine"—the education of the young, the safekeeping of social morality, moral and religious uplift among the poor, municipal housekeeping, bringing the benefits of medical science to bear on family life. Most feminists, especially in the nineteenth century, believed that women should enter public life because they had a unique contribution to make that men could not. A minority of bolder thinkers claimed women's right to participate on the grounds of equality, justice, and the critical importance of satisfying work to proper human development. Many felt that even after women gained full participation in politics, education, and the professions, they would continue to act like women and fortunately would bring their special perspective to their work. Others insisted that once women were properly exposed to public and professional life, they would learn to act more like men, and that was all to the good.

The ranks of women doctors displayed this wide-ranging diversity. Many would not have called themselves feminists. Some were unmoved by the suffrage campaign; there were even a few who opposed female suffrage altogether and spoke against it.[2] They disagreed over strategy and substance. One group concentrated on the building of separate institutions in order to preserve and strengthen female spheres of influence within the profession. Another wished to see women assimilate into male institutions as quickly as possible. Yet however much they differed over specific issues or strategies, women physicians expressed feminism in their behavior. Each of them sought for themselves a closer connection between woman's traditional sphere—the family—and the larger public arena. Each of them believed that entering the professional world by becoming a physician was a perfectly legitimate choice for a woman to make.

If there was a dominant point of view among women doctors in the nineteenth and early twentieth centuries, it was that women belonged in the medical profession by virtue of their natural gifts as healers and nurturers. Most would have agreed with Dr. Ella Flagg Young when she observed that "every woman is born a doctor. Men have to study to become one."[3] By the middle of the nineteenth century, medicine appeared especially suited for women because it combined the alleged authority of science with a dedication to alleviating suffering that seemed inherently female. In a period when the family was thought to be particularly threatened by the crassness and moral depravity of a rapidly industrializing society unprepared for the burgeoning problems of poverty and disease, women physicians seemed exceptionally suited for teaching the practical tenets of family health and hygiene that would both protect and soothe an anxious public. In theory at least, they would be dedicated practitioners, oblivious to selfish motives and sensitive to the wives, mothers, and children who would be their primary constituency. They alone could combine sympathy and science—the hard and soft sides of medical practice. "Medicine is indeed a science," Professor Henry Hartshorne reminded his female students at the Woman's Medical College of Pennsylvania in 1872, "but its practice is an art."[4] To the supporters of women's entrance into the profession, the fact that women would bring cooperation, selflessness, nurturing, purity, and social concern to their work was the strongest possible justification for the continued existence of the woman physician.

Less clearly understood at the time were other forces at work which resulted in the ascendancy of professional and scientific standards distinctly different from, and often at odds with "female" values. In the professionalizing world of late nineteenth- and twentieth-century medicine, individualism, scientific objectivity, rationality, personal achievement and careerism formed a new ethos which one historian has labeled "the culture of professionalism."[5] As women struggled for an equal place in medicine, they came into contact with this ethos, and, as committed professionals, dutifully upheld and transmitted its precepts. At the same time, they were segregated from the larger social milieu by their separate experience as women living in a Victorian culture which did not yield easily to the deliberate blurring of the sexual spheres. Moreover, they remained a tiny numerical minority within the medical profession. As a minority and as women, they viewed professionalism from a different and more critical perspective than the majority of their male colleagues.

Nothing illustrates these subtle tensions better than an examina-

tion of gender and medical treatment in the last third of the nineteenth century. Though women physicians believed that they differed markedly from the men in their respective therapeutic styles,
few of these alleged distinctions in treatment can be found in the
patient records. A comparison of obstetrical management at a
male-staffed and a female-staffed hospital in Boston demonstrated
only negligible differences in the administration of heroic drugs
and the use of intervention techniques, such as forceps. What the
records did reveal were possible differences in the subjective experience of the patients. Women physicians had more contact with
their charges, they exhibited a greater concern for patients' moral
and emotional well-being, and their institutions were slower to
respond to the emerging "modern" professional ethos which discarded traditional holistic methods of care in favor of more technocratic approaches.

Thus, the inherent contradictions in the position of these first
generations of women physicians presented them with an interesting and sometimes painful dilemma. Which values should be given
prominence? The writings of many nineteenth- and twentieth-
century women doctors reveal that they believed it possible to act
on both sets of principles: they could humanize society, raise the
moral tone of the profession, and rationalize the family by bringing
science into the home all at once. In the end they helped to accomplish only the last of these goals—the rationalization of the family.
Moreover, as successive generations of young women entered
medicine and learned the habits of rationality, efficiency, and the
scientific method in an overwhelmingly male professional world,
their distinct female vision was gradually lost.

But first, many women physicians, Elizabeth Blackwell being
only the most prominent among them, successfully mounted a critique of the impersonal, dehumanized standards of scientific medicine and of the career building of modern professionalism. During
periods of liberal reform, they received substantial public support
for their position. From 1880 to 1930, women physicians were
highly visible in this nation's reform movements. They were particularly adept at developing programs for women and children
that became an integral part of the liberal welfare state.

As the political atmosphere became hostile to liberalism in the
decade after World War I, the critical vision of women physicians
became a minority position. Even the period of New Deal reform
was no exception to the pattern. Unprecedented economic hardship generated such a strong national outcry against working

women that women professionals also suffered from public disapproval. In spite of the presence in the 1930s of a handful of women physicians like the Children's Bureau Chief Martha May Eliot, women doctors were generally less conspicuous in New Deal reform than they were only two decades earlier. Moreover, the generations of women physicians who came of age after 1930 were trained in a medical world almost totally bereft of female-run institutions, female support systems, or a traditionally female point of view. Young women physicians learned to accept the prevailing values of the profession without wielding any real power within it.

The revival of feminism in the 1960s came in the wake of a resumption of significant public interest in liberal reform. In recent years American society has witnessed notable increases in the ranks of women in the work force. Married women with school-age children are employed in large numbers. The impressive jump in the percentage of women in professional occupations has also been striking. Women physicians have benefited in substantial ways from these developments, ranging from the dramatic increases in application and acceptance statistics at medical schools across the country, to the reemergence of a national debate on woman's role.

Perhaps not surprisingly, reformers in the 1960s generated a good deal of criticism of the elitism and the masculine orientation of the professional ethos that had prevailed almost unchallenged in American culture since the turn of the century. In medicine especially but by no means exclusively, a new appreciation has appeared for the traditionally "female" qualities of nurturing and cooperation.

It is probably too soon to conclude that this recent admiration will result in a general reorientation of professional values. Therefore, this book will not make any predictions about the prospective role of women physicians or about the possible results of their increasing numbers within the profession. It can, however, like every good history, attempt to provide an accurate picture of their experience in the past. It is my hope that such an accounting will lend a balanced perspective to the present and will provide helpful insights in shaping the future.

CHAPTER 1

Colonial Beginnings:
Public Men and Private Women

Whether sympathy and science and practical energy are incompatible,
time must determine; at any rate, tears and tenderness are more to my
taste than oaths and hard looks. In fact, although it may seem queer, I
had rather have a doctor smelling of rose and ihlang-ihlang, than of
tobacco and whisky!

Augustus K. Gardner, M.D., 1870.

It was an early November morning in 1869, and Dean Ann Preston
of the Woman's Medical College of Pennsylvania, normally a
rather austere woman, could not hide her delight. For several
years she had sought to gain permission for students to attend the
teaching clinics in general surgery at the Pennsylvania Hospital in
Philadelphia. Preston well understood the value of being exposed
to some of Philadelphia's greatest clinicians. Although the Wom-
en's Medical College had its own small hospital, where surgery had
been taught since 1854, the school's meager resources meant that it
could not match the majestic surgical amphitheaters or the distinguished surgical faculties of the renowned major hospitals of Philadelphia. Today she had finally received permission from the Pennsylvania's managers to bring her students to the Saturday clinics.
Preston had no reason to expect trouble, for the women had already been attending clinics at Philadelphia's Blockley Hospital for
almost a year.

Neither she nor the thirty-five students who eagerly accompanied her that day were in the least prepared for the ensuing
events—events that would be reported and rehashed in great detail in newspapers from Boston to New York over the next several
months. Dr. Elizabeth Keller, later senior surgeon at the New
England Hospital for Women and Children, never forgot the experience. Neither did Dr. Eliza Jane Wood, whose scrapbook of
clippings can still be found in her file at the Medical College of
Pennsylvania in Philadelphia.

The men were "determined to make it so unpleasant for us,"

Keller recalled, "that from choice, we would not care to attend another [clinic]." She remembered being greeted by jeers, whistles, groans, and the stamping of feet, while some men actually threw stones.[1] Wood carefully preserved the Philadelphia *Evening Bulletin*'s detailed description of the incident:

> The students of the male colleges, knowing that the ladies would be present, turned out several hundred strong, with the design of expressing their disapproval of the action of the managers of the hospital particularly, and of the admission of women to the medical profession generally.
>
> Ranging themselves in line, these gallant gentlemen assailed the young ladies, as they passed out, with insolent and offensive language, and then followed them into the street, where the whole gang, with the fluency of long practice, joined in insulting them. . . .
>
> During the last hour missiles of paper, tinfoil, tobacco-quids, etc., were thrown upon the ladies, while some of these men defiled the dresses of the ladies near them with tobacco juice.[2]

Although such violent public displays of male opposition were not frequent occurrences in the decades after the Civil War, women physicians who experienced such unpleasantries often remembered them with bitterness.[3] In spite of their discomfort, however, what is most significant about the incident in Philadelphia and those few that occurred in other cities was not the extraordinary nastiness of the male students, or even the more measured protest against female students in the form of a letter a few days later from some faculty members. On the contrary, the event's historical importance was instead to demonstrate that in 1869, public sympathies lay, not with the male students or their recalcitrant teachers, but with the women. The managers of the Pennsylvania Hospital, for example, refused to yield to the coarse behavior and determined that women should continue to be admitted to the Saturday morning clinics in spite of the men's bad manners. Moreover, the *Evening Bulletin,* in conjunction with most of the other newspapers in the Northeast that reported the story, had nothing but contempt for the misconduct. The Philadelphia *Public Ledger,* for example, labeled the response "moral carditis," arguing that "this community has been the victim of an insult which it is compelled to resent to the uttermost." Hinting that women might indeed be the intellectual superiors of men after all, the editors denounced the male students for "seeking to triumph over struggling mind, encased though it was in a female shell."[4]

Besides considerable public sympathy, the women students had also won a number of male physicians to their cause. Only a year after the Philadelphia incident, a prominent New York physician, Augustus K. Gardner, published an article in *Leslie's Illustrated News* proclaiming himself ready to "eat my words" on the subject of women physicians. Acknowledging that twenty years before he had had some "unkind, and, I am now free to confess unjust" remarks to make about them, he wished to set the record straight. Not ashamed to admit publicly that he himself had changed both "in looks" and "in opinions," Gardner observed that he had "lived to see women advanced." No longer a figment of men's imagination, women doctors were now "powers . . . educated, erudite, thoughtful." What this meant to Gardner, and to other supporters like him, was that although one might still harbor notions that females were different and probably "the weaker vessel," one would, nevertheless, be willing to give women their chance at self-improvement. "A woman who feels an irresistible impulse to study medicine," he wrote,

> so strong as to overcome her natural timidity, or to be willing to take the obloquy and covert, if not open, insults from the world in general, and very often her own family and friends in particular—she will make a better doctor than a stupid lout, of whom, being found good for nothing, his father makes either a minister or a doctor. . . . The great limitations to women come from society, and are not from *esssential* inferiorities of the sex.
>
> I say, today, Don't interfere with women. Give them a fair chance. If, side by side with a man, a woman does an equal day's work, pay the two alike. . . . Now, let women study medicine as thoroughly and as freely as men; let them stand equal with male doctors, and let those who want the one or the other employ either, as they may be found capable. I, for one, will give women physicians every countenance; meet with them on equal footing. . . .[5]

Like Dr. Gardner, women who entered medicine in the mid-nineteenth century also believed that things had changed. "Our age is a progressive one," explained Dr. Prudence Saur in her graduating thesis from the Woman's Medical College of Pennsylvania. Women had a new and important role to play in the upward advance of humanity, agreed Angenette A. Hunt.[6] Their dean, Dr. Ann Preston, who had done so much to make the study of medicine a reality for women, felt that the entrance of women into the profession marked the advance of civilization and the "fuller appreciation of the scope of Christianity." "You feel that you have not gone out of your way to seize upon medicine as on some far off thing," she told her students, but with significant social progress, its study "has come to you."[7]

Women physicians' enthusiasm reflected their confidence that they lived in the best of all possible worlds. They were convinced that women's status had changed for the better in the nineteenth century, and that the range of female activity had dramatically broadened in their lifetime. With new conditions had come novel opportunities not available to their predecessors. So they believed, but how historically accurate was this assessment?

Until recently, most scholars would have taken issue with their rosy picture of the nineteenth-century woman's expanded options and life-choices. Researchers, basing their conclusions on the work of Elizabeth A. Dexter, have emphasized the social confinement of Victorian women as compared with the relative flexibility of seventeenth- and eighteenth-century sex roles. They have argued that American women in the colonial and revolutionary periods had experienced a degree of autonomy and independence shared neither by their English counterparts nor their nineteenth-century descendants. They have found that even though most women in the colonies worked within their homes, and in the context of the family economy, they labored in a wide variety of occupations, sometimes exhibiting a considerable measure of status. There were female butchers, silversmiths, and upholsterers; women ran plantations, mills, shipyards, shops, and taverns. They pursued journalism, printing, teaching, tanning, and the healing arts. Most acquired their skills through apprenticeship training, often with their immediate families.[8]

In keeping with this diverse range of female tasks, the colonies also boasted a varied group of women healers who earned part or all of their incomes from medical practice. Some were urban specialists in infant care who came to aid well-to-do mothers after childbirth, and lived six to ten weeks with a particular family before moving on. Resident nurses who were frequently consulted in folk medicine before advanced illness made it necessary to procure the aid of a physician also peopled the ranks of colonial medical practitioners. Teenaged girls, too, were sent to nurse sick relatives or attend childbeds, and many acquired significant knowledge through experience. Cotton Mather, for example, believed in woman's natural affinity for healing and taught medicine to his own daughter.[9] In addition, we know that women were employed as nurses in the American forces during the Revolution, and history has preserved the name of at least one woman, a Mrs. Allyn, who served as an army surgeon during King Phillip's War.[10]

Women were most commonly occupied with medical practice as midwives. So formidable was the custom of using midwives in the management of childbirth in the colonies that a man, Francis Rayns, was prosecuted and fined in 1646 by a Maine court for acting as a midwife.[11] Colonial American women faced the perils of childbirth in the company of a community of other females who provided both companionship and medical assistance. The science of obstetrics as it is now known was still in its infancy. Midwifery in these years was a folk art that remained unquestionably women's work.[12]

A handful of American midwives were formally trained in Europe in the seventeenth and eighteenth centuries. Many more acquired their skill by reading midwifery manuals and apprenticing themselves to more experienced women when they could. But ability varied considerably. It is likely, in fact, that Dr. Valentine Seaman was quite correct when he claimed in 1800 that the "greater part" of these women came to their calling by accident, "having first been catched . . . with a woman in labour."[13]

Still, midwives earned the respect and high regard of their communities. Indeed, of all the women who practiced healing in the colonies, skilled midwives probably enjoyed the highest status. A study of loyalist women's property claims after the American Revolution, for example, found that at least one Charleston midwife, Janet Cumming, testified to yearly earnings of four hundred pounds sterling, an income equivalent to that of a prosperous merchant, lawyer, or government official. Earlier, in Plymouth Colony, the annals of Rehoboth record the arrival in 1663 of Samuel Fuller and his mother, he to practice medicine, she to act as midwife and "answer the town's necessity, which was great." The epitaph of Mrs. Wiat of Dorchester, who died in 1705, testified to her attendance at over one thousand successful births, while the Boston *Weekly News-Letter* in 1730 mourned the death of the "noted midwife" Mary Bradway, who lived to be one hundred years old. Numerous examples of such skilled and revered women exist in colonial records.[14]

The social importance of midwives and the record of female employment in other occupations prompted the notion that these years represented a "golden age" in its tolerance for a wide variation of roles for women. After the Revolution, historians have argued, women's opportunities were gradually constricted. Women presumably lost status and eventually were displaced from professions—like medicine—where they had been active. What was described as an informal equality between men and women fostered by the preindustrial economy allegedly gave way to a rigidification of the sexual spheres culminating in the cult of domesticity and the idealistic glorification of wifehood and motherhood in the nineteenth-century.

Recent research has concentrated more closely on the social context of the greater colonial flexibility in definitions of women's work, however. The result has been a more complex picture of social relations, intimating that earlier interpretations were too simplistic. Newer scholarship suggests, in fact, that Ann Preston and her students at the Woman's Medical College of Pennsylvania may well have been more accurate when they claimed in the 1860s that women's entrance into the medical profession was something wholly new in modern history.

Revisionist historians do not dispute earlier evidence that women in colonial America performed a wider range of economic tasks than their nineteenth-century descendants. Their findings suggest instead that such role flexibility should not automatically be interpreted to indicate high status for women in a particular culture, *unless it holds such meaning for the participants themselves.* In this regard, recent work has demonstrated that in seventeenth- and eighteenth-century America, women's labor was so inextricably tied to household, husband, and children that no one dared challenge the assumption that their lives would be bounded primarily by the domestic circle. In colonial society both men and women knew their place; there was little need to analyze its dimensions. Hence, the historian will search in vain for lengthy treatises on masculinity and femininity, or systematic definitions of women's roles. Such evidence usually appears when commonly held assumptions are breaking down. The absence of a public ideology about gender suggests a range of agreement so broad that the premises could be left unstated. Though a sexual division of labor existed, it was less ideologically defined than it would be in the nineteenth century and remained largely unspoken. Thus, women might perform a multiplicity of economic tasks, but the social meaning of their work would always be found in its relation to the family welfare. The variegated nature of women's production indicated, not the extensive economic opportunity available to them, but rather the length and breadth of their economic responsibility.[15]

In this context, the practice of medicine by women takes on a
meaning different than historians had originally thought. Let us
look, for example, at childbirth. Before 1760 no other event in a
woman's life cycle exhibited greater female control or firmer female bonding. At the beginning of labor, a parturient mother
"called her women together," leaving male members of the household to wait on the periphery in anticipation. The midwife remained in control of the event, while neighbors and friends offered
comfort and support. Only when women were not available did
men participate in delivery, and only in difficult cases were physicians called to intervene. The experience of William Byrd of Virginia was typical. "I went to bed about 10 o'clock," he wrote in his
diary, "and left the women full of expectation with my wife."[16]

A number of historians have acknowledged the central role this
"social childbirth" experience played in strengthening bonds between women and enriching domestic female culture.[17] Yet Laurel
Thatcher Ulrich has rightly cautioned us not to interpret even
premodern childbirth as an event entirely independent of male
jurisdiction. In the colonies two men—the minister and the physician—might occasionally challenge female sovereignty by virtue of
their status as "learned gentlemen." In 1724, for example, the
Reverend Hugh Adams of Durham, New Hampshire, was called to
Exeter by a midwife attending a woman who had been in labor
three and one-half days. Adams, whose scant obstetrical knowledge consisted primarily of reading a few English treatises on
childbirth, claimed in his memoirs to have performed version—the
complicated procedure of turning the fetus in utero—in order to
deliver the child safely. The significance of such a story lies neither
in this man's pompous temerity in plunging ahead, nor even in his
extraordinary luck when the infant lived. Although not common,
this example of male interference still stands as a reminder of the
powerful status of the "learned man" in a society where women
had no learning, and the sanction such status afforded its beneficiaries to intrude if necessary at the last moment on a woman's
event.[18]

In a society where a woman's destiny was to marry, have children, and direct the work of the household, the practice of medicine by women also remained linked to the private sphere. Even
when they did care for the sick, they did not enjoy the same status
as many of their male counterparts, but doctored primarily as
skilled amateurs. Women employed as nurses in the American
forces during the Revolution, for example, were rarely allowed to

administer medicine and received much lower pay than male nurses or physicians.[19] Even "professional" midwives functioned entirely within this context. They were primarily women who needed to contribute to the family economy, or widows without an alternative means of support, and they used traditional skills available to them according to the sexual division of labor. When they had difficulty, they were expected to appeal to physicians. Thus, women who practiced medicine in the colonies were never considered part of the medical profession, in spite of the fact that in these years American medical professionalism was itself in disarray and the medical credentials of many male practitioners left much to be desired.

Originating in the traditions of England, the medical system of the mother country reproduced itself only imperfectly in the colonies. American patterns emerged slowly out of the amalgam of English heritage and colonial experience. In the mother country, only medicine, law, and divinity were recognized as "learned professions," and all of them required a university education. Physicians were drawn from the social elite. Gentlemen and scholars, they neither worked with their hands, as did surgeons, nor, like apothecaries, engaged in trade. These latter came from the middle classes and gained their expertise through apprenticeship. Members of an occupational group rather than learned professionals, they were denied the prestige and status of the physician. Physicians, in turn, took for granted a leadership role in social and governmental affairs.[20]

London distinctions among physicians, surgeons, and apothecaries, however, dwindled as one moved into the countryside, and they had even less practical use in the English colonies. Few formally trained physicians emigrated, and apprenticeship soon became the chief mode of education for those laying claim to professional medical status. In America, among all the professions, specialists became generalists. Thus physicians there would perform surgery, practice dentistry, and sell drugs. It has been estimated that on the eve of the American Revolution, there were approximately thirty-five hundred medical practitioners in the colonies, and only four hundred of them had received formal training.[21]

The fluid state of colonial professionalism lasted until the middle of the eighteenth century. It meant that there was plenty of room for quacks and an occasional lady "doctress." But the presence of women in medicine reflected primarily the shortage of healers in the seventeenth-century colonies. Even in this period lady doctors stood outside the medical *profession*. Whatever the reality of colonial practice, the so-called professional physician, who in England boasted of gentlemanly status and a university degree, was still by definition a *man*. Thus colonial licensing laws need not bother to bar women from the profession, because in the unspoken realm of social ideology a woman *physician* was still a contradiction in terms. Furthermore, women's participation in general medical practice did not last long. The number of female practitioners declined early in the eighteenth century, probably because of both the increasing availability of trained men and the growth of commercial capitalism. This latter development sharply separated public and private life and created a gradual hardening of the social definitions of men's and women's work.

By the middle of the eighteenth century, moreover, the few hundred formally trained American physicians took steps to professionalize their ranks along European lines. After 1730 more and more young men found the means to finance medical study abroad. They returned home impressed not only by European advances in medical science, but by the self-conscious professionalism of European guilds, societies, publications, and hospitals.

Returning with prestigious foreign degrees, these doctors took the initiative in guiding subsequent institutional developments. Social and economic progress in the colonies created a provincial self-consciousness conducive to a genuine medical awakening. Opportunites for genteel practice multiplied in colonial towns and cities. In 1751 Dr. Thomas Bond and Benjamin Franklin founded the Pennsylvania Hospital, patterned on British models and the first American hospital in the modern meaning of the term. Intended to serve both poor and private patients, the new institution also offered clinical opportunities to medical students. Fourteen years later the University of Pennsylvania Medical School was established, followed by King's College (Columbia) in 1768 and Harvard in 1780. All three institutions imitated the Continental-Scottish tradition of a university college. Though this tradition of connecting the medical school to the greater university was challenged briefly by developments in nineteenth-century medical education, it has largely reasserted itself in the twentieth century. The appearance of medical societies lending prestige to the better-qualified practitioners and pressuring provincial legislatures to pass licensing restrictions added a final touch to colonial professional developments.

It is true, of course, that the model of gentlemanly professionalism, which gained increasing acceptance in the colonies, set the tone primarily for the few hundred elite practitioners. The great bulk of the colonies' thirty-five hundred practitioners ranged from the competently apprentice-trained to the ill-trained and even the untrained. Scattered in the towns and countryside, they provided most of the medical care. Women, when they participated in the healing arts, were found among this group as nurses, midwives, and practitioners of folk medicine. Those women in the cities who might have perhaps aspired to something more formal were denied access to a university education and relegated by social ideology more and more exclusively in these years to the home. Such developments slowly but unquestionably excluded them from legitimate practice.[22]

Developments in midwifery in the larger towns and cities of England and America well illustrate this process of professionalization and exclusion. Seventeenth-century ignorance of anatomy, physiology, and surgery put physicians, surgeons, and midwives on a relatively equal plane in the management of parturition. As long as childbirth continued to be defined as a normal process, and all practitioners remained equally ignorant of the physiological mechanisms involved, custom and superstition usually barred men from the lying-in chamber, except to extricate a dead fetus. By the middle of the eighteenth century, however, improvements in the use of the forceps provided a major breakthrough in obstetrical practice and threatened the dominance of midwives, especially in slow and difficult births. Skilled mechanical interference could shorten labor and often meant life instead of death for mother and child. Gradually, with the approval of parturient women themselves and their anxious husbands, determined male accoucheurs defied custom. Among the most important of these was William Smellie, a surgeon who devoted his life to the clinical study of childbirth and became England's leading instructor of midwifery in the eighteenth century.

Technical improvements, however, tell only half the story, for advances in anatomical research, primarily on the pregnant human uterus, also occurred. In 1774 Dr. William Hunter gave physicians their first accurate picture of the progress of the fetus through the birth canal. Taken together, the skillful use of forceps and the improved anatomical familiarity with the birth process opened the door of the lying-in chamber to the male accoucheur.[23]

American expatriates in the middle of the eighteenth century often studied with the founders of the "new obstetrics." William

Shippen, Jr., and Samuel Bard, for example, both attended the lectures of William Hunter in London and apprenticed with students of Smellie. Naturally these young men became caught up in all that was fresh and innovative about English medical practice. Before long the management of childbirth among the urban middle classes on both sides of the Atlantic passed from the hands of the midwife to those of the professional physician. Although tradition, modesty and midwives themselves resoundingly denounced male midwifery, women's fears of death or physical disability made them willing to move away from traditional birthing patterns. While most poor and rural women continued to depend on midwives, the new obstetrics gained increasing acceptance among economically advantaged men and women of influence because it stood for safety, progress, and science.[24]

A few early male obstetricians in England and the colonies were willing to work with the midwife to allow her to retain control over "normal" cases. Indeed, William Smellie hoped to upgrade the quality of midwives' practice by offering formal instruction to women as well as to men. Though no physician would teach a midwife to use forceps, Smellie's writings refer with respect to skillful women, whose work he commended. Despite the fact that his own practice included some normal deliveries, he expected that the male accoucheur would attend primarily to abnormal births, where the dexterous use of instruments, a more precise knowledge of anatomy, and the techniques of version were needed.

In the colonies conservative physicians like William Shippen in Philadelphia and Samuel Bard and Valentine Seaman in New York, offered private instruction to midwives, while early in the nineteenth-century Boston physicians John Collins Warren and James Jackson hired Janet Alexander, a midwife who had trained in Scotland, to handle their normal cases.[25] But this professional tolerance did not last long. Most midwives could not afford to attend private classes and thus remained vulnerable to charges of ignorance. Moreover, more and more physicians believed that professional as well as scientific considerations necessitated their exclusive control over parturition. Midwifery, after all, was an excellent means for the struggling young physician to gain entree into a respectable family. Thus, after a period of intense competition between male and female practitioners, obstetricians sought to gain the upper hand.

In many respects, changes in the management of childbirth merely mirrored more profound shifts in society at large. Between

1750 and 1850, for example, the simple, undifferentiated family economy devoted primarily to subsistence agriculture began to transform itself into the increasingly intricate and complex structures of commercial capitalistic enterprise. The gradual removal of production from the household caused an elaborate shift in the economic and social meaning of women's work.

For some women, changes in the division of labor heralded a variety of new economic options. The development of a market economy allowed the vast majority of farm women to organize at least some of their production around the demands of the market. Farmers' wives learned to sell their surplus products—eggs, milk, or cloth—to nearby merchants for cash. In the late eighteenth and early nineteenth century they also participated in the more formalized manufacture of textiles through the putting-out system.

In cities and towns, wives and daughters participated in the budding commercial enterprises of their husbands and fathers. Some women even kept their own shops and taverns. Others profited by selling their traditional skills as nurses, teachers of young children, or midwives. Finally, women entered domestic service or filled places in New England's nascent factory system.

Yet, however varied was women's actual economic adjustment to these changes, as commercial capitalism gave way to industrial capitalism after 1820, the social ideology accompanying the new economic order decidedly sharpened distinctions between men's and women's work. Capitalism gradually drew men into an increasingly complicated economic system separated spacially as well as socially from the household. Simultaneously, it slowly reduced the time women spent in household production. As a result household labor began to take on a different character, centering more and more on strictly domestic tasks like decorating the home and caring for children. For a growing number of middle-class women this meant that consumption would replace production as an increasingly important part of their daily lives. Accompanying these economic changes was a domestic ideology that glorified the separation between the home and the world and extolled female qualities of nurturing, moral superiority, maternity, and subordination.

Political changes also seemed at first to underscore the sharpening rift between the public and private worlds. Although the republican spirit of the Revolution had a profound effect on some women's political perceptions and self-definition, neither the War for Independence nor the new Federal Government recognized women as political beings. Indeed, their political stature relative to men actually declined in the decades after the establishment of the Constitution, as the achievement of universal white manhood suffrage highlighted as never before women's exclusion from politics. Although they had not formally participated in political decision-making in the colonial period, networks of neighbors and kin had given them greater access to the seat of power, which was still primarily local. When the Constitution centralized the political process, making it more formal and remote, women were removed even further than they had been from the political realm.[27]

No one described the results of these developments better than the acute French eyewitness to American life, Alexis de Tocqueville. Commenting in the 1830s that democracy had not led Americans to the erroneous doctrines prevalent in some parts of Europe that "would give to both [sexes] the same functions, impose on both the same duties, and grant them both the same rights," he went on to explain:

> The Americans have applied to the sexes the great principle of political economy which governs the manufactures of our age, by carefully dividing the duties of man from those of woman, in order that the great work of society may be the better carried on.
>
> In no country has such constant care been taken as in America to trace two clearly distinct lines of action for the two sexes, and to make them keep pace one with the other, but in two pathways which are always different. American women never manage the outward concerns of the family, or conduct a business, or take a part in political life; nor are they, on the other hand, ever compelled to perform the rough labor of the fields, or to make any of those laborious exertions which demand the exertion of physical strength. No families are so poor as to form an exception to this rule. If, on the one hand, an American woman cannot escape from the quiet circle of domestic employments, she is never forced, on the other, to go beyond it. Hence it is, that the women of America, who often exhibit a masculine strength of understanding and a manly energy, generally preserve great delicacy of personal appearance, and always retain the manners of women, although they sometimes show that they have the hearts and minds of men.[28]

Although we need not accept all Tocqueville's observations at face value, he does suggest that the political and social changes of the late eighteenth and early nineteenth centuries threw the separation of the sexes into sharper focus. As a result, a small but significant portion of the female middle-class experienced a growing sense of confinement. By the late eighteenth century, for example, the writer Judith Sargent Murray complained that girls who were raised exclusively for matrimony were denied both a strong sense of their own identity and the personal resources to resist a bad union. To remedy the situation, Murray strongly advocated women's education, arguing the intellectual equality of the sexes. "Should it still be vociferated," she wrote, " 'Your domestick employments are sufficient'—I would calmly ask, is it reasonable, that a candidate for immortality, for the joys of heaven, an intelligent being . . . should at present be so degraded, as to be allowed no other ideas, than those which are suggested by the mechanism of a pudding, or the sewing of the seams of a garment?"[29] Others joined Murray in advocating schooling for girls, while the decline in home production created a greater willingness on the part of middle-class families to part with the labor of their daughters for the sake of education.

This movement to educate women demonstrated as no other event would that even as a new theory of womanhood arose to sequester women more securely in the private sphere, it began almost at once to be eroded by the weight of its own contradictions. The historian Linda Kerber has skillfully located the origins of the ideology of separate spheres—the nineteenth-century cult of "domesticity"—in the notion of "Republican motherhood." At first, women's customary absence from civic culture meant that during the intensely political time of the Revolution and after, they lacked both a vocabulary and an outlet for their patriotism. But even as political independence gave rise to structures which further banished women from the political process, it also became the catalyst for a theory of women's roles which simultaneously worked to justify their limited participation in the public sphere.[30]

Naturally, at a time when women's major role in household production was being gradually supplanted by the factory, the new theory would seek as much as possible to preserve women's integral connection with the domestic circle. If the result of such a theory was to emphasize the widening gap between public and private life, republicanism, with its passionate concern for an educated citizenry, itself intervened to bridge this growing separation. Ironically, the social theory of democracy connected the public and private in a particular way—through the politicization of women's role in the family. Creating a civic culture that allegedly depended for its healthy existence on the virtue of its people, American democracy gave a central place to motherhood, now defined as a device to insure the perpetuation of a responsible citizenry. For the

first time what women did with their children in the home had
relevance for and an impact on the public process. Once women's
role as educator became politicized in such a manner, the future of
women's education was assured, though the radicalizing effects of
the educative process that resulted from women's schooling were
hardly intended by many and would not be witnessed for several
generations to come.

The ideology of domesticity did not merely reaffirm, it exaggerated woman's traditional connection with the private sphere. Dictating a limited and sex-specific role for women in the home, it
reflected the real subordination in marriage and in society that was
still their lot in the early nineteenth century. Accompanying this
shift in emphasis between 1780 and 1820 was an ideology of female
prudery which has been labeled "passionlessness." A belief in exaggerated female delicacy became decidedly more prevalent in
public ideology as woman's image shifted from that of a being
innately sensual to one who was naturally moral. Disarming the
older Puritan notions of female carnality, this new emphasis on
woman's intellectual and spiritual power replaced the conviction
that women were the inheritors of Eve's questionable legacy with
assertions of female purity and superiority. Some women embraced the shift as a means of enhancing their status, gaining control over indiscriminate male lust in the sexual arena, and depre-
ciating the sexual characteristics that had served as a justification
for their exclusion from public life. But eventually this change in
emphasis from female physiology to female spirituality would so
distort notions of female modesty that it would foster a dangerous
ignorance of physiology among women.[31] Both feminists and male
physicians would question the negative aspects of this ideology of
"passionlessness" once it became entrenched, but they did so in
different ways and for different motives. Many women would also
come to understand that in surrendering too easily to an image that
defined their sex in terms of innate purity and moral righteousness
they had traded one congeries of exaggerated female characteristics for another. Although the ideology of domesticity allowed
them some gain in social and familial power, the concept could
also be used to confine radically their circle of activity.

And yet, although the ideology of domesticity implied for social
conservatives the inequality of the sexes and the subordination of
women in the public realm, some women—especially educated
women—took it to mean for themselves not only more power in
the private realm, but a broader definition of woman's sphere. As

a consequence, the period after 1830 was a turning point in women's public participation and social visibility. In emphasizing the socially transforming aspects of woman's role in the home, educated middle-class women used their learning and newly acquired self-confidence to assert themselves in public. Making the home a model for social interaction, they played an unprecedented part in what eventually became the reformist critique of industrial America. The ideology of domesticity, though seemingly contradicted by the appearance of feminism, emerged historically from the same social and economic roots as women's rights, drawing moral and ideological power from the glorification of women's new domestic role. Indeed, it is even likely that the conservative proponents of domesticity became increasingly more shrill and demanding as they observed that many women used the cult of domesticity, not to separate themselves off from the world of men, but to participate as women in selected aspects of social and economic life.[32]

If we look again briefly at the decline in female midwifery among the middle class, we can see how these important economic, social, and ideological shifts could simultaneously limit female activity in one way while potentially expanding female opportunity in another. First came the particularization of the economy and the beginning of the professionalization of medicine in America between 1780 and 1835. These occupational changes were accompanied by the growing popularity of the ideology of separate sexual spheres. In obstetrics, because of real advances in anatomical knowledge and medical technology, what had been exclusively an event in the family guided by female custom and folk art began to move slowly toward greater professional control. The cult of domesticity kindled a greater ceremonial appreciation of women, and male obstetricians frequently argued that they were demonstrating their respect by applying their knowledge to reduce both the dangers and the pain of childbearing. Yet there were also feminist possibilities inherent in the cult of domesticity, especially the emphasis on women's transforming power in the social realm. These possibilities inspired some women to assert their influence in matters of sickness and health in a far more comprehensive manner than they previously had—by training as professional physicians.

An apology for male midwifery published in 1820 by an anonymous Boston doctor, reputed to be John Ware, serves as a measure of just how far these complicated social and ideological shifts had progressed. Young general practitioners like Ware apparently depended on midwifery cases to win the confidence and patronage of middle-class families. Yet, in opposing female midwifery, Ware moved well beyond a defense of his pocketbook. He was also concerned to divert women's attention from the idea of studying medicine, and, in the course of twenty-two pages, he touched on most of the arguments that would be leveled against women physicians in the decades to come.[33]

Ware's confident assertion that probably in no other city in America were midwifery cases "so entirely confined to male practitioners" unwittingly reveals that in many parts of the country the "new obstetrics" would not so quickly eradicate deep-seated, cultural objections to men in the lying-in room. For almost a century, the enemies of male midwifery had argued that the practice threatened the moral fabric of society by compromising female modesty. The transition from the midwife to the male accoucheur was not accomplished without severe protest, not just from midwives themselves, but from social conservatives who saw it as an outrage to female modesty. From the end of the eighteenth century on, both English and American critics railed against the moral depravity of the new obstetrics. Doctors were accused of taking advantage of innocent female patients. Horror stories about modest women who were so shocked by the presence of a strange man in the bedchamber that they ceased to labor appeared repeatedly in opposition literature.[34]

As the belief in female "passionlessness" gained ground in the nineteenth century, it often turned the virtues of innocence and purity into the less desirable traits of ignorance and prudery. Victorian delicacy threatened to make it difficult for physicians to treat their women patients at all. Doctors themselves often found it hard to balance the competing claims of professionalism and delicacy. Many of them, like Charles Meigs, Professor of Obstetrics and Diseases of Women and Children at Jefferson Medical College in Philadelphia, shared an exaggerated conception of womanhood. Although Meigs worried constantly that female delicacy often prevented doctors from giving their women patients adequate treatment, his remarkable ambivalence became apparent when he observed in 1848 that,

> It is best, upon the whole, that this great degree of modesty should exist, even to the extent of putting a bar to researchers. . . . I confess I am proud to say that, in this country . . . there are women who prefer to suffer the extremity of danger and pain, rather than

waive those scruples of delicacy which prevent their maladies from being fully explored. I say it is an evidence of the dominion of a fine morality in our society.[35]

Meigs's private conflict between professional concerns and emerging cultural norms was common. In the nineteenth century, portions of the medical establishment accepted the idea of female "passionlessness" so thoroughly that they moved the grounds for its conceptual defense from religion to science. Only when the role of doctors in this transformation is thoroughly noted can the import of Meigs's observations be fully understood.[36]

Of course, not all physicians and not all women found comfort in Meigs's remarks. In 1817 Dr. Thomas Ewell had proposed that the American government sponsor schools of midwifery modeled after those in Europe.[37] His reasons stemmed from his belief that male doctors treating parturient women engendered social depravity. Like William Shippen, Jr., and Samuel Bard before him, he hoped to upgrade the quality of midwifery practice in normal cases, while retaining for the physician control of difficult and dangerous deliveries. Although his program met with scant success, a generation later in 1848, Samuel Gregory, a lay health reformer, repeated Ewell's arguments with considerably more practical results. Paradoxically, feminists by this time had begun to understand the inherently confining aspects of the idea of female "passionlessness" and modesty. Seeking to expand women's control in health matters they joined Gregory in an uneasy alliance to establish a medical school for women in Boston.[38]

John Ware was quite willing to appreciate in passing the fact that women exhibited noble qualities of delicacy and spirituality. Indeed, in the best of all possible worlds, he admitted that "the circumstances, which would render females agreeable and most desirable as attendants . . . are obvious." But for him, as for most of his colleagues, the choice was one of delicacy of feeling versus safety, with "safety . . . the first circumstance to be regarded."[39]

In order to defend professional physicians' claims to providing greater safety for women, Ware next attempted to discredit the older notion of childbirth as a natural or "mechanical" event. Childbirth was complicated, he warned, and "no one can thoroughly understand the nature and treatment of labour, who does not understand thoroughly *the profession of medicine as a whole.*" Of course, this excluded midwives. Ware cautioned that midwives, ignorant as they were of general physiology, could not even detect,

much less cope with, placenta previa, shock, convulsions, or puerperal fever. "Mere manual adroitness," according to him, was
hopelessly inadequate. Thus, for Ware the choice clearly lay "between the true and legitimate practitioners of the professions, and
ignorant and assuming pretenders."[40]

The presence of male physicians in the lying-in chamber initiated
a significant transformation in the social and scientific definition of
childbirth. Over the next century and a half, parturition evolved
from an event in the female life cycle that was managed by a
community of women to a more private experience confined to the
immediate family and shared almost exclusively by a woman and
her doctor. In time childbirth gradually ceased to be viewed as
natural and increasingly became defined by doctors as a disease.
Moreover, the medicalization of parturition in the nineteenth century set the stage for its transferal in the twentieth century from
the privacy of the home to impersonality of the hospital. At first
the shift remained confined to middle- and upper-class Americans,
but today the change has become universal. One reason for the
transition was surely a new social appreciation of women and a
desire to minimize the risks of childbirth. But the new obstetrics
was also tied to the determined efforts of physicians to professionalize, and as such signaled the diminution and disparagement of
laywomen's participation in this area of medical practice.[26]

But why not teach women medicine? With the growing popularity
of female education, Ware could not successfully ignore this possibility, and so he moved to the second part of his argument. Reflect-
ing on the nineteenth century's new respect for woman's intellect,
Ware was quick to deny "any intellectual inferiority or incompetence in the sex." He admitted quite simply that his objections to
women becoming doctors were "founded rather upon the nature of
their moral qualities, than of the powers of their minds, and upon
those very qualities, which render them, in their appropriate sphere,
the pride, the ornament, and the blessing of mankind."[41]

According to the Victorian stereotype, women were distinguished from men by their inability to restrain their "natural tendency to sympathy" as men could and as physicians must. "The
profession of medicine," Ware observed, "does not afford a field
for the display and indulgence of those finer feelings." It was "obvious" to him that "we cannot instruct women as we do men in the
science of medicine; we cannot carry them into the dissecting room
and the hospital." He admitted that medical training required men
to subdue many of their "more delicate feelings" and their capacity

for "refined sensibility" but went on to say that "in females" such sensibilities would be destroyed. He concluded by stating that "a female could scarce pass through the course of education requisite to prepare her, as she ought to be prepared, for the practice of midwifery, without destroying those moral qualities of character, which are essential to the office."[42]

Ware's elaborate protestations well demonstrate the limitations of the ideology of female moral superiority in effecting female emancipation. Too great an emphasis on female moral purity gave credence to the formulation of an idea of separate spheres which encouraged men like Ware to use Victorian sexual stereotyping to keep women out of medicine, as well as out of other public or professional activities for which they might find themselves distinctly suited.

Ironically, the emergence of Victorian prudery encouraged some social conservatives, such as the health reformer Samuel Gregory, to support the movement to train women in medicine. More important, however, were the socially transforming elements in the cult of domesticity that inspired many middle-class women to take control of their own health and the health of their families. The result was the emergence of a popular health movement with feminist overtones which in time would help to sanction a new role for women as medical professionals. Little did John Ware dream, when he published his pamphlet in 1820, that fifty years later Dean Ann Preston of the Woman's Medical College of Pennsylvania would receive both public and professional approval when she brought her students to attend the surgical clinics at one of the oldest and most prestigious hospitals in America.

CHAPTER 2

The Middle-Class Woman
Finds Health Reform

The true Physician bears not the least resemblance to the *small pretenders* who swarm over the land. . . . The true Physician deeply feels the great responsibilities resting upon him & in order to prepare himself for the discharge of his duties invokes the aid of science. . . . I have used the masculine pronoun in describing the Physician but . . . public opinion is beginning to prove that there is a female side to *this subject*. . . . It is certain that the health of the world, depends on the women of the world and at least, some of the qualities needed in the medical profession—as gentleness, patience, quick perceptions, natural instinct which is often surer than science, deep sympathy . . . all these belong to the sex in an eminent degree. . . . With proper education these qualities *may* be called into exercise and rendered available in a higher sphere than formally been accorded to woman—one not bounded by the kitchen & the nursery.

Dr. Angenette A. Hunt, 1851

While economic and social changes reworked the traditional patterns of men's and women's lives, the medical profession struggled with the results of its own version of technological and intellectual innovation. Advances in medical science in the first half of the nineteenth century aroused skepticism regarding the efficacy of traditional heroic therapeutics, making the medical profession extremely vulnerable to criticism of several different kinds. "The time is passing," warned Ann Preston in her 1851 graduate medical thesis on "General Diagnosis," "when . . . the licensed graduate whose lancet is sprung for every head-ache and *heart-ache* that he may meet can obtain public confidence." Preston, soon to become dean of her alma mater, the newly established Female Medical College of Pennsylvania, gave voice to what was by 1851 a lively public issue. Her fellow classmate, Angenette A. Hunt, echoed Preston's admonition when she observed in her own thesis that the present public criticism of the medical profession was well deserved: "The merit of the Physician," she declared vehemently, "is not now estimated by the quantity of medicines he prescribes, but by the effect produced, and the public throat is rebelling against swallowing nauseous drugs for the pleasure and profit of the doctors."[1]

By midcentury dissatisfaction with established medical practice had reached astonishing proportions; doctors had good reason to feel on the defensive. "The practice, or so-called *science* of medicine, has been little else than one of experiment," observed the health reformer Mrs. Marie Louise Shew in a scathing indictment. Standard medical therapeutics, she claimed, had hitherto been characterized by "uncertainty" and "chance." Little progress had been made in alleviating the sufferings of mankind.[2] "Why," asked Shew's colleague Mary Gove Nichols, "are we sick? Why cannot the doctors cure us?" Men, women, and society had sought a cure so long in vain that they began to distrust their doctors. "We are tired of professions and promises."[3]

Heroic methods of treatment—bleeding, purging, and puking—were indeed painful and dangerous, and the American public, sick to death of bloodletting and calomel, had reason to rebel. Yet for decades regularly trained physicians could muster only a weak and ineffectual response. Between 1800 and 1840, innovative research was being conducted in Europe, most notably in France by the so-called Paris school. Investigators painstakingly correlated bedside symptoms with lesions observed during autopsies. For the first time, they began to distinguish clearly between various diseases. Indeed, French clinicians became so skeptical of accepted therapeutics that they helped to discredit the assumptions of heroic medicine, which relied on monistic approaches to disease—the assumption that every sickness could be attributed to one ultimate cause—and distinguished only among symptoms rather than discrete illnesses. Unfortunately, in taking the first hesitant steps toward a concept of specific etiology, these physicians undermined public and professional confidence in older therapies before they were able to put anything in their place. This "relatively cold-blooded" approach to human illness, as Richard Shryock has wryly pointed out, was "of little aid to the sick."[4] The eventual result was occasional therapeutic nihilism among doctors and public revulsion against the harshness of regular practice.

The discovery of anesthesia at the end of the 1840s compounded the profession's difficulties by calling into question older concepts of professionalism. If professionalism is defined as involving not only licensing and standards but also a set of values and prescriptions for behavior that help people to balance conflicting occupational demands, we can see why this occurred. Nineteenth-century

professional ideas reflected the social structure, values, and technical capabilities of the age.[5] As researchers have shown, before
anesthesia the possible necessity of inflicting physical pain on patients was a part of the daily reality of professional practice and
constituted an integral feature of the self-image and ideology of
physicians. Physicians and surgeons sought to balance empathy
with cool detachment; the best surgeon knew that the physician's
first responsibility was to cure, not to soothe. One author has
observed that the two professional prerequisites for a surgeon were
a strong stomach and a willingness to "cut like an executioner."[6]

John Ware used this need for detachment as an argument against
teaching women medicine. According to him, females could not
achieve such emotional distance. Ware's views were so typical that
women themselves occasionally shared them. "The Past, with the
lancet, and poison, and operative surgery," wrote Mary Gove Nichols, a hydropathic physician, feminist, and health reformer, "did
not insult woman by asking her to become a physician; and the
Past has not asked her to become hangman, general, or jailer. We
may well excuse all believers in Allopathy, if they judge woman
unfit for the profession."[7] The use of ether and chloroform, however, would quickly undermine a major objection to women practitioners while "feminizing" medicine by calling into question the
"heroic" image of the physician.[8]

These important changes in medical science and technology were
accompanied by institutional growing pains. Efforts to raise standards floundered in the antebellum period. One factor contributing
to the problem was the proliferation of proprietary medical schools,
which were set up by private physicians to provide an educational
program, not for its own sake, but for their profit. The ensuing
intense competition for students lowered educational quality. Clinical facilities remained meagre or nonexistent. Eventually, even the
university-affiliated colleges of medicine could not attract students
without reducing their requirements. It became possible to turn
oneself into a doctor in less than a year merely by attending two
terms of didactic lectures. Scores of young men held a medical
degree with little or no clinical experience and often without ever
having witnessed a single childbirth. The degeneration of medical
education in the first half of the nineteenth century made a mockery
of physicians' claims to superior skill in the lying-in chamber.

Jacksonian antielitism added to the profession's difficulties, as
hostility to all professional distinctions became a featured aspect of
American political rhetoric. Beginning around 1830, most states

responded by abolishing restrictive licensing legislation, which already had proved difficult to enforce. Although the American Medical Association and the New York Academy of Medicine were founded in 1846 to counter such trends, there was only slow progress in medical education until the end of the century.[9]

Probably none of the aforementioned problems bothered physicians as much as the rise of sectarianism and the proliferation of quackery. Although these two phenomena were different, regular physicians often defiantly lumped them together. Physicians looked on helplessly as the habit of self-dosing encouraged the small-scale patent medicine industry to adopt aggressive methods of advertising and thus emerge as a million-dollar business at the end of the nineteenth century.

Sectarians presented a different challenge. Responding in part to the growing dissatisfaction with heroic medicine, the followers of several new medical systems began to compete with the regular profession for public patronage, legitimacy, and authority. Some of these sects opposed the physician's heroic methods and use of drugs and substituted for them the belief that only nature should do the healing. Hydropaths, for example, used only water internally, and externally in the form of baths and hot and cold compresses, shunning surgery and drugs altogether. Others, like the Botanics, later known as Eclectics, substituted so-called natural remedies for chemical and mineral ones. Homeopaths, although they used a variety of drugs, believed in such miniscule doses that their prescriptions had no deleterious effect—and possibly no effect at all. Like other sectarians, they too believed strongly in the healing powers of nature.[10]

In time these sectarians formed their own professional institutions—schools, journals, and societies. Favoring the popular diffusion of professional knowledge, and respecting women's enhanced responsibilities in the family, their schools often welcomed women students, and consequently middle-class women initially gravitated to sectarian medicine. Many of the first generation of women doctors received their degrees from sectarian institutions. The challenge posed by sectarian medicine to older concepts of professionalism worked in favor of women. Paradoxically, in the mid-nineteenth century the abandonment of licensing legislation and the ease of access to a medical degree actually served to maintain a professional identity for all medical practitioners by conferring the title of doctor on a large proportion of them. This temporary fluidity allowed women who wished to achieve professional status to do so before definitions of professionalism crystallized once more.[11]

The health-reform movement provided a different alternative to a dissatisfied public, and it grew and flourished in the atmosphere created by vociferous debate between sectarians and regulars over more humane methods of treatment. Beginning in the antebellum period, self-help in health matters, public hygiene, dietary reform, temperance, hydro-therapy, and physiological instruction merged as ingredients in a coherent and articulate campaign to save the nation by combating the ill-health of its citizenry. Although such attention to personal health and hygiene was not wholly original, never before had the regard for good health given rise to such widespread public activity.[12]

In the modernizing world of the nineteenth century, health reformers played a critical role in promoting the assumption that men and women were responsible for their own health, the health of their families and the health of society at large. Itinerant speakers lecturing to enthusiastic audiences and dedicated to furthering common knowledge of health and hygiene traversed the cities and towns of the North and West. Hundreds of heuristic tracts instructed eager readers in the "laws of life." A handful of journals kept men and women informed of new developments. The popular *Water-Cure Journal,* for example, boasted 10,000 subscribers in 1849, the second year of its publication.[13]

The concern with hygiene was an integral part of the antebellum reformist world view. The popularity of both sectarian medicine and health reform helped to shape the character of the midnineteenth-century reform consciousness. Indeed, the health crusade converged with several better-known radical concerns. Historians have been quick to point out this identity of ideas and personnel. Abolitionist speakers, for example, lodged at health-reform boarding houses, and a large number of women's-rights advocates followed some form of Sylvester Graham's vegetarian diet. Oberlin College, familiar as a breeding ground for abolitionism and women's rights, adopted strict vegetarianism in its dining-room in 1835. Asa Mahan, the college's president, put a "reformation in food, drink, and dress" high on the list of important causes.[14]

A cursory glance at the men and women who actively promoted the health revolution suggests that, like other reformers, they came from the Northeastern, predominantly middle-class sectors of the American population. Sylvester Graham began his career in New Jersey as a Presbyterian minister and temperance lecturer. William

A. Alcott, cousin of Bronson, was a thoughtful, Yale-trained physician. Joel Shew and Russell Trall graduated from regular medical schools in New York. James Caleb Jackson was the son of a yeoman farmer in upstate New York. Mary Gove Nichols became a teacher in Maine. Rachel Brooks Gleason graduated from New York's Central Eclectic School of Medicine and ran a water-cure establishment with her physician husband. Paulina Wright Davis and Elizabeth Oakes Smith both hailed from prominent New York landholding families. Harriot Hunt's father, a skilled navigator, invested his small capital in Boston's commercial shipping industry. Lydia Folger Fowler, wife of the phrenologist publisher Lorenzo, was the second woman to receive a medical degree in the United States. A descendant of the Puritan settlers of Nantucket and a distant cousin of the astronomer Maria Mitchell, Lydia's father was a manufacturer, a ship-owner, and a selectman of his native town. An intensive study of the rank and file of the Boston Ladies Physiological Society found that the large majority were predominantly the wives and mothers of Boston's middle class.[15]

A shared theme of all health advocates was the inhibition of disease through the teaching of the laws of physiology and hygiene. Over and over again they argued that disease was *preventable;* that it was up to the individual to keep himself well. No longer were sickness and death to be tolerated with a stoicism and resignation that contrasted the limited moral choices of man with the all-powerful inscrutability of God. "Many people," Mary Gove Nichols observed, "seem to think that all diseases are immediate visitations from the Almighty, arising from no cause but his *immediate* dispensation. . . . Many seem to have no idea that there are established laws with respect to life and health, and that the transgression of these laws is followed by disease."[16]

Sylvester Graham, Nichols's mentor, agreed that before people attributed disease to the Supreme Being who loved them, they must look to their own bad habits. Graham's disciple Marie Louise Shew, whose husband edited the *Water-Cure Journal,* similarly warned against the "unwise, irrational, and unphilosophical" tendency of mankind to regard illness as "the *infliction* of Divine Providence." God's true design was for man "as a rule" to live in good health to a ripe old age. Human beings could affect the future by manipulating the environment according to nature's laws and by gaining conscious control of themselves.[17]

Implicit in the health reformers' theory of sickness was the idea of self-help. Disease resulted from the remedial effort of Nature to overcome or cast out of the body some impurity or poison which interfered with the functions of life.[18] Since man was naturally healthy, to keep well he needed only to avoid unwise practices, such as eating the wrong foods and losing control of his "passions." Knowledge of his own physical nature would make men free. "People," announced Mrs. Shew, "must learn to think for themselves." Ignorance could no longer be offered as an excuse for illness, agreed Nichols.[19]

Reformers accused the regular medical profession of making "no effort to remove the causes of disease," while "vainly" endeavoring "to cure conditions, while causes remain. We even have reason to believe," argued Dr. Ellen M. Snow, "that they have greatly multiplied disease by the use of poisonous drugs." In a chilling denunciation of the dependence of the people on physicians, she declared:

> They do not aim to enlighten mankind in regard to their physical well being, but rather seek to envelop their processes of cure in deep and impenetrable mystery. This mystery possesses a magic charm for the uninitiated and ignorant. You have only to look about you to become aware of the credulity and superstition with which the Medical Profession is regarded. . . .[20]

In a flurry of antielitist rhetoric, health reformers deplored the complicated language of most medical journals. "Reader," warned the editor of the *Water-Cure Journal,* "if you cannot understand what an author is writing about, you may reasonably presume he does not know himself." "I would have the *highest science,* clothed in words, that the people can understand," wrote Aurelia Raymond, in her graduate thesis at the Female Medical College of Pennsylvania. "I have studied medicine because I am one of the people . . . to enter my protest against the exclusiveness, which sets itself up as something superior to the people. . . ."[21]

Such accusations did scant justice to the more enlightened members of the regular medical profession. Physicians had long since recognized the value of increasing public knowledge of anatomy, physiology, and hygiene. Yet the rhetoric of the health reformers proved more congenial to the public temperament than the somber empiricism of the regulars which at the moment lacked application to treatment while it discredited heroic methods. Borrowing from the vocabulary of Christian perfectionism to make their point, popular lecturers like Sylvester Graham, William Andrus Alcott, and Mary Gove Nichols succeeded in making health reform a moral imperative.[22]

Public lectures on physiology and hygiene became an important tool in the campaign to combat ignorance. In 1837 the American Physiological Society was founded in Boston to promote health and longevity by dispelling ignorance of physiological laws. William Alcott was the society's first president, and other prominent health reformers, including Sylvester Graham and David Cambell, were also involved. During its first year the society sponsored a number of lectures given by prominent physicians and reformers, including Graham and J.V.C. Smith, a regular physician and the editor of the *Boston Medical and Surgical Journal.*[23]

Although the health-reform movement attracted both men and women, it was to the middle-class woman, by virtue of her new role in an increasingly complex society, that many of the health reformers addressed themselves. Almost a third of the members of the American Physiological Society, for example, were women. At its second annual meeting the new organization acknowledged women's central role in promoting good health in the following resolution:

> *Resolved,* That woman in her character as wife and mother is only second to the Deity in the influence that she exerts on the physical, the intellectual, and the moral interests of the human race, and that her education should be adapted to qualify her in the highest degree to cherish those interests in the wisest and best manner.[24]

Women took to the field as lecturers. Ladies' Physiological Societies appeared throughout the Northeast and West. The names of Mary Gove Nichols, Harriot Hunt, and Lydia Folger Fowler are only the most familiar of the dozens of women who taught enthusiastic female audiences the "laws of life."

The spread of female education received the enthusiastic support of health reformers, who eagerly espoused the tenets of Republican motherhood. They understood that American mothers confronted new responsibilities in a reformed and reconstituted family, which they hoped would serve as the ideological model for social institutions and for society as a whole. Many of women's new tasks fell under the rubrics of physiology, hygiene, and health. Women would be taught to practice domesticity as a science. Health reformers desired to elevate and professionalize the domestic sphere as a means of seeking an effective and practical role for women in a new and unpredictable social setting. "Now who," asked a typical contributor to the *Practical Educator and Journal of Health* in 1847, "is the best qualified to supervise a household? She who has been thoroughly trained . . . or she who knows practically nothing about it. . . . Let woman be intellectually educated as highly as possible."[25]

The "cult of domesticity," then, gave women new authority in the private sphere. The separation of home and work reduced the father's role in domestic life while allowing increasing numbers of women to become primarily wives and mothers for the first time. At the same moment, changes in religious ideas enhanced the importance of parental nurture over predestination. The harsh doctrine of infant depravity bowed to a new belief in the malleability of young minds. Children and childhood were romanticized. The ideal of the modern family—small in size, emotionally intense, and woman supervised—made its appearance as a distinctive emblem of middle-class culture.

Many reformers noted these changes with satisfaction. In a letter to the *Water-Cure Journal* in 1854, the reformer Frances Dana Gage observed:

> Steam power suggested steam power, [sic] and one invention gave leisure for another; mind was released from physical labor, and gained time and leisure for higher and nobler development; woman was obliged to keep sight of the age. She was a help-meet, suggesting, striving, planning, and executing; thinking for the young, and leading them to the depots of usefulness. . . . Woman . . . thirty years ago seldom went from the home, because she *could not be spared,* now that spinning-jennies and patent looms do the spinning and weaving, and sewing machines are doing the needle-work, steam-power does the knitting, and garments are made so cheap . . . it seems an idle waste of time to use "Her needle". . .[26]

Health reformers gave to their female constituents a justification for devoting their full-time efforts to woman's traditional role of homemaking, recast, it is important to note, in a modern and "scientific" setting.

Because her procreative role often made a woman's health more precarious than her mate's, reformers devoted much attention to the state of female health. "If a plan for *destroying female health,* in all the ways in which it could be most effectively done, were drawn up," announced Catharine Beecher in a discussion of what she judged to be middle-class women's new idleness, "it would be exactly the course which is now pursued by a large portion of this nation, especially in the more wealthy classes." Dr. James C. Jackson, founder of the Danville water cure, agreed. "American girls," he lamented, "are all sickly." "You are sick," wrote Mrs. S. M.

Estee to the feminine readers of the *Water-Cure Journal,* "and have been for months, years, and some of you your whole lives."[27]

We cannot know for sure whether or not this generation of women was sicker than their mothers and grandmothers. What is certain, however, is that they *thought* they were. Indeed, they well may have been. Fashionable dress took its toll on female health; the corset and tight lacing did much to damage female anatomy. Increased urbanization brought crowded and unsanitary living conditions. More and more middle-class women were denied the fresh air and exercise available to the rural housewife out of necessity rather than by choice. And the psychological strains of dislocation may have prompted some women to opt for ill-health, rather than stand and face changes which they could still barely comprehend.[28]

It soon became apparent to health reformers that only healthy, vigorous women could meet the challenges thrust upon them by a society in transition. Health reformers believed that woman was in the process of creating a new role for herself. "Woman . . ." wrote Dr. James Jackson to his associate Dr. Harriet A. Judd, "is a new element in society just emerging from her hybernation . . . and so much better fitted to take to herself *new* ideas, and develop them." Good health was essential to woman's new self-expression and improved status. "Let mothers be educated in all that concerns life and health. . . ." insisted Mrs. Eliza de La Vergue, M.D. "Let them learn that *knowledge gives the highest order of power.*"[29]

Good health became a prerequisite to woman's new place in the world. "Woman was neither made a toy nor a slave, but a help-meet to man," wrote "A Bloomer to Her Sisters," "and as such devolves upon her very many important duties and obligations which cannot be met so long as she is the puny, sickly, aching, weakly, dying creature that we find her to be; and woman must, to a very considerable extent, redeem herself—she must throw off the shackles that have hitherto bound both body and mind, and rise into the newness of life."[30]

Women could achieve none of these goals until they learned to dress properly. Health reformers made dress reform a symbol of women's new aspirations. Impractical clothes immobilized women and kept them from their responsibilities. Some regular physicians had linked fashionable dress to female ill health, but health reformers succeeded in making dress reform a moral imperative. Good health was doomed, they argued, as long as women clung to the dictates of French fashion. They called upon women to liberate their souls by freeing their bodies from the harmful effects of tight lacing and long, heavy unhygienic skirts. "How . . . glorious," mused Rachel Brooks Gleason, M.D., "would it be to see every woman free from *every* fetter that fashion has imposed! Such a day of 'universal emancipation' of the sex would be worthy of a celebration through all coming time." Healthy bodies might even lead women into new arenas of accomplishment. "We can expect but small achievement from women," warned Mary Gove Nichols, "so long as it is the labor of their lives to carry about their clothes." "How in the name of common sense," asked Edith Denner, "is a woman with long, full skirts, ever to become a practical Ornithologist, Geologist, or Botanist?"[31]

Health-reform journals pressed the issue. Lengthy technical descriptions of the damage wrought to female anatomy by the corset appeared, complete with diagrams. Pictures entitled the "Allopathic Lady, or Pure Cod Liver Oil Female, Who Patronizes a Fashionable Doctor, And Considers It Decidedly Vulgar to Enjoy Good Health," were published side by side with those of women in reformed dress. A typical picture caption read "A Water-Cure Bloomer, Who Believes In The Equal Rights Of Men And Women To Help Themselves And Each Other, And Who Thinks It Respectable, If Not Genteel, To Be Well." Not content merely to admonish their readers, some journals printed instructions for sewing bloomers. A modest sum could buy a pattern from the *Laws of Life*.[32]

In a society where women were expected to play in increasingly complex role in the nurture of children and the organization of family life, health crusaders brought to the bewildered housewife, not just sympathy and compassion, but a structured regimen and way of life. In 1839 William A. Alcott took for granted the mother's primary responsibility in child rearing and the father's extended absence from the home. "All, or nearly all," he wrote in his book *The Young Mother,* "must devolve on the mother. The father has not time to attend to his children."[33]

Burdened by this reorienting of their family responsibilities, many ordinary women found in the health-reform movement a means of coping with an imprecise, undependable, and often hostile environment. Lectures, journals, and domestic tracts provided friendly advice and companionship in an era characterized by weakening ties between relatives and neighbors. Women found a means to end their isolation and make contact with others of their sex. In study groups and through letters to the various journals, they shared their common experiences with other women. No longer must woman bear her burden alone. This collective sensitivity to the community among women was symbolized by the frequent references to "sisterhood" in health-reform literature.[34]

"I wish," wrote Mary Gove Nichols of her motives in becoming a health reformer, "to teach mothers how to cure their own diseases, and those of their children; and to increase health, purity, and happiness in the family and the home."[35] For some women, Mrs. Nichols and her fellow reformers achieved these goals.[36] Numerous articles on cookery, bathing, teething, care of infants, childhood sexuality, cleanliness, and domestic economy carefully taught women how to manage their households properly. Itinerant physiological lecturers assaulted women's widespread ignorance of their bodies. Nichols relied heavily on discussion of anatomy and physiology in her lectures. She instructed her listeners in the formation of bone structure, the role of respiration and circulation, the anatomy and physiology of the stomach. The process of digestion was described in detail. The remainder of her course involved information on dietetics and the importance of physical education. The alleged evils of "tight lacing," and dire warnings against the harmful effects of masturbation—the "solitary vice"—also proved popular topics of discussion.[37]

Advice on the supervision of pregnancy and childbirth was more "conservative" than that given by regular physicians and especially resisted the nascent definition of childbirth as a disease. Health reformers questioned this novel approach to the process of parturition, calling regular treatment "unnatural and often outrageous." "Here," observed Thomas Low Nichols,

> where august nature should reign supreme, her laws are too often violated, and all her teachings set at naught. Instead of preparing a woman to go through the process of labor with all the energy of her vitality, she is weakened by medication and blood-letting. Instead of being put upon a proper regimen, and a diet suited to her condition, she is more than ever pampered and indulged. And when labor comes on, the chances are that it will be interfered with in the most mistaken, the most unjustifiable . . . manner. The uterus will be stimulated into excessive and spasmodic action by the deadly ergot; the mother, at this most interesting and sacred hour of life, will be made dead drunk with ether or chloroform . . . and if a weakened and deranged system does not act as promptly as the doctor wishes, he proceeds to deliver with instruments, with the risk, often the certainty of destroying the child, and very often inflicting upon the mother irreparable injury.

"Under the popular medical orders of the day," agreed Russell Trall, "pregnant females are regarded as invalids, and are bled, paregoric'd, magnesia'd, stimulated, mineralized and poisoned, just as though they were going through a regular course of fever." In contrast, health reformers viewed conception, gestation, and parturition as natural functions. They rejected the notion that pain in childbirth was inevitable, labeling such a belief "an insult to Providence." They urged exercise, fresh air, proper diet, and cleanliness. Daily bathing was advised for infants, who were to be dressed in loose-fitting, comfortable garments to give plenty of opportunity for movement. No drugs were allowed for mother or child. Such attention to hygiene and diet probably improved the health of many, if we can believe the numerous testimonials from satisfied individuals to be found in the back pages of health-reform journals.[38]

When the middle-class woman took possession of her life and the lives of those around her in the area of health, she sometimes gained the self-confidence to effect other changes within the family and in society. One doubts if this process was always conscious. But the psychological acceptance of various domestic responsibilities could lead often to subtle shifts in the power relationship between the sexes, giving rise to new attitudes toward what was and what was not acceptable in marriage. Nowhere was this process more apparent than in the health reformers' attitudes toward sexual intercourse.

While some health reformers subscribed to the theory of female passionlessness, almost all were among the first nineteenth-century thinkers to prescribe restraint in sexual matters. Believing that good health required constant control, vigilant self-discipline, and vigorous dominion over man's animal nature, they warned that of all the sensual passions, "the sexual element" was the most difficult to subdue. "No other element in our own nature," wrote Henry C. Wright, "has so much to do in . . . forming our character and shaping our destiny. . . . But what is done . . . to bring the sexual element under the control of an enlightened reason and a tender conscience?"[39]

Reformers clearly intended sexual restraint to benefit women and urged them to assert their rights in the sexual sphere. Much of female ill-health and infant mortality, they argued, could be attributed to husbands' sexual abuse of their wives. Asserting that the male's passion for copulation far outdistanced his wife's, thinkers and educators urged men to follow the sexual rhythms of their more delicate spouses.[40]

Excessive childbearing allegedly endangered female health while it drained most women of the energy needed to perform the duties of educated motherhood. Hence, health reformers linked their insistence on sexual restraint to family limitation. They were among the first to advocate birth control publicly. Children, they argued, must never be the result "of chance, of mere reckless, selfish passion." When, asked Henry C. Wright, "will men and women show a rational, conscientious, loving forethought, in giving existence to their children as they do in commerce, politics, and religion?" Every child should be a welcome child. "Welcome" became a code word for "planned." The "great object" of sexual intercourse, continued Wright, was the *"perpetuation and perfection of the race."* Couples not ready to have children should remain sexually continent.[41]

In an era when many people were still largely ignorant of or opposed to artificial means of contraception, women benefited from such cautious attitudes in numerous ways. Historians have already documented many women's profound fears of pregnancy in this period. Less frequent childbearing did improve female health. The desire to avoid conception probably colored women's enjoyment of coitus. Some undoubtedly shared the common belief that failure to achieve orgasm would prevent pregnancy. Moreover, lovemaking techniques were often brutal and aggressive. Even nineteenth-century physicians, although aware of the female orgasm, knew very little else about the intricate nature of female sexual response. One suspects that middle-class women spoke to their husbands and sons of the laws of sexual continence with a degree of enthusiasm and a measure of self-defense.[42]

While exalting the rewards of parenthood and elevating the motherly role, health reformers enjoined couples to limit the number of their offspring. The ideal of educated motherhood proved antithetical to large families. Women were simply incapable of achieving either the emotional intensity or the domestic expertise required of them when caring for a large brood. The injunction that parents should have fewer and better babies had its origins in the antebellum period, among these "enlightened" sections of the middle class.[43]

Educated motherhood, with its approval of smaller families, preserved women's importance while it emphasized their central role in the task of human betterment. Improvement of female health could lead to social regeneration. Woman was invested with awesome responsibilities. "There are no duties on earth so nearly angelic as those which devolve upon women." declared Alcott. "If all wives loved and delighted in their homes as Solomon would have them, few husbands would go down to a premature grave through the avenues of intemperance and lust, and their kindred vices." *The Lily,* a feminist and temperance journal, emphasized woman's moral power. "Woman's influence is truly kingly in general society. It is powerful in a daughter and a sister; but it is the mother who weaves the garlands that flourish in eternity." The gravity of woman's influence went even beyond her own family, for health reformers shared a contemporary belief in the inheritance of acquired characteristics. "For the sake of the race," explained Mary Gove Nichols, "I ask that all be done for woman that can be done, for it is an awful truth that fools are the mothers of fools." James C. Jackson was even more blunt: "God punishes as well as rewards mankind *through woman.* . . . She is appointed to dispense divine retributions as well as divine blessings . . . through her does God visit the iniquities of the father on the children to the third and fourth generations."[44]

Though such attitudes gave women genuine responsibility and power, they also exacted a large measure of anxiety and even guilt. "Women are answerable, in a very large degree," admonished Paulina Wright Davis, "for the imbecilities of disease, mental and bodily, and for the premature deaths prevailing throughout society—for the weakness, wretchedness, and shortness of life—and no remedy will be radical till reformation of life and practice obtains among our sex."[45] Such a psychological burden might well have been unbearable had not health reformers given to women fellowship, moral support, and practical information.

By the end of the nineteenth century, reform ideas about personal cleanliness, public health, and family hygiene had become familiar axioms of middle-class American culture—a badge of distinction by which members could set themselves off from "illegitimate" immigrant groups, many of whom retained distinctly premodern daily habits and attitudes toward disease.[46] Holding out to confused wives and mothers the prospect of improving the quality of life, not merely by changing the environment, but by gaining control of themselves, health reformers promised women that they could raise healthy children and keep husbands moral by cooking the right foods, and promoting exercise, cleanliness, and fresh air. The health-reform regimen established new standards by which middle-class women could measure their respectability and self-worth. Elevating the art of domesticity to a science, reformers restored to their followers a sense of purpose and direction, while, unwittingly perhaps, preserving in a new form traditional assumptions about woman's role which were deeply imbedded in the culture.[47]

At the same time, the middle-class bias of the health reformers offered little support to working-class women. The cult of domesticity encouraged married women who had to work to aspire to an impossible goal—full-time motherhood—helping to make them undependable allies in labor disputes. Believing that their primary commitment should be to the family, they often accepted low pay and low status jobs, insisting that their situation was only temporary. The domestic ideology could also deepen women's perceptions of class differences. Middle-class women were often advised to be cautious about the health of hired servants. Advice literature, for example, warned of the dangers of immigrant girls infecting the household.[48]

Despite these drawbacks, health reform still represents an important chapter in the development of feminist domestic reform in America. Domestic feminism provided those women who were chafing under a too narrowly defined domesticity a practical approach to improving their status. Conservative domestic reformers such as Catharine Beecher concentrated primarily on "professionalizing" women's traditional tasks in the home. More radical feminists like Caroline Dall, Paulina Wright Davis, and Elizabeth Blackwell attempted to construct out of the attention to preventive hygiene and physiological science a social ideology which chipped away at the edges of the public/private dichotomy that had emerged from the separation of home and work. These theorists found convincing justification for women's public activity.[49] Although some historians draw a sharp distinction between domestic reformers and suffragists, suggesting that only the latter were truly radical and that domestic reformers "could aspire merely to modify women's subordinate status, never to eliminate it," such an approach obscures both the potential radicalism of many domestic feminists as well as the conservatism of a number of suffrage advocates.[50]

Health reformers attracted both types of women to its ranks. For many it provided a means of moving into the public world without wandering too far from traditional womanly concerns. Yet though health reformers shared with conservative nineteenth-century Americans the belief that a woman's role was invested with cosmic moral significance, they subscribed to the widest possible definitions of woman's sphere. They understood that to purify society some women might indeed have to enter it. For bolder thinkers in the antebellum period, the movement's protective shelter sanctioned not only the exploration of professional roles for women, but the search for a radical alteration in the relationship between the sexes.

Health reformers did not welcome the changing social and economic patterns which seemed to accentuate the separation between men and women, and they often longed in their rhetoric for a lost age of harmony.[51] As members of a small group among the middle class who were in many respects social innovators, they benefited early from the increase in leisure and the spread of education to women which resulted in more uniform attitudes toward the socialization of the sexes. These developments worked to narrow the gap between men's and women's experience, even as work patterns between the sexes became more sharply distinct. Thus, they preached a degree of male-female mutuality and companionship which spoke to their own experience as reformers but did not take hold among larger segments of the population until well into the twentieth century.

Openly rejecting traditional authoritarian concepts of marriage, they favored a relationship based on mutual love, common interest, and affection. Men were urged to pattern themselves after their wives, while women were told to imitate the strength and conviction of their husbands. Groping toward a redefinition of masculinity and femininity, James C. Jackson, the founder of the Danville Water Cure, observed,

> while it never looks well to see a *masculine* woman, or an *effeminate* man, it *does* look well to see a *manly* woman, and a *feminine* man, the one wearing over her delicacy decision and consciousness of purpose, the other over his massive strength, those soft and kindly touchings which polish but weaken not, yet rather serve to give his essential characteristics thorougher relief.

The phrenologist Orson Fowler boldly condemned the "Odd Fellows, Free Masons, and Young Mens' Christian Associations" for excluding women. "What woman does not help do," he declared, "is but miserably done; what she may not help do should never be done."[52]

Fathers were urged to forsake the pursuit of money and reinvolve themselves in the wholesome atmosphere of family life; the spiritual rewards of parenthood were emphasized. Married couples should learn to share each other's concerns. Indeed, the pursuit of a "companionate marriage" led many young men and women to advertise for like-minded mates in the *Water-Cure Journal,* which for a number of years devoted an entire section to matrimonial advertising. One such ad, placed by "Henry Homes" paints an inviting scene of the mutuality inherent in the reformers' ideal of domestic life:

> I seek a congenial spirit, if she is of the EARNEST, BRAVE, and TRUE, with well developed brain and body, a warm heart and willing hand; in other words, INTELLIGENT, SYMPATHIZING, and PRACTICAL. Am 22, medium height, size of brain 23 inches; temperament, nervous-sanguine; a RADICAL thinker and truth seeker, with untrammeled mind; anti-rum, slavery, drug, tea, and coffee, and am a vegetarian; am identified with the cause of human progress; a great lover of home, and warmly attached to friends, and those who cherish my sentiments. Shall be happy to communicate with any one interested. Address Greenville, Darke County, Ohio.

Women advertised as well. "I am thirty years old," wrote "Victoria,"

> five feet two inches high, healthy, and considered good looking, black hair and eyes, weigh 150 lbs; am just the one that knows when the household duties are done right or not; can spin, weave, teach school, and if necessary work in the meadow, too; am economical in all matters, I think; am anti-slavery, temperance, and a strong believer in phrenology, hydropathy, and advocate the rights of women, and have adopted the Bloomer dress . . . will exhange miniatures if requested. . . .[53]

Victoria would not have mixed well with a group of fashionable nineteenth-century ladies. Indeed, it was their ineffective and ornamental role that health reformers repeatedly deplored.

Of course, they never claimed that men and women were the same. Their vision of companionate marriage, in typical nineteenth-century fashion, depended on their high valuation of women's moral superiority. Women were indeed different from men, and their special abilities were much too important to confine to a narrow sphere. Thus, only a short step from their assessment of women's natural abilities in matters of health lay the argument that women should study medicine.

Indeed, the entrance of women into the medical profession received powerful stimulus from the health-reform movement. "In sickness there is no hand like a woman's hand," the *Water-Cure*

Journal reminded its readers. "The property of her nature," argued a contributor to *Godey's Lady's Book,* "which renders her the best of nurses, with proper instruction, equally qualifies her to be the best of physicians. Above all is this the case with her own sex and her children." Enthusiastically, health reformers applauded the early acceptance of women as medical students at sectarian institutions, chiding the regulars for their conservatism. "What," asked the editor of the *Water-Cure Journal,* "will our Allopathic doctors say to this? We pause for a reply. In the meantime, our women are buckling on the armor for a struggle which must ultimately prove successful."[54]

Women interested in health reform and medical study did not, however, confine themselves only to sectarian medical institutions. Ann Preston herself gave physiological lectures for many years after she received her degree. So, too, did Drs. Hannah Longshore and Angenette Hunt, two of Preston's classmates from the Woman's Medical College of Pennsylvania. Samantha Nivison, who received her degree there in 1855, went on to found a water-cure institute near Ithaca, New York—not far, as a matter of fact, from a similar establishment owned by Dr. Cordelia Greene, who graduated from Western Reserve Medical School in the same year that Nivison finished in Philadelphia. Clemence Lozier, on the other hand, began her health-reform career as a teacher and lecturer before she entered the Eclectic Medical College of Syracuse for a medical degree. Finding homeopathy the most congenial of all the medical persuasions, she established the New York Medical College and Hospital for Women in 1863. Lozier eventually became an active figure in New York reform circles, where she maintained a long and intimate relationship with Elizabeth Cady Stanton. Mary Gove Nichols also founded a medical school in New York—The Hygeio-Therapeutic Institute—after a decade-long career as a health reformer. Indeed, the close relationship between feminists, health reformers, and pioneer women physicians clearly illustrates their common goals. In time these early women physicians, who were attracted to medicine out of an ardent desire to fulfill their destinies as superior moral beings with natural abilities to cure, would be transformed into full-fledged professionals by their contact with an increasingly scientific and empirical discipline. They, as well as their system of values, would be permanently altered in the process.

CHAPTER 3

Bringing Science into the Home: Women Enter the Medical Profession

That women have a natural feeling and talent for the vocation of physicians is proved by innumerable instances . . . and it is a shame and pity that men have not hitherto permitted these to be developed by science.

Fredrika Bremer, 1868.

> Young ladies all, of every clime,
>   Especially of Britain,
> Who wholly occupy your time
>   In novels or in knitting,
> Whose highest skill is but to play,
>   Sing, dance, or French to clack well,
> Reflect on the example, pray,
>   Of excellent Miss Blackwell! . . .
>
> How much more blest were married life
>   To men of small condition,
> If every one could have his wife
>   For family physician;
> His nursery kept from ailments free,
>   By proper regulation,
> And for advice his only fee
>   A thankful salutation.

Punch, 1849. On the occasion
of Elizabeth Blackwell's graduation
from Geneva Medical College.

When the young audience attending the fall session of Geneva Medical College in upstate New York listened to the dean of the faculty one morning in 1847, they probably only dimly comprehended the historical significance of the gentleman's words. In quavering tones, he spoke to them of a letter from a prominent physician in Philadelphia and sought their response to the writer's unconventional request.

For several months the physician had been preceptor to a lady student who had already attended a course of medical lectures in

Cincinnati. He wished her to have the opportunity to graduate from an eastern medical college, but his efforts in securing her acceptance had thus far ended in failure. A country college like Geneva, he hoped, would prove more open-minded. If not, the young woman's only other recourse would be to seek training in Europe. As the dean spoke, a silence fell upon the room. For several moments the students sat transfixed as he concluded his remarks with the comment that the faculty would accede to the request only if the students favored acceptance unanimously.

The students themselves did not realize that the faculty was emphatically opposed to the admission of a woman. Not wanting to assume the sole responsibility for denying the request, they had thought the students would reject the proposal, and they planned to use the actions of a united student body to justify their own response.

Steven Smith, then a bright young member of the class and later a prominent New York physician and public-health advocate, witnessed the ensuing events. Over half a century later at a memorial service for his longtime friend and colleague, Elizabeth Blackwell, he recalled:

> But the Faculty did not understand the tone and temper of the class. For a minute or two, after the departure of the Dean, there was a pause, then the ludicrousness of the situation seemed to seize the entire class, and a perfect Babel of talk, laughter, and cat-calls followed. Congratulations upon the new source of excitement were everywhere heard, and a demand was made for a class meeting to take action on the Faculty's communication. . . . At length the question was put to vote, and the whole class arose and voted "Aye" with waving of handkerchiefs, throwing up of hats, and all manner of vocal demonstrations.
>
> A fortnight or more had passed, and the incident . . . had ceased to interest any one, when one morning the Dean came into the class-room, evidently in a state of unusual agitation. The class took alarm, fearing some great calamity was about to befall the College, possibly its closure under the decree of the court that it was a public nuisance. He stated, with trembling voice, that . . . the female student . . . had arrived.
>
> With this introduction . . . a lady . . . entered, whom he formally introduced as Miss Elizabeth Blackwell. . . . A hush fell upon the class as if each member had been stricken with paralysis. A death-like stillness prevailed during the lecture, and only the newly arrived student took notes. She retired with the Professor, and thereafter came in with him and sat on the platform during the lecture.[1]

Blackwell studied medicine for two full terms at Geneva, but in an insulting footnote to the story, the school closed its doors to women soon after she received her degree. Such was the inauspicious start of the formal movement to train women as physicians.

Undaunted, women continued to seek medical training. Within two years three more graduated from the eclectic Central Medical College in Syracuse, the first coeducational medical school in the country. In Philadelphia a group of Quakers led by Dr. Joseph Longshore pledged themselves to teach women medicine and established the Woman's (originally Female) Medical College of Pennsylvania in 1850. The following year eight women were graduated in the first class. A Boston school, founded originally by Samuel Gregory in 1848 to train women as midwives, gained a Massachusetts charter in 1856 as the New England Female Medical College. Here Marie Zakrzewska, former medical associate of Elizabeth Blackwell, early female graduate of the Cleveland Medical College, and the influential founder of the New England Hospital for Women and Children, came to teach in 1859.

Meanwhile, in New York the Homeopathic New York Medical College for Women, established in 1863 by still another early graduate, Clemence Lozier, enjoyed such success that by the end of the decade it had matriculated approximately one hundred women. Five years later Elizabeth Blackwell, now joined in practice by her sister Emily, also a doctor, opened the Women's Medical College of the New York Infirmary.

Armed with the conviction that medical science needed a woman's influence, hundreds of women received medical training in the decades following Elizabeth Blackwell's graduation from Geneva Medical College.[2] By 1880 a handful of medical schools accepted women on a regular basis. But female pioneers, still dissatisfied with what they believed to be the slow progress of medical coeducation, founded five "regular" and several sectarian women's medical colleges. They built dispensaries and hospitals to provide clinical training for female graduates. By the end of the nineteenth century, female physicians numbered between 4 and 5 percent of the profession, a figure that remained relatively stable until the 1960s.[3]

The movement to teach women medicine developed logically from the denigration of regular heroic practice, the structural growing pains of a profession in transition, and the appearance of the popular health crusade which gave women a central role in health matters. In addition, as we have seen, the changes in the organization of family life provided middle-class women with education, while their declining role in productive labor allowed them to search for new ways of performing traditional tasks. The feminist movement contributed the belief in the centrality of scientific hygiene to female emancipation and an evolving notion of woman's right to participate in the public world beyond the home.

Women entered the profession as part of a broad effort toward self-determination in which all reformist women, from conservative social feminists to radical suffrage advocates, played varying parts. Like these, women doctors sought to redefine womanhood to fit better the demands of an industrializing society. Medicine, indeed, attracted more women votaries in the nineteenth century than any other profession except teaching, and female physicians took seriously their role in health education.

Although they remained a small minority of the profession, women doctors were conspicuous because they violated nineteenth-century norms for female behavior in a way that teachers did not. No wonder they became the focus of a debate over women's proper role in and relationship to public and private health. Whereas amateur instructors of physiology could be dismissed as objects of public ridicule, professionally trained women physicians were another matter entirely. By the end of the 1860s, protest against them mounted from within the profession, requiring them to refine and elaborate an ideological defense of their cause.

One can see from examining their arguments that women physicians were at once ideological innovators and conservators of the past. They shared this role with other women of their era who sought an expansion of female activity, and their ideas fell well within the mainstream of feminist thinking. They used these ideas to give each other encouragement and support and to convince others to enlist themselves in the cause. The process of developing an ideology itself exerted a powerful influence on their perception of reality, shaping it and giving it meaning within the context of nineteenth-century values. We shall see that, although their reasoning was often brilliant and effective, and their practical work important, their arguments remained almost always some variation on the theme of domesticity. Indeed, they as well as their opponents depended on the tenets of the cult of domesticity to buttress their case. Though such a justification for female public activity would later prove self-limiting, this was neither true nor apparent in the nineteenth century, when only a handful of women physicians understood the dangers that lurked for them in this line of reasoning, dangers which would by the turn of the twentieth century hamper their progress within the profession.

The opponents of medical education for women, of course, were not interested in the socially transforming aspect of the new reverence for the female character. Placing women on a pedestal located firmly within the confines of the home, they justified an emotional preference for sequestered women by making them the moral guardians of society and the repositories of virtue. Fearing that women who sought professional training would avoid their child-rearing responsibilities, they reminded their colleagues in overworked metaphors that "the hand that rocks the cradle rules the world." Woman, argued a spokesman, held "to her bosom the embryo race, the pledge of mutual love." Her mission was not the pursuit of science, but "to rear the offspring and ever fan the flame of piety, patriotism and love upon the sacred altar of her home."[4]

Rational legitimation of the female role often veiled less rational preferences: the home represented for nineteenth-century Americans a refuge from an immoral and often brutalizing world. A woman who dared to move beyond her sphere was "a monstrosity," an "intellectual and moral hermaphrodite." Nevertheless, insisted Dr. Paul de Lacy Baker, women controlled society, government, and civilization through the "home influence." Home was

> the place of rest and refuge for man, weary and worn by manual labor, or exhausted by care and mental toil. Thither he turns him from the trials and dangers, the temptations and seductions, the embarrassments and failures of life, to the one spot beneath all the skies where hope and comfort come out to meet him and drive back the demons of despair that pursue him from the outside world. There the sweet enchantress that rules and cheers his home supports his sinking spirits, reanimates his self-respect, confirms his manly resolves and sustains his personal honor.[5]

While revering the purity and repose of the home, doctors, like other Victorians, feared the animal in man and dwelt on the significance of female moral superiority in curbing man's most brutal instincts. Woman's venturing out into the world boded ill for civilization, for women kept men respectable. In imitating men, they ran the risk of demoralizing both sexes. Men, confessed Dr. J. S. Weatherly to his colleagues, were "little less than brutes," and "where men are bestialized, women suffer untold wrongs." Woman's great strength and safety, he concluded, was in the institution of marriage, and "everything she does to lessen men's respect and love for her, weakens it, and makes her rights more precarious; for without the home influence which marriage brings, men will become selfish and brutal; and then away go women's rights."[6]

Conservatives also worried that teaching women the mysteries of the human body would affront female modesty. "Improper exposures" would destroy the delicacy and refinement that constituted women's primary charms. John Ware's conviction that medical education with its "ghastly" rituals and "blood and agony" in the dissecting room would harden women's hearts and leave them bereft of softness and empathy reappeared in elaborate guise.[7]

Despite the popularity of this defense of female delicacy, conservatives compromised their case when they readily admitted that women's special sympathy made them excellent nurses. Praising Florence Nightingale's achievements in the Crimea, they credited her work primarily to her ignorance of scientific medicine. Medical education, they argued, would surely have hardened her heart, leaving her bereft of softness and empathy.[8]

Supporters of female education quickly discovered that respect for feminine delicacy could work in their favor. Was the mother who nursed her family at the bedside ever shielded from the indelicacies of the human body? they asked. If the issue was female modesty, then why should men—even medical men—*ever* be allowed to treat women? As the use of pelvic examinations became part of ordinary practice, male physicians posed a greater threat to feminine delicacy than women practitioners. Indeed, the doctrine of "passionlessness" gave rise to such elaborate exaggerations of womanly delicacy that some social conservatives and some feminists alike viewed the training of women physicians as a necessary solution to the problems arising from female reluctance to disclose symptoms to male practitioners. Elizabeth Blackwell, for example, admitted in her autobiography that her first encounter with the idea of studying medicine arose from the agonized suggestion of a friend, dying of what was probably uterine cancer, that her sufferings would have been considerably alleviated had she been "treated by a lady doctor."[9] Although many feminists remained ambivalent about the practical value of extreme modesty to women doctors or to women themselves, Blackwell always used the concern about the potential compromise of female delicacy generated by male treatment as an argument in favor of training women in medicine.[10] It was in response to such a point of view that Boston feminists joined with the health reformer Samuel Gregory in 1848 to establish a school of midwifery that would be incorporated in 1856 as the New England Female Medical College.

But male physicians alleged other unsuitable character traits against women besides their innocence. Many agreed that Nature had limited the capacity of women's intellect. Women were impulsive and irrational, unable to do mathematics, and deficient in judgment and courage. Their passivity of mind and weakness of body left them powerless to practice surgery. And if these disadvantages were not enough, there remained the enigmatic side of the female temperament. Dependent, "nervous," and "excitable," women, "as all medical men know," were subject to uncontrollable hysteria. "Hysteria," regretted J. S. Weatherly, M.D., "is second Nature to them."[11]

Even more subtle and insidious was the fear that the influx of women would alter the image of the profession by feminizing it in unacceptable ways. "The primary requisite of a good surgeon," insisted Edmund Andrews, "is *to be a man,*—a man of courage." Few physicians were prepared to surrender their masculinity gracefully, especially when technical developments like the discovery of anesthesia actually were rendering harsher images of the doctor obsolete. One Boston doctor taunted women physicians with the remark, "If they cannot stride a mustang or mend bullet holes, so much the better for an enterprizing and skillful practitioner of the stern sex."[12]

The editor of the *Boston Medical and Surgical Journal* continually grumbled about women becoming an economic threat in a profession already burdened with an oversupply of practitioners. When the graduates of the orthodox female medical colleges sought admission to local and national medical societies in the 1870s, they were rejected on the grounds that their training was either irregular or of poor quality. Opponents held women's allegedly inferior schooling against them, yet denied them access to the type of education that was acceptable and often refused to consult with them or ostracized those male practitioners who did. These insults were perpetrated despite the fact that a fair number of medical women received excellent training in the nineteenth century. As we shall see in the next chapter, a comparative study of curricula and clinical offerings in several nineteenth-century medical schools revealed that those women who earned their diplomas at the orthodox women's colleges endured a vigorous, demanding, and refreshingly progressive course of study. Other women, self-conscious about their inadequacies and determined to procure proper preparation, sought postgraduate instruction in Europe.[13] Complaints about inferior education and economic competition arose out of disgust with the multiplication of proprietary schools in the 1830s and 1840s which sharply increased the number of practitioners. But what remains most striking about such objections is that they took for granted women's success in practicing medicine, as well as their ready acceptance by the public.[14] Indeed, there was a desperation about this rhetoric that suggests that complaints about the entrance of women into the medical profession reflected, not the hardening of social lines between men and women, but the increasing permeability of those social boundaries.

The majority of women physicians' professional opponents were, therefore, neither scientific nor consistent. They praised women's abilities to nurse, but rejected their competence in medicine; they offered their arguments for female inferiority, vulnerability, and dependence alongside claims for women's moral superiority and domestic power. But it was the group of physicians who managed to cloak their prejudices in the guise of science that proved the most injurious to women's free development. In the 1870s and 1880s these physicians transferred the grounds for the argument over "female nature" from the spiritual to the somatic.

Rallying around a book entitled *Sex in Education: A Fair Chance for Girls,* published in 1873 by the Harvard professor Dr. E. H. Clarke, they based their case against women almost entirely on biological factors. Menstruation was depicted as mysteriously debilitating and higher education in any subject, as sapping the energy needed for the normal development of the reproductive organs. The results, lamented Clarke with total seriousness, were "those grievous maladies which torture a woman's earthly existence: leuchorrhoea, amenorrhea, dysmenorrhea, chronic and acute ovaritis, prolapsus uteri, hysteria, neuralgia, and the like."[15] He concluded that higher education for women produced "monstrous brains and puny bodies; abnormally active cerebration and abnormally weak digestion; flowing thought and constipated bowels."[16]

When they chose to emphasize the devitalizing and still-ambiguous effects of menstruation, traditionalists were indeed effective. Physicians knew little about the influence of women's periodicity, and the culture treated menstruation as a disease.[17] Reasoning that only rest could help women counteract the weakness resulting from the loss of blood, complete bedrest was commonly prescribed. Thus even if opponents appeared willing to concede women's intellectual equality—and many were prepared to do so—women's biological disabilities seemed insurmountable.[18] Since menstruation incapacitated women for a week out of every month, could they ever be depended on in medical emergencies?

The biological argument proved particularly vexing to feminists. As M. Carey Thomas, the indomitable president of Bryn Mawr and a fierce supporter of women physicians, recalled years later, "We did not know when we began whether women's health could stand the strain of education. We were haunted in those days, by the clanging chains of that gloomy little specter, Dr. Edward H. Clarke's *Sex in Education*."[19]

Female physicians helped to dispel doubts about the effects of menstruation by functioning skillfully in their own professional lives. Many joined with the feminist community to launch a full-scale counterattack against the Clarke thesis. Outraged by the influence of Clarke's book, a group of women in Boston cast about for a woman doctor with the proper credentials to call its thesis into question. In 1874 they gained the opportunity for a public forum when Harvard Medical School announced that the topic for its celebrated Boylston Essay would be the effects of menstruation on women. Writing to Dr. Mary Putnam Jacobi in the fall of that year, C. Alice Baker urged her to take up the "good work," and "win credit for all women, while winning for yourself the Boylston Medical Prize for 1876." Jacobi met the challenge. Because the essays were submitted anonymously, the judges did not know that the author was female. Her essay "The Question of Rest for Women During Menstruation" won the prize, to the opposition's chagrin. The study challenged conservative medical opinion on the subject with sophisticated statistical analyses and case studies, concluding that there was "nothing in the nature of menstruation to imply the necessity, or even the desirability, of rest for women whose nutrition is really normal."[20]

In 1881 Emily and Augusta Pope, graduates of the New England Female Medical College, and Emma Call, an early alumna of the University of Michigan Medical School, published a survey of women physicians sponsored by the American Social Science Association. While serving as staff physicians at the New England Hospital for Women and Children, they summarized the results of their findings on the health of 430 women doctors and concluded that "some unnecessary anxiety has been wasted on this point." They went on to say, "We do not think it would be easy to find a better record of health among an equal number of women, taken at random, from all over the country."[21] Similarly, women physicians who held resident positions at the various women's colleges painstakingly monitored the physiological effects of higher education on their charges. Several of these women published studies that added to the growing body of scientific literature seriously questioning Clarke's thesis. Indeed, one of the important contributions women physicians made to the feminist movement in the late nineteenth century arose from their willingness to challenge on scientific and empirical grounds the somatic definition of woman's nature and to push toward innovative and less biologically constricting approaches to female health and hygiene.[22]

To those Social Darwinists who used the Clarke thesis to raise the spector of race suicide by arguing that sickly women would give birth, if they did so at all, to sickly children, women physicians and their supporters responded with optimistic eugenic reasoning. They depicted themselves as living examples of the transition to higher life forms. They joined with their critics in denouncing the frivolity of the leisured woman, "crushed beneath the despotic power of relentless Fashion." Warning that increased leisure accruing from technological advances demanded that women be given noble work to do, they urged society to check the notorious aimlessness of the civilized woman's life. Women's boredom was notorious: "For one case of breakdown from overwork among women," quipped Dr. Ruffin Coleman, "there are a score from ennui and sheer inanition from doing nothing." Professional careers, they contended, might prove essential to prevent the deterioration of women.[23]

Along with most American scientists of the period, physicians accepted the neo-Lamarckian concept of the inheritance of acquired characteristics. Women doctors drew the logical object lesson: if mental as well as physical characteristics were inherited, the race would steadily improve, but only if women could uplift themselves. Their arguments remained a warning as well as a prophecy: Hold back your women—your mothers—and you retard the race.[24]

Much like their opponents, female physicians took seriously the idea of their own moral superiority as women and their abilities as natural healers. They rarely quarreled directly with the concept of separate spheres, although their interpretation of this concept was quite different from that of the conservatives. Like other social feminists, women physicians defined "woman's sphere" as broadly as possible and connected it quite directly with the surveillance of and participation in public life. Examining the ethical implications of the scientific method for medicine and society, women physicians claimed for themselves the task of integrating Science and

Morality. In a letter to Dr. Harriot Hunt in 1855, Sarah Grimké expressed to her friend her own conviction that medical study held important rewards for women and for society:

> It seems to me the Medical profession opens more than all other things a highway of improvement to woman—it is so peculiarly her sphere to minister to the sick it affords such an extensive field to physiological research to an investigation of all that pertains to the structure & uses of our organs to the injury sustained by those organs from the abuses to which they are subjected, it will bring women into such intimate relation with families, afford such an opportunity of knowing the true condition of men & women in the marriage relation and let them into those secrets which must be known & canvassed in order to be remedied—what an unspeakable blessing it will be to the world, if women of the right stamp . . . capable of becoming acquainted with the science of medicine are spread . . . over the land.[25]

A glance at the titles of the popular health manuals of the period reveals the pervasiveness of the concept of Woman as Natural Healer.[26] Supporters of women physicians elaborated on such cultural assumptions to buttress their argument. "Is not Woman man's Superior?" asked Dr. J. P. Chesney of Missouri. "It is an idea extremely paradoxical," he continued, "to suppose that woman, the fairest and best of God's handiwork, and practical medicine, a calling little less sacred than the holy ministry itself, should, when united, become a loathsome abomination . . . from which virtue must stand widely aloof." Women needed the tools of modern medicine. Women *would* attend in the sickroom, and instinct and sympathy were increasingly insufficient to fit them for this role. Women's "affections need truths to guide them," Harriot Hunt explained to a receptive audience at the Worcester Women's Rights Convention in 1850. "It has begun to occur to people," agreed Dr. Emmeline Cleveland of the Woman's Medical College of Pennsylvania in 1859, "that perhaps the fullest performance of her own home duties" required of woman "a more extended and systematic education . . . especially in those departments of science and literature which have practical bearing upon the lives and health of the community."[27]

Like their opponents, supporters constantly connected womanhood with the guardianship of home and children. Women were morally superior to men, claimed Elizabeth Blackwell, because of the "spiritual power of maternity." The true physician, male or female, she argued, "must possess the essential qualities of mater-

nity." For Sarah Grimké, this quality was a "love spirit." Like
Blackwell, she deplored for women the study of science for its own
sake. No woman could be called a physician who could not minister to the spirit as well as to the body, and she confessed that her
deepest fear was the proliferation of women doctors "unblest with
this gift and whose highest attainment is a scientific knowledge of
medicine."[28]

Everyone agreed, however, that vigorous medical training for
women was necessary for the promotion of scientific motherhood.
Ignorance of her own body and scant knowledge in child management were taking their toll on American mothers and offspring
alike. "What higher trust could be dedicated to the wife and
mother," asked Dr. Joseph Longshore in his introductory lecture
to the first class at the Woman's Medical College of Pennsylvania,
"than guardianship of the health of the household?" His colleague
Emmeline Cleveland, a brilliant gynecological surgeon, affirmed
the necessity of giving to all women knowledge of the human body.
She reminded her students that their high vocation "as nature's
appointed guardians of childhood and youth," meant they would
"become the conservators of public health and in an eminent degree responsible for the physical and moral evils which afflict
society."[29]

Medical women like Cleveland intended to play a central role in
the elevation of their sisters. As science was brought to bear on
domestic life, women physicians would become the "connecting
link" between the science of the medical profession and the everyday life of women.[30] To accomplish this purpose, each of the female medical schools offered courses in physiology and hygiene to
nonmatriculants, mostly mothers and teachers hoping to gain
knowledge in health education.

When critics charged that medical training was wasted on women
who would eventually marry and have children, female physicians
responded by pointing out that medical knowledge was important
for any woman, even if the skills acquired would not be used to
practice. Competence in medicine made women better mothers. A
few women adopted a bolder stance by denying that motherhood
necessarily conflicted with general practice. This recognition of the
possibility of combining marriage and career marked a radical departure from nineteenth-century thinking. "A woman can love and
respect her family just as much if not more," asserted Dr. Georgiana Glenn, "when she feels that she is supporting herself and
adding to their comfort and happiness." Dr. Mary Putnam Jacobi

agreed. Conceding that marriage complicated professional life, she nevertheless felt that "the increased vigor and vitality accruing to healthy women from the bearing and possession of children, a good deal more than compensates for the difficulties involved in caring for them, when professional duties replace the more usual ones, of sewing, cooking, etc."[31]

Medical women also insisted that they had special contributions to make to the profession. Feminization could enhance the practice of medicine, whose goal was the eradication of suffering. Association with female colleagues would "exert a beneficial influence on the male," making men more gentle and sensitive in their practice. Combining the best of masculine and feminine attributes would raise medical practice to its highest level. Occasionally supporters carried the implications of this reasoning even further. Female physicians expected to challenge heroic therapeutics directly. As the "handmaids of nature," women would place greater value on the "natural system of curing diseases . . . in contradistinction to the pharmaceutical." They would promote a "generally milder and less energetic mode of practice."[32]

Some women physicians in the earliest generation consciously did spurn heroic medicine. The husband of Hannah Longshore, the first female physician to establish a practice in Philadelphia, recorded the following in a biographical sketch of his wife:

The Woman's Medical College claimed to be an entirely regular or old school institution and its faculty had a testimony to bear against homeopathy and eclecticism or in any irregularity of its graduates from the established old school practice. But many of its alumni [*sic*] discovered that the growing aversion to large doses of strong and disagreeable medicine among the more liberal and progressive elements in society and that many intelligent women had become tinctured with the heresy of Homeopathy and gave a preference to the physician who would prescribe or administer their milder and pleasant remedies, and especially for the children who would take their medicines voluntarily. This discovery led the woman doctor to an investigation of their remedies and theories of therapeutics and to partial adoption of their remedies and methods of treatment. This conformity to the demands for mild remedies gave the women doctors access to many families whose views were in accord with the reform movements that recognized the growing interest in enlarging the sphere of woman. The woman doctors who saw that the door was opening for this reform of regular practice and prepared themselves accordingly were the first to get into successful business.[33]

Marie Zakrzewska, who, as founder of the New England Hospital for Women and Children in Boston, earned the respect of even the most stubborn members of the male opposition, also remained skeptical of heroic dosing. In a letter to Elizabeth Blackwell she confessed that her whole success in practice was based on the cautious use of medicine, "often used as Placebos in infinitesemal [*sic*] forms." Her reputation, she wrote, had been built largely on her careful use of medicine and her preference for teaching her patients preventive hygiene. "This subject is a large theme," she concluded, "and I am thankful from the innermost of my emotions . . . that nobody has ever been injured, if not relieved by my prescriptions."[34]

In keeping with this interest in prevention rather than cure, friends claimed that women physicians would become zealous advocates of public health and social morality. Emmeline Cleveland noted that women were naturally altruistic, while Elizabeth Blackwell expected her female colleagues to provide the "onward impulse" in seeing to it that human beings were "well born, well nourished, and well educated." Dr. Sarah Adamson Dolley urged women doctors to bring to the profession their "moral power." "Educated medical women," wrote Dr. Eliza Mosher of the University of Michigan, "touch humanity in a manner different from men; by virtue of their womanhood, their interests in children, in girls and young women, both moral and otherwise, in homes and in society." Most of their male supporters agreed. Dr. James J. Walsh admitted that men did not recognize their social duties as readily as women. "Therefore," he confessed, "I have always welcomed the coming into the medical profession of that leaven of tender humanity that women represent."[35]

Women physicians sincerely believed that they would behave differently from men and that they had their own special contribution to make to society. Certainly many chose a career in medicine for more private reasons than these. Many even saw medical practice as a lucrative means of self-support. But whatever their personal motives, such women belonged to a movement that justified itself in larger terms, and they gained their self-image from the social context in which they acted. After wishing the New York Infirmary graduating class of 1899 financial success—"We are always glad to hear of a woman's making money"—Dean Emily Blackwell urged her students to remember, "There are other kinds of success that . . . we hope you will always consider far higher prizes." These, she continued, were "the consciousness of doing good work in your own line, of being of use to others, of exerting an influence for right in all social and professional questions." Readily conceding that her students "doubtless all entered upon medical study from individual motives," she hoped that they had learned "that the work of every woman physician, her character and influence, her success or failure, tells upon all, and helps or hinders those who work around her or come after her."

Forty years earlier, a younger Emily Blackwell confided similar sentiments to her diary when she thanked God that she was only twenty-five and not yet too old to commence a life's labor full of "great deeds." Newly decided on a medical career, she prayed that at life's close God would grant her the ability to look back on a "woman's work done for thee and my fellows." Opportunities were then appearing for women to live a "heroic life," and Emily desperately wished to avail herself of them.[36]

While both sides in the debate over women's role in medicine claimed to be seeking moral progress and civilization's advancement, female physicians, like the health reformers who cleared them a path, diverged fundamentally from their conservative opponents in their commitment to using women's abilities systematically and scientifically. Women doctors hoped to reform society by feminizing it, a task that required the professionalization of "womanhood." Acknowledging that their goals required a broader interpretation of woman's sphere, they felt this a small price to pay for a morally righteous and civilized America.

Nineteenth-century women doctors never drifted too far out of the ideological mainstream. As proponents of the expansion of women's role, they perceived gradual change to be the only kind the public would tolerate. Slowly they succeeded in creating a positive image for the female physician. A minority proved that wives and mothers could handle a professional career, and the inevitable interaction with male colleagues eventually convinced many critics that women could be competent doctors and still maintain their femininity.

Female physicians largely confined themselves to what became feminine specialties—obstetrics and gynecology in the nineteenth century, pediatrics, public health, teaching, and counseling later on. Such specialization was not due solely to resistance from male professionals, although women doctors occasionally blamed discrimination. Women practitioners also gravitated to these specialties because they were conscious of their "special" abilities. They concerned themselves with the health problems of women and children because they hoped to raise the moral tone of society through the improvement of family life.

But confining themselves to women's concerns also circumscribed women physicians' professional influence. A few even willingly advocated an informal curtailment of their medical role, hoping to gain support by taking themselves out of competition with men.[37] Others disdained this approach. Such women were converted early to the modern and empirical world of professional medicine, and their first love was science. Uneasy in the moralistic world of their medical sisters, they exhibited a toughness and clarity of vision that set them apart from those women who used medicine primarily as a moral platform. Physicians like Mary Putnam Jacobi and Marie Zakrzewska insisted from the beginning that medical women needed to be of superior mettle. Fearing that specialization in diseases of women and children would mean a loss of grounding in general medicine, they warned that women would be justly relegated to the position of second-class professionals. Eventually their performance even within their specialty would become second-rate. If women would succeed in medicine, they asserted, they had to be thoroughly trained.[38] Despite such predictions, specializing remained popular throughout the nineteenth century and into the next because it continued to provide advantages in blunting the resentment of male colleagues.

Those who stressed women's peculiar adaptability to medicine risked perpetuating an exaggerated concept of womanhood, and their arguments proved less applicable to less obviously "feminine" pursuits. Dr. Frances Emily White attributed women's great success in medicine compared with other professions to a "peculiar fitness" for the work and the lack elsewhere "of equal opportunities for the exercise of those qualities that have become specialized in women"[39] Pursuits like teaching and nursing fit the pattern well, but law did not. Though women lawyers justified their legal work in a similar fashion, it was harder for them to prove that law was an extension of women's natural sphere; indeed, few women preferred law to medicine in the nineteenth and early twentieth centuries. The reasons for this disparity remain complex, but the "natural sphere" argument did exhibit vexing limitations as women moved out of the home and into the world.[40]

A few individuals struggled uncomfortably with the implications of such reasoning. The journalist Helen Watterson, for example, denounced the woman movement's emphasis on "woman's qualities." Mary Putnam Jacobi quipped that "recently emancipated people are always bores, until they themselves have forgotten all about their emancipation." And Marie Zakrzewska frowned upon women who chose medicine out of female "sympathy." The only motives the profession permitted its votaries, she maintained, were "an inborn taste and talent for medicine, and an earnest desire and love of scientific investigation."[41]

Jacobi remained particularly sensitive to the psychological disadvantages that hampered women physicians from attaining equal status within the profession. Society was still against them, impairing both their own confidence and that of other women in them. Because society refused to judge medical women by their achievements, women doctors were in danger of setting lower standards for themselves. In the nineteenth century any woman who ventured beyond the domestic role was considered an anomaly. To spur them on, Jacobi insistently urged her students to measure themselves by the highest standards of professional excellence: "If you cannot learn to act without masters," she warned them prophetically, "you evidently will never become the real equals of those who do."[42]

By the late nineteenth century, thousands of young women would wrestle with the meaning of Jacobi's words, and for none of them would success come without a price.

CHAPTER 4

Separate but Equal: Medical Education for Women in the Nineteenth Century

Women practiced freely in medicine so long as the practice of medicine was free, and entrance upon it was decided merely by natural taste for dealing with the sick and ministering to their infirmities. When, however, instruction in medicine began to be systematized, when universities took charge of it, and legal standards of qualification were established, women were excluded, because, at the time, no one thought of them as either able or willing to submit to the new conditions imposed. . . . Women are now merely endeavoring to reenter the stream, by adapting themselves, whenever they are allowed to do so, to the changed conditions of things.

Mary Putnam Jacobí, "Shall Women Practice Medicine?" 1882

Fourteen years after Elizabeth Blackwell received her degree from Geneva Medical College in 1849, Virginia Penny, author of *The Employments of Women: A Cyclopedia of Women's Work*, wrote to her regarding the possibilities for women's medical study in the United States. Blackwell's reply reflected both her tough-minded perception of the importance of superior training in breaking down professional barriers against women and her still-vivid memories of her own difficult struggle to obtain such an education. "It is almost impossible," she answered, "for a lady to get a *good* medical education without going to Europe." The women's medical schools that existed in Philadelphia and Boston gave students the "legal right" to practice, but did not yet offer much by way of "theoretical instruction." "There is a real necessity for women physicians; therefore, in course of time they will be created," she ventured confidently. "But," she added, "the imperfect efforts and most inadequate preparation of those who now study, rather retard the movement, and the creation of practice is a very slow thing."[1]

A year later Mary Putnam [Jacobi] took a degree at the Woman's Medical College of Pennsylvania. Hoping to supplement her meager theoretical teaching with clinical experience, she spent several subsequent months at the New England Hospital for Women and Children in Boston.[2] In the end her dissatisfaction with both institutions confirmed Blackwell's assessment of the opportunities then available to women. She chose in the fall of 1866 to seek advanced study in France. There she lived and studied until 1871, when she became the second woman to receive a degree from the École de Médecine in Paris, graduating with high honors and winning a bronze medal for her thesis.[3]

Other women also studied in Europe. In August 1860 Emmeline Cleveland, a member of the faculty of the Woman's Medical College of Pennsylvania since her graduation in 1855, was sent to the school of Obstetrics at the Paris Maternité for postgraduate work by a group of Quaker women planning to endow a hospital at the college. After a year she received her diploma, along with five prizes, two of them firsts, and an honorable mention for excellence in clinical observation. She then briefly toured wards and lecture rooms in London and Paris, returning to Philadelphia with advanced professional training and newly acquired skills in hospital management. There she took up the chief residency of the Woman's Hospital, newly chartered by the medical college. Years later, Jacobi judged Cleveland a "woman of real ability" and the "first adequate teacher to appear in the school."[4]

Until the end of the nineteenth century, orthodox medical schools remained frustratingly slow to admit women. By 1893 only 37 out of the 105 regular institutions accepted them. Many of these were part of the major state universities, most of which were founded after the Civil War and were obligated by their charters to provide coeducation.[5] Impatient with the sluggishness of the profession's response, women founded five orthodox colleges and a handful of sectarian women's medical schools between 1850 and 1900. Separate education, however, was not the preference of leaders of the movement, who insisted on equal access with men to professional training. Consequently, each of the five most successful female medical colleges was established in response to the exclusionary policies of men's schools in the area.

As we have seen, women physicians generally advocated their own conception of the conventional doctrine of separate sexual spheres, claiming that women had a role in medicine by virtue of their special abilities to nurture, abilities that would compensate for and be complementary to the role and achievements of men. "The meaning of the medical movement amongst women in America," wrote Elizabeth Blackwell in 1860, "is the felt necessity for the education of women in Science. . . . It is the full cultivation of the natural powers of a large number of intelligent women, for the purpose of occupying positions which men cannot fully occupy, and exercising an influence which men cannot wield at all."[6] Such women intended to create a professional role that could bridge the gap between public and private life. This entailed applying domestic values to larger communal concerns and utilizing the scientific and technical advances made in the public realm for improving life in the home.

On the issue of coeducation, however, regular women physicians—who became the primary publicists for women's medical education after the Civil War—were much less willing to comply with convention.[7] As the profession itself grew more acutely conscious of the status and quality of medical care in the United States and worked systematically to limit sectarian activity and to gain control over definitions of professional status, these women responded by carefully scrutinizing the quality of women's medical education. They worried that separate institutions for women, lacking in facilities and experienced teachers, would prove inferior and thus established them with considerable reluctance and internal conflict. When debating the state of women's medical education in 1860, the trustees of the New York Infirmary for Women and Children argued that "no system of separate institutions," could ever be as valuable as giving women the opportunity to share "the accumulated experience of the profession in public institutions and receiving the stimulus and guidance and companionship of men in the acquisition of knowledge."[8]

Four out of the five major women's medical colleges were founded only after existing male institutions failed to accept female students. In New York, for example, Elizabeth Blackwell and the trustees of the New York Infirmary worked vigorously to convince established schools to take female applicants. Uneasy at the pending appearance of a homeopathic woman's medical college in the city, prestigious physicians who favored regular medical education for women urged Blackwell to start her own school. Blackwell decided to go ahead with plans for a Woman's Medical College attached to the New York Infirmary, but she regretted the necessity for the move. She and her female colleagues at the hospital "felt very strongly the advantage of admission to the large organized system of public instruction already existing for men; and also the benefits arising from associating with men as instructors and companions in the early years of medical study."[9]

Mary Putnam Jacobi, a teacher for the next several decades at the Infirmary Medical School and probably the most highly respected woman physician of her time, was even more blunt about the rewards of coeducation. "There is no manner of doubt," she wrote, "that . . . coeducation in medicine is essential to the real and permanent success of women in medicine. Isolated groups of women cannot maintain the same intellectual standards as are established and maintained by men. The claim of ability to learn, to follow, to apply knowledge, to even do honest original work among the innumerable details of modern science, does not imply a claim to be able to originate, or to maintain by themselves the robust, massive intellectual enterprises, which, in the highest places are now carried on by masculine strength and energy."[10]

Indeed, the women's medical colleges labored under a stigma of inferiority which was sometimes internalized and perpetuated by women doctors themselves. Bethenia Owens-Adair, who in the early 1870s had attended Penn Medical University, a sectarian institution in Philadelphia, decided after a few years' practice in Oregon that she needed a regular medical degree to advance her status. She decided to return to Philadelphia to attend Jefferson Medical College, a bastion of male privilege which did not open its door to women until 1961. When Owens-Adair arrived in the city, she sought an interview with Samuel Gross, a well-known surgeon and distinguished member of the Jefferson faculty. Hearing of her plans, Gross cordially regretted that although he would "gladly open the doors of Jefferson" to her, the board of regents had the power "and they are a whole age behind the times. . . . Why not go to the Woman's College?" he queried. "It is just as good. The examinations . . . are identically the same." Owens-Adair's reply spoke volumes: "I know that, Professor Gross," she answered, "but a Woman's College out West stands below par, and I must have a degree that is second to none." "Then the University of Michigan is the school for you," Gross concluded.[11]

Owens-Adair took Gross's advice and went to Michigan, as doubts about women's capacity to withstand the rigors of medical training plagued other female medical educators. Given their mistrust of female abilities, it is a wonder they pressed so hard for coeducation. Once the women's medical schools were established, for example, they attempted to provide compensatory education to students, reasoning that women were not yet used to the discipline of science. "It was realized . . ." remembered Jacobi of the New York Infirmary, "that the best way to compensate the enormous disadvantages under which women physicians must enter upon their work, was to prepare them for it with peculiar thoroughness. Women students were almost universally deficient in preliminary training: their lesser physical strength rendered a cramming system more dangerous to health and more ineffective as a means of preparation. . . ." Blackwell, too, was aware of what she termed "intimate sources of difficulty." "Women have no business habits: their education is desultory in its character, girls are seldom drilled thoroughly in anything; they are not trained to use their minds any more than their muscles; they seldom apply themselves with a will and a grip to master any subject."[12]

The decades after 1860 were regarded as a trial period in which women, barred for the most part from men's schools, would prove that they were, in Jacobi's words, made of "superior mettle."[13] All but one of the woman's colleges struggled valiantly and for the most part successfully in these years to establish and maintain professional standards that would remain beyond the reproach of male colleagues. The task was a monumental one, especially when the profession itself was taking a long, hard look at the deficiences of medical education.

As proprietary medical schools founded to turn a profit multiplied in the midnineteenth century, these institutions drastically reduced the standards of medical education in the fierce competition for students. Some faculties shortened lecture sessions to enable students to receive the degree after nine months of attendance; other schools virtually abolished preliminary educational requirements, and clinical training at all but a select few remained scant. Although technically most schools still demanded one year of clinical apprenticeship with a private physician before issuing the degree, the preceptorial requirement had virtually broken down by 1850, so that in many places students were no longer obligated to submit preceptor's certificates.

The multiplication of colleges, the decline in standards and the consequent decrease in the quality of medical practice worked to undermine the prestige of physicians as a group. In his opening address to the American Medical Association in 1869, president William O. Baldwin spoke of a deteriorating system of education. "Any man can enter a medical college in this country without having gone through even the jest or mockery of spending a year in a private preceptor's office," he complained. Many colleges admitted students for "simply paying the fees required." Those who so desired would "attend the lectures and hold private quiz-clubs to familiarize themselves with the material," while many of the other students attended the "lager-beer saloons and theatres at night." Because of low standards, he concluded, it was "but a short step from the plough-handles to the diploma." Similarly, Steven Smith recalled that it was a common saying among the townsfolk of Geneva, New York, where he took his degree "that a boy who proved to be unfit for anything else must become a Doctor."[14]

The founding of sectarian institutions that admitted women students exacerbated already bitter feelings in the regular profession regarding allegations of poorly trained men. The Penn Medical University in Philadelphia, for example, boasted several prominent eclectic physicians on its faculty, and graduated well over a hundred women from its Female Department between 1853, when it was founded, and 1881, when it finally succumbed to financial pressures. Even more distasteful to the regulars was Russell T. Trall's New York Hygieo-Therapeutic Medical College, chartered by the state legislature in 1857. Trall, the editor of the *Water-Cure Journal*, trained dozens of hydropathic physicians every year, many of them couples who left for the West to found water-cure establishments. His school also recruited women students in the pages of the feminist journal *The Revolution* and offered them scholarships.[15]

This situation prompted a reform-minded minority to take steps to deal with the problems facing the entire medical community. Concerned professionals had organized the American Medical Association in 1846, and shortly afterward members formed a committee on medical education to study the problem and recommend measures for improvement. Investigation of the regular schools revealed a dismal picture. A report stated that only twenty-two of the thirty-eight colleges had seven or more professors; a mere four had terms of six months or longer, less than half required dissection, only a handful demanded hospital attendance, and at least ten schools had abolished the required certificate from a preceptor.[16]

In 1847 and again in 1867 the AMA Committee on Medical Education published a series of guidelines for its member colleges. In the first report the committee recommended a six and one-half month term, three years of study, required dissection, clinical instruction, a faculty of at least seven members, and more stringent preliminary education standards. Twenty years later a second report added to its recommendations a graded curriculum, yearly examinations, and an increase to nine in the number of required professors.[17]

It was in the midst of this crisis over medical education that the women's medical schools were founded. Thus, the debate over women physicians almost naturally became intertwined with the one over raising medical standards. The connection in the minds of many male physicians became apparent particularly in discussions in the 1860s and early 1870s surrounding the admission of women to membership in the medical societies. Opponents claimed that women were poorly trained, and that the lowering of professional standards involved in admitting inferior members hurt the status of their professional organizations. Jealously guarding their professional image, many physicians used inadequate schooling as an iron-clad excuse for barring women from membership.[18]

Lurking beneath the surface of the debate over raising standards was the more elusive objection to men and women studying medicine in mixed classes. Although some men undoubtedly supported separate women's schools as an excuse to exclude females from the mainstream of the profession, others gave every evidence of a genuine respect for female achievements. Not all male opposition to coeducation can be attributed to the irrational disapproval of women doctors. Many like Henry I. Bowditch and James Chadwick of Boston were more than willing to see women educated, so long as it was done in separate institutions of comparable quality. "To say that men and women should be educated in medicine separately," wrote an anonymous Chicago correspondent to the *Boston Medical and Surgical Journal* in 1878 "is no disparagement to women students, nor is it opposition to the free and equal entry of women into the profession. It is simply a deference to an almost universal feeling of the sexes toward each other—a feeling with which from childhood up we are indoctrinated by the civilization of our time." Like Bowditch, this commentator was quite satisfied to see men and women doctors working together as clinicians, but only *after* they had received the M.D. degree, for only then was it possible for physicians to "meet each other on a basis of high ethics and science and forget sex." The problem, explained the writer, was that "students are not physicians." Male students in particular needed "time . . . to develop," and for that reason, he claimed, Chicago's experiment in coeducation had proved short-lived. Instead, Chicago had done much better by establishing a separate but equal school for women. To nineteenth-century ladies and gentlemen, the question of men and women studying the human body together in the same classroom remained a delicate issue and a deterrent to admitting women to existing schools on an equal basis with men. Even at Michigan—the first university to admit women in a coeducational atmosphere—women attended some classes separately, and well into the first decades of the twentieth century many coeducational schools arbitrarily "excused" women from their all-male urology clinics.[19]

Though women physicians generally remained unwilling to challenge too many Victorian sensibilities, they had few second thoughts about the importance of coeducation to the future of women in medicine, and demonstrated little tolerance for such arguments when discussing them among themselves. Yet careful strategy dictated that they give due respect to objections raised on the grounds of delicacy. Marie Zakrzewska, who wanted to see women integrated into most of the classes at Harvard much as they were at Michigan, stubbornly hung back from making unrealistic demands in order to keep key supporters like Henry Bowditch and James Chadwick, prominent members of Boston's medical elite, in her camp. Thus, she upbraided the feminist Caroline Dall in 1867 for the publication of an overly aggressive article demanding the admission of women to Harvard Medical School. Dall had proposed the erection of new classrooms and dissecting laboratories to accommodate women, and Zakrzewska warned that her ill-conceived remarks "thrown out to the public" would give both physicians and laymen an excuse for opposing the admission of women. Better to concentrate on the right of women to study, she cautioned, and "keep quiet about all minor arrangements until the admission is effected."[20]

But the complicated and contradictory arguments raised by the opposition to women physicians condemned female medical educators in this period to the thankless task of maneuvering themselves in and around objections put forward by the more vocal members of a profession that collectively proved to be decidedly less than cordial to their efforts. Yet the bitterest irony in this story concerns women doctors' successful efforts to establish medical colleges of their own. In the 1860s they had pleaded to be admitted to men's institutions on the grounds that the fledgling women's schools that existed were producing ill-trained physicians. When their efforts failed, women like Elizabeth Blackwell and Mary Putnam Jacobi, who had themselves been so critical of opportunities for women to study, solved the problem by founding new schools and improving the old ones. By the 1880s students at the regular women's medical colleges were receiving an education comparable to men at the best schools.

Though some male physicians had opposed coeducation on the grounds of Victorian delicacy, by far the most common argument hurled against women physicians by the medical societies in the 1860s and 1870s was their inferior training. When the women's schools started to succeed, the opposition perversely switched ground. In a series of articles in 1879 expressing mock surprise at women physicians' self-confessed inferiority, the *Boston Medical and Surgical Journal* berated them for demanding to be admitted to Harvard Medical School. Now, however, the editors opposed such a move, not on the grounds of women's inferior instruction, but rather because of the "universal opinion of the profession," which was "decidedly and strongly against the coeducation of the sexes in medicine." The editor went on to examine carefully the curricula at the women's medical colleges in New York and Philadelphia, declaring that they exhibited a "standard of examinations as good as that at the best colleges." Women did not need to be admitted to Harvard, he concluded, because they had first-rate institutions of their own.[21]

The fact was that the editor of the *Boston Medical and Surgical Journal* was correct in his evaluation of the women's schools. By the end of the 1880s four of the five most successful of them offered what must be judged an adequate or even superior medical course, particularly when compared to the other vanguard contemporary institutions which were slowly responding to AMA guidelines.

From the day the Woman's Medical College of the New York Infirmary opened its doors, for example, it complied with almost all of the AMA's suggested reforms. The Blackwell sisters founded the school in 1868, ten years after they set up the Infirmary itself, a small but efficient woman's and children's hospital originally located on the edge of the Five Points district in New York City.

The Infirmary had grown gradually out of Elizabeth Blackwell's struggles to establish herself as a woman practitioner in the city. In 1852 she began there after two years' study in France and England. Patients materialized at a snail's pace, and Blackwell's mounting discontent with both a desultory practice and the lectures on physiology she gave to women and girls to fill up her time and pocketbook led her to approach several of the city's dispensaries, hoping to win a place in the Women's Department. No one would hire a woman physician, and medical friends urged her to establish her own institution.[22]

Blackwell gathered support for the endeavor from many prominent Quakers and reformers in the city. Her friends included the lawyer Charles Butler, journalists Charles A. Dana and Horace Greeley, Theodore Sedgwick, the lawyer son of the prominent Federalist of the same name, publisher Stacy B. Collins, reformer Marcus Spring, and the Reverend Henry Ward Beecher.

The dispensary opened in 1854. Blackwell was joined by her sister Emily, and later by Marie Zakrzewska, an immigrant German midwife who would soon earn a medical degree and subsequently found the New England Hospital for Women and Children. In time Zakrzewska also became a leader among women physicians in America.

In 1857 the original dispensary was expanded into a full hospital, according to Blackwell's ambitious plan to give fledgling women physicians bedside clinical experience. In the next decade the Infirmary received a number of graduates from Philadelphia and Boston who stayed for six months to a year for clinical training. Several of these women—Mary H. Thompson and Annette Buckel, for example—went on to found their own hospitals patterned after the Infirmary in cities in the Midwest and West. All such hospitals shared a threefold purpose: to provide medical and surgical assistance to women and children in need, to train an efficient body of nurses for community service, and to provide a clinical atmosphere where newly graduated women physicians could receive bedside instruction.[23]

The Blackwell sisters understood the importance of maintaining the highest professionalism in all their endeavors, and were careful not to allow any of their activities to be tainted with accusations of sectarianism. Marie Zakrzewska recalled constant applications from students for clinical experience, many from people she termed "all sorts of extremists . . . such as women in very short Bloomer costume, with hair cut also very short, to whom patients objected most strenuously." Others had been trained in water-cure establishments "and wished to avail themselves of our out-door practice in order to introduce their theories and methods of healing." All such candidates were refused on the grounds that "popular prejudices could be overcome only in the most careful and conservative manner."[24] Later, the New England Hospital for Women and Children would bar homeopathic women physicians for similar reasons. Indeed, Blackwell's contempt for sectarian women practitioners is particularly pronounced in her private correspondence, especially when she speaks of Clemence Lozier and the New York Medical College for Women. Lozier was extremely active in women's rights circles, and her homeopathic medical school, founded a few years before Blackwell's, competed with the Infirmary for students. Certainly some of Blackwell's hostility can be attributed to personal pique at being upstaged, but equally important was her hardheaded assessment of the most efficacious way for women to make their way in the profession.[25]

In the early years before the establishment of the medical school, the Infirmary enjoyed the support of a number of prominent physicians in New York City. Valentine Mott, a leading surgeon at Bellevue Hospital, became a consulting physician until his death in 1865. Another consultant was Dr. John Watson, an attending surgeon at New York Hospital. Willard Parker, Steven Smith, and Isaac E. Taylor, all conspicuously active in the Academy of Medicine and the New York County Medical Society, not only served as consulting physicians to the hospital for many years, but also held places on a special Board of Examiners created with the establishment of the medical school. Thus, although medical opinion had not yet reached the point where women could be admitted as residents to existing dispensaries, women physicians in New York were not without medical friends.

The Infirmary's Annual Report of 1862 reveals dissatisfaction on the part of Blackwell and other trustees with the medical training of the women students who came to work there. After a lengthy discussion, the Board of Trustees decided to create a fund that could be used to "procure a thorough course of medical lectures for women in connection with some well-established college." Members felt this to be the "most economical means of securing a complete education," believing a separate school for women to be too expensive and hoping that the major contribution of the Infirmary would be "to gain the attention and respect of the community and win that confidence from the profession which will induce them to receive its students into their wider opportunities."[26]

Attempts to use the fund at New York schools were rebuffed, however, and when rumors began circulating that New York City would soon have a new homeopathic medical school for women, Blackwell's professional friends urged her to found her own college, pleading that women's "medical education should not be allowed to pass into the hands of . . . irresponsible persons."[27]

When the Infirmary's medical school opened six years later, it reflected Blackwell's high standards of medical education. It introduced a number of curricular innovations—a required three-year course; a progressive, graded curriculum; a Board of Examiners consisting of some of the most distinguished male physicians in the city which passed on every student graduating from the school; the first course in Hygiene (preventive medicine) offered anywhere in the country; and obligatory hospital residence or medical work under the supervision of various clinics for all candidates for graduation. The faculty included seven male and three female physicians for a student body numbering seventeen. Not until 1871 did Harvard make similar innovations in its course offerings, and the University of Pennsylvania did not follow suit until 1877.[28]

Faculty minutes suggest that the institution never wavered from its original high standards. Students were barred from graduation if they failed their examinations, and occasionally were asked to leave if their preliminary education made it clear that they could not perform adequately.[29]

By 1874, when the term was lengthened to six months and a three-year course became obligatory, the school stood at the forefront of the movement for higher standards. The college continued to make curriculum changes throughout the century and its clinical teaching proved innovative. Meanwhile, few of the male medical schools altered their policies in accordance with AMA standards because when they did they invariably lost students. Only five medical schools—Chicago Medical College, Harvard, the University of Pennsylvania, Syracuse, and the coeducational University of Michigan—managed to lengthen their terms and institute a three-years' graded course by the end of the 1870s.[30]

Blackwell deemed it essential to preserve friendly relations with male physicians. "It must not be taken for granted," she reminded her supporters, "that the exclusion of female students from medical colleges and public institutions indicates a settled hostility to the movement." The new medical school would continue to help women form "links with the profession." And indeed, many prominent medical men spoke highly of the college. In 1911 Dr. Steven Smith reminisced that during the same years that he was a member of the Infirmary's Board of Examiners he was also a professor in a men's medical school. "As to the qualifications of the two classes, both technical and practical," he confessed, "the graduating classes of the women's school generally averaged the highest." He felt the Infirmary "took rank with the best medical schools of the country."[31] William Welch, also a member of the Examining Board in his early career, admitted years later to Dr. Josephine Baker, "I am now ashamed of the type of questions we required those young women to answer. I am sure no one would have tolerated them in our own colleges. But our excuse must be that Dr. Blackwell demanded more difficult questions than could be submitted to our students, for she was determined that all women graduated from her college should be a carefully selected group."[32]

Because they labored under greater financial burdens, three of the four major women's medical colleges were slower than their sister school in New York to improve curriculum, but all of them boasted a respectable program well in advance of the majority of medical schools. In 1850 a group of liberal Quaker physicians and businessmen founded the Woman's Medical College of Pennsylvania. Several of the doctors—N.R. Moseley, Hiram Corson, Bartholomew Fussel, and Joseph Longshore—had already been acting as medical preceptors to a sizeable group of Quaker women who wished to study medicine. When it became clear that no medical school in the city would admit female students, the doctors founded a college of their own. The semester opened with six faculty members teaching forty matriculants. A year later eight students received M.D. degrees.[33]

The Woman's Medical College of Pennsylvania labored under the collective hostility of the Philadelphia medical community for almost two decades. Until 1871 the state medical society refused to recognize its graduates, adhering to a resolution passed in 1860 barring members from consultation with the school's faculty or alumnae.[34] Though members deliberately ignored this resolution, and no violating physician was ever formally disciplined, the repeated efforts of friends of the school to gain admission and recognition for female graduates on both the county and state level met with defeat until the middle of the 1870s. "For a medical man to be connected at that time with the Woman's Medical College required pluck." recalled Dr. Henry Hartshorne, a professor at the school and in the 1880s a faculty member at the University of Pennsylvania as well. Dr. C. N. Pierce, an original incorporator of the school confirmed Hartshorne's recollection when he reminisced to Dean Clara Marshall in the 1890s:

> With the exception of a few annual donations from interested friends, there was not a dollar in the treasury for compensation of professors or illustration of lectures; not a medical journal in the land would publish our advertisement, or do other than grossly misrepresent the college; no hospital could admit our students for clinical advantages without danger of their being insulted by both professors and students. So intense was the feeling on the part of the profession against the men who were willing to accept professorships

in the school or give instruction in medicine to women, that it was with difficulty that good teachers could be obtained.[35]

In spite of the problems, the small but respectable faculty determined to prove that women could study medicine and were as careful as Elizabeth Blackwell in New York to make the institution professionally acceptable. The school rid itself of the suspicion of sectarianism when two members, regularly trained but partial to eclecticism, resigned in 1854. Female professors took their places on the teaching staff as soon as properly educated women became available. In 1866 Dr. Ann Preston, a member of the first class, was appointed dean. As we have already seen, another professor, Emmeline Cleveland, was sent to Europe for training in surgery, gynecology, obstetrics, and hospital management.[36]

Maintaining high standards was a constant concern. The college announced a graded curriculum only a year after it was offered at the New York Infirmary in 1868, although the change did not become obligatory until 1881. In 1871 students were urged to attend an eight-month term, although again a lengthened course was not required until ten years later. Entering students were required, however, to present a diploma from an advanced preparatory school or to take an entrance examination. A three-year course was instituted only four years after it was required by the University of Pennsylvania, while trustees added new laboratory equipment as needed. As late as 1895, for example, the Woman's Medical College of Pennsylvania was the only school besides Johns Hopkins to require work in the physiology laboratory. The faculty began yearly examinations for course work early in the college's history and joined with five other schools—Harvard, Michigan, Chicago Medical College, and the New York Infirmary—in requiring a four-year course as early as 1893.[37]

The dean's correspondence also displays evidence of the desire to maintain high standards. Letters to Harvard and the New York Infirmary in the 1880s and the 1890s inquiring about educational policy indicated a concern to be at the forefront of educational innovation. The college was an early member of the Association of American Medical Colleges and sent two delegates to its convention every year.[38]

Indeed, the school did a remarkable job despite its persistent handicap of limited funds. But lack of money was always an irritant. Writing to Charlotte Blake Brown, a distinguished graduate who settled in San Francisco and founded the Woman's and Children's Hospital there, Dean Clara Marshall responded in 1890 to some friendly criticism Brown had offered on a recent visit to Philadelphia:

> What we . . . need most . . . is not criticism, but *money*. . . . The college is not sufficiently "fashionable" to awaken the interest of those who are working in the direction of Johns Hopkins [reference to a group of women working to raise money to open the Baltimore school to women]. The substantial aid has heretofore come from Quakers who through careful business managers, number few very rich men. When we compare the position of the college with that of the University of Pennsylvania which is receiving its thousands [bequests] every year it seems a wonder that we have done so well. At this moment, poor as we are, our entrance examination is much more severe.[39]

By the mid-1870s the early opposition to women physicians in Philadelphia had abated slightly. One conspicuous change was the admission of women students to clinical opportunities elsewhere in the city. In 1869, for example, Alfred Stillé, the distinguished surgeon and later president of the AMA, welcomed women to his lectures at the Pennslyvania Hospital, remarking publicly, "I not only have no objection to seeing ladies among a medical audience, but, on the other hand, I welcome them." Women were admitted to private classes on the medical wards at Blockley in 1878. Early in the 1880s they began attending regular weekly clinics at the Pennsylvania, Wills' Eye Hospital, the Bedford Street Mission, and the Eye and Ear Department of the Philadelphia Dispensary. Clinical positions also became possible to obtain for the first time. Emmeline Cleveland was appointed gynecologist to the Department of the Insane of the Pennsylvania Hospital in 1878, and two years later her student Alice Bennett took a job as the first female medical superintendent in the Department for Women at the Norristown State Hospital. Blockley began accepting women interns after 1883, and in the next decade women became assistant physicians and pathologists at other city and state institutions.[40]

The desire to develop a special role for women in medicine also led the New York Infirmary and the Woman's Medical in Philadelphia to important clinical innovations. A recent study of the teaching of obstetrics has revealed that this branch of medical education lagged pitifully behind other subjects. In most institutions midwifery teaching consisted solely of didactic lectures. In contrast, Dr. Anna Broomall organized an out-patient department connected to the Woman's Hospital of the Woman's Medical College of Pennsylvania in 1876. Eventually this department offered the first prenatal care in the country. Each medical student was responsible for the independent management of at least six obstetric cases before she was graduated. The New York Infirmary provided a similar experience in obstetrics and gynecology. The 1888 faculty minutes refer to a requirement demanding that every student attend at least twelve cases before graduation.[41]

The city of Chicago gained a woman's medical college in 1870, after an inconsistent history on the question of women physicians. In 1851 Emily Blackwell was accepted as a student at Rush Medical College and attended classes for a year, but when the medical society put pressure on Rush, the school denied Blackwell readmission to finish the two-year course. No other women gained acceptance to regular schools in Chicago until Mary Harris Thompson arrived there during the Civil War. Thompson had earned a medical degree from the New England Female Medical College and had settled in Chicago because it seemed to offer still-unexplored opportunities for a woman physician in practice. In 1863 Thompson befriended Dr. William G. Dyas and his wife Miranda, both actively engaged in service as members of the U.S. Sanitary Commission. Thompson soon became interested in the plight of war widows and orphaned children, and with the help of the Dyases she founded a small hospital patterned after the New York Infirmary, where she had interned.

Dissatisfied with the medical training she had received in Boston, Thompson also planned to enter Rush Medical College for postgraduate work. When her attempts to gain admittance failed, she turned to Dyas, who put her in touch with a sympathetic faculty member at Rush's rival medical school, the Chicago Medical College. Through the influence of Professor of Obstetrics and Gynecology William H. Byford, who rapidly became a loyal supporter of female medical education in Chicago, Mary Thompson and two other women who were just beginning their training were admitted for the 1869–1870 sesion at Chicago Medical.

Thompson completed her work in a year and received a second diploma, but the other two women were not as fortunate. Complaints from male students that mixed classes hampered the teaching of important but delicate subjects prompted the college to ask the remaining female students to leave before they could begin their second year. Byford, who had become a close friend of Thompson's, was mortified, and together they formed a committee that organized the Woman's Hospital Medical College in 1870. The

faculty of the new school consisted primarily of the consulting staff
of Mary Thompson's hospital. Its Board of Trustees numbered
several prominent Chicago reformers and clergymen, and a handful of physicians sympathetic to women.[42]

Like the Woman's Medical College of Pennsylvania, the Chicago
school labored under a small endowment and struggled valiantly to
provide adequate training. The faculty contained several respectable male physicians, including Dyas and Byford himself, who retained an active interest until his death in 1890. Despite the
school's handicaps, it managed to turn out a whole generation of
prominent women physicians in Chicago who ultimately took
places on the faculty: Marie J. Mergler, Sarah Hackett Stevenson,
Frances Dickinson, Mary E. Bates, and many others.

Like their counterparts in New York and Philadelphia, Byford
and Thompson were careful to comply with AMA guidelines as
quickly as possible. The school opened with a large faculty of
seventeen. It required both dissection and clinical instruction from
the start, and although a graded curriculum was not made obligatory until 1876, students were strongly advised to take a progressive course, which was conveniently divided into "Junior" and "Senior" sections. Yearly examinations were adopted. The term of
study remained only five months initially, but was lengthened to
seven in 1883. The faculty urged students to pursue a three-year
course, though it required only two years until 1890. Clinical and
laboratory work, including practical obstetrics, pathology, chemistry, and histology was required early in Chicago, as in all but one
of the women's colleges.[43] By the 1880s, the school had gained
such a worthy reputation in the city that Cook County hospital
opened its competitive examinations to women, and a few, including Mary E. Bates and Jeanette Kearsley, won appointments,
though the hospital remained reluctant to accept more than one
woman at a time. In 1892 the school merged with Northwestern
University, continuing to train competent women physicians until
it was closed by Northwestern's trustees in 1902.[44]

In Baltimore a woman's medical college was established in 1882
when a group of female philanthropists met with seven male physicians, including the uncle of the indomitable future president of
Bryn Mawr, M. Carey Thomas, to open a school they hoped would
offer "all the opportunities for the pursuit of knowledge that are
offered to men," within an "unrestrained" and "unembarrassed"
atmosphere. The faculty immediately set the term at seven months,
required final examinations at the end of each year, and instituted

a graded course of instruction with the mandatory completion of a "creditable" dissection. In 1888 the course was extended from two to three years, and in 1895, to four.[45] According to Abraham Flexner, who visited the school in 1909, laboratory facilities were "scrupulously well kept." They showed, he thought, a desire to do "the best possible with meager resources." Although clinical opportunities existed, Flexner found these to be inadequate, but not more so than the majority of medical institutions at the time. Because no adequate history of the school exists, comparatively less is known about it than what is known of Chicago, New York, or Philadelphia. Still, its catalogues indicate that its curriculum compared favorably to the others. Unfortunately, the Woman's Medical College of Baltimore remained dominated by men; only a few women appear on its faculty lists even as educated women professionals became available. Despite this drawback the school graduated seventy-three students by 1900. How well it did its work is evidenced by the fact that in 1890 two of its graduates won internships in Blockley hospital in Philadelphia following a stiff competitive examination.[46]

The only major regular woman's medical college that in any way deserved the accusations of inferior teaching hurled by the medical opposition was the New England Female Medical College in Boston, founded as a school of midwifery in 1848 by Samuel Gregory, an idiosyncratic and opinionated health reformer, who had no formal medical training. A Yale graduate, Gregory made his living as an itinerant lecturer and pamphlet writer. In the late 1840s he became obsessed with the growing popularity of male midwifery, and published several articles and pamphlets terming the new custom an affront to female modesty and to civilization itself. Arguing that only women should attend other women in childbirth, Gregory managed to rally to his support a mixed assortment of New England reformers, lawyers, teachers, clergy, and businessmen, including Samuel Sewall, Emerson Davis, and James Freeman Clarke. Together they organized the Female Medical Education Society, which first offered courses primarily in nursing and midwifery. In 1856 a woman's medical school, consisting of a faculty of six men, with one woman as demonstrator of anatomy, was chartered by the Massachusetts legislature. Though two of the faculty were members in good standing of the Massachusetts Medical Society, the school's health-reform connections were also strong: William Mason Cornell, professor of physiology, hygiene, and medical jurisprudence, also edited the *Practical Educator and Jour-*

nal of Health, a health periodical that was the official organ of the Massachusetts State Teachers Association.[47]

The New England Female Medical College also had solid feminist ties. A Board of Lady Managers, consisting of some of the most prominent "reform" women in Boston—Mrs. Lyman Beecher, Abby May, Lucy Goddard, Ednah Dow Cheney, Harriet Beecher Stowe—actively raised money on the school's behalf. In 1859 they enticed Marie Zakrzewska to leave the New York Infirmary to become Professor of Obstetrics and Diseases of Women and Children at the school. Zakrzewska was also appointed resident physician in a proposed hospital planned by the lady managers. Thus, the new decade opened with promise. Yet a few years later it became apparent that the New England Female Medical College would prove a disappointment to medical women everywhere.[48]

One historian has suggested that the cause of failure lay primarily with "the resistance of the medical world to women." However, a careful reading of the school's history suggests that the explanation is not that simple. Of course all of the women's medical schools struggled mightily with male hostility, but most of them achieved the profession's grudging respect. The New England, unfortunately, was also burdened with Samuel Gregory's difficult personality and his antiquated ideas about medical education. Gregory's presence dominated trustee meetings. Minutes suggest that he devoted most of his time to school affairs, taking them up as his own private cause. He resented interference from any source on policy or financial issues and clashed with faculty, students, lady managers, and trustees over the future of the school. At issue particularly, especially with some of the faculty, was the question of standards and medical curriculum.[49]

The school's catalogues, for example, written by Gregory himself, were amateurish and rambling, lacking the professional veneer of those of the other women's institutions.[50] Handicapped for years by a small faculty, the college could offer only a short term of study: four months. There is no evidence of a graded curriculum. Clinical facilities remained meager. Zakrzewska, fresh from the New York Infirmary, where she and the Blackwell sisters had given a great deal of thought to educating women physicians, was dismayed from the start by the lack of even the most rudimentary laboratory equipment. When she petitioned for the purchase of a microscope after her first year, Gregory rejected the request on the grounds that such equipment represented "new fangled European notions." In 1860 such a reaction represented the most extreme form of medical conservatism.[51]

Zakrzewska's autobiography chronicles her gradual disenchantment. She found that not only did physicians in Boston deny the school support because of low standards, but even women physicians educated elsewhere kept their distance from the New England. Many feared that its very existence gave women in medicine a bad name. Years later Mary Putnam Jacobi commented that "there was no one connected with [the school] who either knew or cared what medical education should be. . . . It offered a curriculum of instruction, so ludicrously inadequate for the purpose, as to constitute a gross usurpation of the name."[52]

As Zakrzewska received more encouragement from several prominent male physicians in Boston, including Henry I. Bowditch and Samuel Cabot, she realized that Gregory and the New England could become a severe liability, not only to her own career, but to the reputation of women physicians as well. Gregory consistently did battle with Boston's medical elite. Particularly disturbing to Zakrzewska was his monograph, *Man Midwifery,* where he "not only challenged the prevailing method of practice but abused even the best physicians by intimating the grossest indelicacy, yes, even criminality in their relations with their patients. This was the reason," she concluded, "why no physician in Boston would openly acknowledge me as long as I remained in connection with the New England Female Medical College."[53]

Equally frustrating was her campaign to raise the school's standards, especially when she realized that she would not be supported by a united faculty, some of whom believed that they were already "teaching all that a woman doctor ought to know." Zakrzewska also criticized the poor preparatory education required from entering students. While a few had the "best of education," too many others fell far below standard. These latter she could not in good conscience "consider . . . fit subjects to enter upon the practice of a profession which requires so much knowledge in various scientific directions as well as a broad education, so as to enable one to comprehend the effects of all kinds of environment upon the individual patient." In addition, Zakrzewska had difficulty convincing such students of the importance of clinical training, something which she had come to consider, particularly because of her association with the Infirmary, as absolutely essential. Yet the trustees continued to make entrance requirements as lenient as possible in order to attract students.[54]

When her position became "tedious in its teaching duties and unendurable in its relation to the students," Zakrzewska resigned. In 1862 she left the school, taking with her a number of students and trustee supporters who helped her establish the New England Hospital for Women and Children. In doing so she surrendered her hopes of teaching undergraduate medical students, and devoted herself instead to building a hospital which would offer coveted clinical instruction to women medical graduates for the next half century.[55]

Years later Zakrzewska lamented her difficulties with Gregory, complaining that "had the originator of the school . . . been a man of higher education and broader views, the school might have been taken up by the men standing highest in the profession. The prevailing sentiment among these men seemed to be that if women wanted to become physicians, the trial should be made by giving them the same advantages as were offered to men students." For herself, she viewed the struggle over higher standards in the early 1860s as "the beginning of the end of the college." She stubbornly refused to grant women medical diplomas simply because they were women, arguing that "perseverence alone does not entitle persons to receive a diploma."[56]

Acutely sensitive to the reputation of women physicians, Zakrzewska steadfastly held back from open disagreement with the trustees, understanding that any public controversy would involve the school in a "notoriety absolutely fatal to the whole cause." When she resigned in 1862, however, she wrote them a bitter letter, summing up the feelings of many concerned women educators. If it were the intention of the trustees, she observed, "to supply the country with underbred, ill educated women under the name of physicians in order to force the regular schools of medicine to open their doors for the few fitted to study, so as to bring an end to an institution from which are poured forth indiscriminately 'Doctors of Medicine,' I think the New England Female Medical College is on the right track."[57]

After she left, internal dissention continued to cause problems for the school until Gregory's death. Shortly afterward, financial problems forced the institution to merge with Boston University and become homeopathic, a move that drew contempt from female regulars. Mary Putnam Jacobi, for example, could not hide her delight when the New England was finally "extinguished as an independent institution" in 1873.[58]

Female medical educators articulated by word and by deed two primary goals. On the one hand they strove to make women physicians as "professional" as possible, demanding that students comply with, if not surpass, the highest standards of excellence for men. On the other, they sought to preserve for women a "special" role in medicine, hoping to channel their intellectual energies into service appropriate to nineteenth-century conceptions of woman's sphere.

Most women physicians clung to a belief in the necessity of coeducation largely because they doubted women's ability to create separate institutions commensurate with male standards. Although a retrospective study of the major women's schools suggests that such doubt was unfounded and that most of these institutions performed valiantly despite their enforced isolation from the mainstream of American medicine, the majority of female educators established the women's colleges as "cautious experiments." Most women physicians came to view them as valuable merely as a temporary means of proving women's competency in medicine. Only the Woman's Medical College of Pennsylvania seemed curiously oblivious to such short-term goals and quite certain of its own future significance in remaining a woman's school.[59]

Other women's schools, however, were profoundly influenced by the opening of Johns Hopkins medical school in 1892. The establishment of the Baltimore school marked the beginning of an era of considerable consequence in the history of American medicine, while its willingness to admit women on the same terms with men marked an even more crucial event for the history of women in the profession.

The Johns Hopkins University had come into being in 1876 very much because of the vision and foresight of a benefactor and namesake whose educational philosophy was as innovative as his financial contribution was vast. Reviving and improving on the eighteenth-century Scottish tradition of university medical schools, Hopkins wanted a hospital subordinated to the needs of a medical school with both institutions intimately connected to a university. Medical teaching was to utilize and depend on the resources of an up-to-date hospital, while the university itself would be modeled after the system of German higher education. Hopkins's first president, Daniel Coit Gilman, was instructed to canvass and recruit the best teachers and scholars in the United States and western Europe. The result was a highly cosmopolitan group in the original faculty of philosophy: not one man was a native Marylander, and two, the mathematician J. J. Sylvester and the brilliant young physiologist H. Newell Martin, came from England.[60]

Initially, the University's trustees had agreed with President Gilman that coeducation would unquestionably threaten the goals of the new institution, and women were consequently barred from admission. Although several midwestern institutions had reluctantly succumbed to the financial pressure of declining enrollments and recently accepted women students, the larger endowments of eastern private universities, coupled with the establishment of a handful of excellent women's colleges after the Civil War, allowed schools like Harvard, Princeton, Columbia, and Yale to delay the admission of women indefinitely. In 1882 this policy forced Martha Carey Thomas, a graduate of Cornell and the daughter of an influential Hopkins trustee, to obtain her Ph.D. in Zurich, when a year of unsuccessful negotiations could not move the trustees to grant her permission to earn a Hopkins degree. Thomas, proud and imposing, never forgave the university for her humiliation, and it was not long before events conspired to grant her a measure of revenge while opening up a unique opportunity for all women.

The new Johns Hopkins Hospital, designed by Dr. John Shaw Billings and infused with an innovative intellectual spirit by Dr. William Welch, opened its doors in 1889, thirteen years after the founding of the university. Only the completion of the medical school was now awaited to fulfill the vision of its benefactor. But funds intended for this purpose, which since 1880 had been tied up in the fluctuating fortunes of the Baltimore and Ohio Railroad, were not readily forthcoming between 1889 and 1891. In the year the hospital opened, the railroad had ceased to pay dividends at all to its stockholders. Though the key figures of the medical faculty—Welch, Halsted, Osler, and Kelly—had all been appointed, naysayers worried that there would be no school of medicine.

It was at this point that the future of the most innovative institution in the history of modern American medicine became intertwined with the advance of feminism. Under the rigorous and determined leadership of M. Carey Thomas, now dean and professor of English at Bryn Mawr College, four Baltimore young women—all of them the daughters of Hopkins trustees—seized upon the school's financial dilemma as a means of promoting the cause of women.

Thomas and her friends Mary Elizabeth Garrett, Mary Gwinn, and Elizabeth King proposed to take on the task of raising the money needed. Within a year, a national Woman's Fund Committee had been set up throughout the country to tap existing female networks—both women of family and wealth and women of intellect—and to establish new ones.[61]

Partly through the $50,000 contribution from Miss Garrett, the shrewd daughter of the president of the Baltimore and Ohio and his trusted advisor in business affairs, the Woman's Committee in 1890 was able to offer the trustees the sum of $100,000, providing only that women were admitted to the medical school on the same terms as men. Both President Gilman and William Welch opposed the proviso, but Osler, Kelly, and Dr. Henry Hurd, the new superintendent of the hospital, won them over. In the end the trustees voted to accept the offer, and soon afterwards Welch retracted his initial opposition.

One hundred thousand dollars was a good start, but it was still far from the five hundred thousand dollars actually needed to open the school, so the Woman's Committee went back to work. It was only the generous contribution of an additional three hundred thousand dollars from Mary Garrett during Christmas of 1892 that finally enabled the school to begin preparations for its first class the following year. In retrosepct the school owes its existence as much to Mary Garrett as it does to Johns Hopkins himself.

Along with her second donation, Mary Garrett made the demand that the school maintain the highest possible entrance requirements. Embarrassed by her attempt to bind them too closely to what they feared was an impractical goal, Welch and Gilman objected. Although they believed in the abstract principle that entering medical students should be college graduates, they worried that such a requirement would effectively bar eligible candidates. Garrett, however, would not budge, and in the end she forced the innovators at Hopkins to live up to their own high standards. The result was that Johns Hopkins Medical School became the first in America to require a bachelor's degree for admission. The significance of the decision for the future of medical education can be at least partially summed up by recalling William Osler's puckish remark to Welch. "Welch," he admitted, "we are lucky to get in as professors, for I am sure that neither you nor I could ever get in as students."[62]

One indirect result of the admission of women to Johns Hopkins was that, with the exception of the Woman's Medical College of Pennsylvania, the women's medical colleges closed their doors one by one. Plagued by mounting financial burdens engendered by the costs of medical education in a new scientific age, and genuinely excited and hopeful about opportunities at quality institutions like Hopkins, female medical educators optimistically predicted women's greater integration into the profession.[63]

Coeducation, however, would ultimately prove disappointing. For many reasons, including strong cultural resistance to career women in general, the contradictions in their own ideology, and various and subtle forms of institutional discrimination, female enrollments at coeducational institutions remained scattered and generally scanty in the twentieth century. What is more, women at these schools found themselves isolated from the experience of a self-supporting and self-directed female community, something that the women's colleges, despite their handicaps, had managed to provide. Medical professionalism and medical education remained unquestionably dominated by men. Indeed one wonders, given female educators' awareness of the extreme sex-role stereotyping of their culture, how they could have ever expected otherwise?

Equally puzzling is the tenacity with which women physicians clung to the belief that women could be educated to play a special and compensatory role in medicine at coeducational institutions, where they would inevitably be outnumbered. That women physicians held to this conviction suggests the degree to which some of them were still committed to elaborate cultural and biological explanations of gender differences. Even at the end of the century most still found themselves in agreement with Elizabeth Blackwell when she mused to her friend Barbara Bodichon about the role of women physicians:

> I do not look on a good medical training as having power to make men of women, but as a most valuable educator of their own natures, making their benevolence, intelligent, and their activity to the purpose. It is very possible that women so trained, will not act just as men would nor supply the place now occupied by medical men—but they will find their own place and work, & I think it will be very valuable work.[64]

Hardly welcomed into the profession, women entered medicine in spite of male opposition. They did so by founding creditable and occasionally outstanding medical schools in the nineteenth century. Still they could not integrate themselves as a significant group into the medical mainstream. Always suspicious of the rewards of separate institutions, they viewed them as temporary expedients, and in the process overlooked the dangerous pitfalls of coeducation. Their belief in woman's special role in medicine and their gnawing worry that all alone, women simply could not train themselves to be good doctors led them to undervalue the enormous potential benefits of separate professional schools in a culture where extreme sex stereotyping was prevalent. Though the women's institutions had proved that females could be competent, even outstanding physicians, American society was not prepared to come to grips with these achievements. Although successful in the narrow sense, the movement to educate women in medicine in the nineteenth century failed to alter significantly timeworn beliefs about the role of women in the professions.

CHAPTER 5

Women and the Profession:
The Doctor as a Lady

What young woman in this large and attentive audience has not found
herself on a higher plane of being, as she has listened to this recital of
woman's service for humanity and the Divine Master? . . . They are
not perhaps persuaded to become physicians, but they are persuaded
that womanhood of the noblest type can rise to the full possession of all
its powers, and yet lose nothing in sweet grace or womanly dignity, lose
nothing in love of husband or of children, or of friends, friends worthy
of the name of friends. . . . If it be true as our statistics have shown,
that an earnest purpose in life transforms invalids into healthy women,
if it extracts the sting from morbid grief, if it renders that unholy thing,
a marriage of convenience, inexcusable, and leaves every woman free
to enter the estate of matrimony from the purest motives only, then
how desirable is the possession of such a purpose? . . . Who shall say
that they who have toiled in this good work, whose fruition in part, our
eyes have beheld today, toiled in vain!

Rachel Bodley, 1880

The generations of women who entered the medical profession in
the nineteenth and early twentieth centuries struggled tirelessly
with personal and professional problems from which their male
colleagues were spared. Although they were not always conscious
of the most subtle ways in which their womanhood colored their
experiences, they knew that they were breaking new ground. Yet it
is only the modern reader with the benefit of hindsight who can
truly understand the variety and persistence of the obstacles that
they faced. Certainly when one ponders the records of these
women's lives, one cannot help but be struck by their independence, determination, and patience.

In the last third of the nineteenth century, female medical educators began to take stock of their situation and progress. When
statistics became fashionable they took a number of surveys on the
status of women in the profession. Such reports boosted sagging
spirits by demonstrating the success of female medical practitioners. It was no mere accident that Rachel Bodley, the dean of
the Woman's Medical College of Pennsylvania, delivered the first

of these surveys in the form of a valedictory address to the graduating class of 1880. After all, pioneer female educators and their male supporters were championing an unorthodox cause; it was comforting to learn that early battles had not been fought in vain. Taking stock also became both a source for pride in past accomplishments and a reason for hope that the future would fulfill its promise. Finally, such surveys also sought to prove both to male colleagues and to a suspicious public that, as Dr. Marion M. Grady put it in a report to the Woman's Medical College of Pennsylvania Alumnae Association in 1900, "Medical women are now accepted as a fact of civilization."[1]

Bodley's survey on women medical graduates was the first to be completed. She found that of the 189 women out of the 244 polled who responded to her questionnaire, 166 were still in active medical practice and averaging an income of almost $3,000 a year. Eight had quit medicine because of the pull of domestic duties, six because of ill health, and one because of full-time involvement in philanthropic work. Three were retired. Sixteen of the women had some form of surgical practice; the others were general practitioners with a heavy emphasis on gynecology and obstetrics. Sixty were or had been employed by an institution—either a hospital, an asylum or a school for girls. About a third of the group were actively engaged as medical teachers, either as professors in women's medical colleges, as popular lecturers, or as instructors of hygiene in girls' schools. Many expressed deep gratification in such work. One hundred fifty of the respondents reported "cordial social recognition" in their communities, while only seven complained of discrimination. A little under half of the women belonged to one or more medical societies. Only sixty-one of the respondents answered Bodley's last question, "What influence has the study and practice of medicine had upon your domestic relations as wife and mother," although 129 were married. Ten found marriage an impediment to practice. Most cautiously expressed the opinion that medicine had enhanced their personal lives, but many admitted to occasional strain.

For Bodley, the results proved a matter for rejoicing. For the historian, the information gathered in these studies helps to paint a more accurate picture of women physicians' collective experience. But statistics are useful only in assessing the larger picture, they paint meager and unsatisfying portraits of the substance of human endeavor. We may learn from the surveys that a high percentage of women doctors were in practice and doing modestly well, but we hear very little else about the texture of their lives.

Even women physicians themselves understood the poverty of statistical data. Their own special needs for mutual support and encouragement led them to keep abreast of each other's doings as best they could. Friendships formed in medical school bridged the gulf of time and distance through faithful correspondence. Alumnae associations at the women's medical colleges loyally kept records on colleagues and maintained ties with new graduates. Yearly meetings often served as a means of catching up on the news as classmates and teachers gathered in person for the exchange of personal and professional information and listened as the corresponding secretary read letters from colleagues and friends living too far away to attend.[2]

This kind of qualitative evidence can answer more personal questions. What attracted such women to medicine? How did family and friends react? Did their experiences in medical school differ, and what parameters determined their life choices when they graduated? Were husbands supportive? Did women who chose not to marry condemn themselves thereby to a lonely and impoverished emotional life? Of course, the answers must necesssarily be personal and idiosyncratic. And yet the life stories of individual women physicians are at once unique *and* representative. Women entered medicine for a wide variety of personal reasons, but once they committed themselves to its pursuit, their lives were shaped by social options and conventions that moved well beyond personal preferences. Thus, every woman's private choices were eventually monitored by what was socially possible in the climate of late nineteenth- and early twentieth-century America.

Impressionistic evidence suggests that generalizations about the experience of women physicians are indeed possible, even about the uniquely personal. But to say that the broad outlines of the lives of women physicians during this period exhibit characteristics in common is not to claim that their lives were the same. What is here revealed about women doctors will be more useful when compared both with similar studies for women professionals in other fields and for male physicians.

The number of women physicians grew from about two thousand in 1880 to roughly seven thousand in 1900. Common threads permit a few comments about their family backgrounds. Like their male counterparts, the majority came from the middle and upper middle class. In the years before 1880, most of these families were concentrated geographically in the Northeast until medical schools in Washington, D.C., Maryland, and the Midwest and West began

accepting women. Quaker and reform families were also noticeably prominent, especially among the earliest generations. The
Woman's Medical College of Pennsylvania, it will be recalled, was
founded in Philadelphia by Quakers who wished to give their
daughters an opportunity to study medicine.

Because many such families held liberal attitudes on the position
of women, a significant minority of women physicians received an
excellent education for the time; some even attended college. Ida
Richardson, for example, one of the founders of the West Philadelphia Hospital for Women and Children and an 1879 graduate of
the Woman's Medical College of Pennyslvania (WMCP) studied at
Wesleyan College in Delaware. Charity Jane Vincent (WMCP,
1882) gained a good classical education at Westminster College
and then Franklin College in Ohio, where her father was the
President.[3] Edith Anna Barker (WMCP, 1897) attended Smith
College. Emmeline Cleveland, the brilliant gynecological surgeon
who was the first Chief Resident at the Philadelphia Woman's
Hospital and Professor of Obstetrics and Diseases of Women at
the Woman's Medical College, graduated in 1853 from Oberlin
College, as did many of her later students. Charlotte Blake Brown,
founder of the San Francisco Children's Hospital, attended Elmira
College in upstate New York. The father of Mary Hancock
McLean, a pioneer St. Louis woman physician, sent her to Vassar
for two years before she matriculated at the University of Michigan
medical school in 1880. Other women physicians studied at female
seminaries and respectable preparatory schools. By the beginning
of the twentieth century, more and more of them were meeting the
rising standards of at least two years of college preparation.[4]

Not infrequently, there was already a physician in the family,
usually a father, brother, or uncle, but, as the century wore on,
occasionally a mother as well. Agnes Margaret Gardiner (WMCP,
1899) and Cordelia Greene, one of the first women to graduate
from Cleveland Medical College in 1856, both read medicine with
their fathers before seeking formal training.[5] Harriet A. Kane,
whose mother had attended the Women's Medical College in
Philadelphia in 1854, entered the school twenty-seven years later,
settling in the city accompanied by her mother and two brothers,
both of whom simultaneously attended Jefferson Medical College.
Mary McLean's father, a zealot regarding his daughter's education,
was one of the first physicians to open a practice in Washington,
Missouri. And finally, the fathers of Jeannie Sumner, Eugenia
Reyburn, and Clara Bliss Hinds, all graduates of Washington,

D.C., medical schools in the 1880s and 1890s, were prominent medical professionals.[6]

Besides providing important educational opportunities, families could be supportive in other ways as well. Charlotte Blake Brown, who studied medicine in Philadelphia after having married and given birth to three children, managed to leave her home and family in California in the competent and willing hands of her mother. Even her grandparents supported Brown's decision to study medicine, and in 1872 Daniel Farrington registered his approval of his granddaughter's venture in a letter to his daughter. "I hope," he wrote, "she may be prospered in her great undertaking & be the means of doing a great deal of good in her chosen walk of life."[7]

Anna Broomall, Professor of Obstetrics for many years at the Woman's Medical College in Philadelphia, originally had expressed an interest in the law, perhaps because her father was a lawyer and a congressman. When such a professional course proved unfeasible, it was her father who encouraged her to "be a good doctor."[8] Similarly, Anita Newcomb McGee's father Simon Newcomb, an astronomer at the U.S. Naval Observatory, took great pride in his daughter's intellectual accomplishments and enthusiastically supported her decision to enter Columbian University Medical School in 1889, despite the fact that she was already married and the mother of a small child. Cornelia Kahn (WMCP, 1887) enjoyed like support from her father, a wealthy businessman who was "particularly proud of his eldest daughter," and enthusiastically encouraged her medical career. Mary Hood's minister father longed to have one of his children become a doctor. When both sons chose the ministry he pushed his daughter into medicine in the early 1870s.[9]

Available correspondence between relatives and female medical students indicates that advice and emotional support proved significant. When Margaret Butler, later professor of otolaryngology at the Woman's Medical College of Pennsylvania and one of the first women fellows of the American College of Surgeons, became an assistant in Laryngology at the Polyclinic Hospital shortly after her graduation from the Woman's Medical in 1894, her father wrote:

> You need not pitty us when you think us at work and yourself idle, we expect you will be quite as closely employed at your Studies as we are at our business. You are now at the beginning of a career, either of usefulness—or Something worse, and as you labor, and build So will your life be, if you expect to be of use in this world, you

will have to struggle to be above the common herd—but this need not alarm you as it is employment that makes life pleasant and useful, we were not created to rust out as drones, You know did we not plant and till the Earth it would bring forth noxious weeds and our beautiful country now verdant and covered with grain fruit and flowers became a desert, it is even so with the mind if not properly used for seeds falling will germinate and in after life bring fruit either of usefulness or bitterness. Remember that yours is the Springtime of life and as you Sow of the same kind will you reap. The harvest and Autumn is yet to come if you labor—you will be able to over-come all difficulties and may expect a bountiful harvest in after life, the Almighty, has not created us without a purpose. Try not to live in vain.[10]

Such parental interest eased the burdens of medical students, especially those far from home. Sarah Ernestine Howard, whose mother Emily Pagelson Howard had graduated from the University of Michigan Medical School in 1882 and whose father was the superintendant of the Peter Bent Brigham Hospital in Boston, wrote chatty responses to her parent's inquiries almost daily during the years between 1913 and 1917 when she attended Johns Hopkins. A favorite topic of discussion was the women students—how they were faring in the male world of professional medicine. The correspondence makes it clear that parental concern helped sustain her through the difficult times.[11]

While a student in Baltimore at the turn of the century, Florence Sabin, the first woman to receive a faculty appointment at Johns Hopkins and later the first woman Fellow of the Rockefeller Institute, wrote often to a favorite uncle about Hopkins matters. Sabin had lost her mother when she was only a child and for a time lived with her uncle Albert and his family in Chicago. A teacher, a lover of music, nature, and good reading, this warm and urbane ex-New Englander gave Sabin the security and encouragement that she had missed by her mother's early death. Years later it was with her uncle Albert that she discussed her frustrations, and it was Uncle Albert who always responded with love and encouragement. In 1907, for example, he wrote her in reference to a particularly discouraged letter:

I think you are grand. You have sized up the problem in all its dimensions and are not appalled. You will do your whole duty as you see it. You will be serene through it all. Whether you make or break with the faculty north, south, east, or west, your old uncle will love you still and believe you are the best of the pack.[12]

Familial aid often came regardless of parents' initial reservations about their daughter's chosen career. Despite his belief that medicine was a "repulsive pursuit," especially for a lady, Mary Putnam Jacobi's father rendered her invaluable emotional and psychological support. In 1867 she wrote to him, "You have always been such a dear good father. . . . The more I see of other people's way of doing, the more highly I value the large liberty in which you have always left me. It has occasioned certain mistakes, but on the whole, the advantage has infinitely outweighed the disadvantage. I do not see how I could have lived without it."[13] Similarly, the parents of Martha May Eliot, subsequently director of the United States Children's Bureau and a 1918 graduate of Hopkins with Ernestine Howard, had hoped that she would become a teacher. When she chose medicine instead, they continued their interest and pride in her accomplishments. Their enthusiasm did not go unappreciated. In 1918 Martha wrote gratefully to her mother:

> This is to be a little private letter for you and Papa, to try and tell you in a very poor way, I am afraid, how very much I have appreciated what you have given me during these past four years. They have been, as really would go without saying, the most wonderful years yet for me and it makes me very humble when I think that it was you two working all the time at home who made it all possible for me. I can never thank you enough and I don't really think you would have me try, for it would be attempting what cannot be done.[14]

The positive response of at least some family and friends attests to the fact that a small but perhaps significant number of parents nurtured identical aspirations for both male and female children. Such evidence may suggest that historians must be careful not to view the socialization of girls in the nineteenth century as entirely uniform or monolithic. Less apparent and more difficult to glean from the evidence is an answer to why certain parents treated their daughters so evenhandedly.

When it was forthcoming, family approval and material aid eased the burdens of many aspiring physicians. But others struggled alone. Indeed, some families simply did not have the resources to finance a daughter's unorthodox aspirations. Medical educators estimated that in the late 1860s a two-year medical course cost between six hundred and seven hundred dollars. The expense and duration of medical education reflected both its class and gender bias. Structured to suit the conventions of male experience, medical training was easier for men than for women to finance in the burgeoning economy of nineteenth-century America.[15]

Nevertheless, many women sought outside employment. Like many of her own future students at the Woman's Medical College of Pennsylvania, Emmeline Cleveland became a teacher in her district school in order to earn enough money to further her education. Hundreds of women doctors in the next several generations would follow her example. Teaching remained both respectable and accessible to young women in the nineteenth century, despite the fact that they earned only one-third the salary of men. As the century progressed, many of them, dissatisfied with the poor financial rewards or seeking something more challenging, opted for medicine as opportunities in the field began to open up for women in the years after the Civil War. Others saw teaching merely as a stepping stone to the long-cherished goal of a medical degree.[16]

For young women like M.S. Devereaux, studying medicine was the logical culmination of motives that had drawn them to teaching in the first place. In 1881 Devereaux wrote for advice to Dr. James B. Chadwick, a warm supporter of women physicians and a professor at Harvard Medical School. Her letter reveals thoughts that must have been common for many like her. She began by confessing that she had often dreamed of being a doctor, but hesitated chiefly because she was already a teacher. Yet she wished to utilize her teaching ability to "lift the cloud of ignorance and carelessness that hangs over the subject of hygiene and Physiology—especially among women. I am sure," she continued, "that the subject should be presented in a thorough, simple and earnest manner in lectures and classroom work—especially with the interest and cooperation of physicians. There is sufficient sense of moral obligation to be arroused to the preservation of the health and strength of the body; and sufficient common sense to make people ready to listen." The papers of Clara Marshall and Rachel Bodley, both deans of the Woman's Medical College of Pennsylvania, contain fascinating letters of inquiry of just this sort from other teachers wishing to study medicine.[17]

Some women moved from nursing to medicine. Cordelia Greene financed her medical education with earnings received from nursing jobs in several water-cure establishments. Annette C. Buckel nursed soldiers during the Civil War.[18] Indeed, the resourcefulness of women students, faced with what Mary Putnam Jacobi termed "homely struggles," gave, she believed, "a solidity, a vitality to the movement." Women seeking a medical education have "starved on half rations . . ." she wrote in 1891, and "have resorted to innumerable devices,—taught school, edited newspapers, nursed sick people, given massage, worked till they could scrape a few dollars together, expended that in study—then stepped aside for a while to earn more. After graduating, the struggle has continued—but here the resource of taking lodgers has often tided over the difficult time."[19]

Correspondence to the dean of the Woman's Medical College of Pennyslvania contains numerous letters of inquiry from potential students, all requesting financial aid or placement in part-time work to defray the expenses of medical study. Typical of the latter, for example, was a note to Clara Marshall from Mattie A. Long, writing in 1890 from Bloomington, Illinois, to inquire as to "whether I can do shorthand to pay my expenses." Similarly, Rosa Dean, a senior at Wellesley College in Massachusetts, explained:

> I have my own way to pay and do not wish to ask for pecuniary aid. The aid of some self-supporting work in the city which would allow me to take one course of lectures, or if such a thing were possible some work in connection with the college itself would be my desire. If such are not attainable, I must wait and earn something in other ways and places first.[20]

Occasionally requests came, not only from potential students, but from interested friends and supporters. In 1891 Charles C. Thompson, a teacher, wrote Clara Marshall from Staunton, Virginia, on behalf of a former pupil, "a young lady who teaches as her only means of support and has made a good woman of herself by her own efforts." Her people, he explained, were "honourable but poor." The mother was a widow. When Thompson first met her, the girl was working for fifty cents a week "doing drudgery for a family." Recognizing her ability he found her a teaching position. But, Thompson explained, "she . . . wants to take medicine." Voicing his own admiration for her courage and grit, he concluded, "If your college offered anything special to deserving women you cannot go amiss in her case."[21]

It often happened that the dean was able to arrange employment for some of these women. Occasionally networks of female reformers willing to sponsor the medical education of young and poor aspirants came to her aid. Emmeline Cleveland had hoped to become a missionary, and as her plans crystallized while at Oberlin she corresponded with Sarah Josepha Hale, editor of *Godey's Lady's Book* and the recently elected secretary of the Pennsylvania

Ladies Missionary society. Hale advocated separate medical educa-tion for women, especially for the purpose of preparing them for missionary work. In the 1850s and 1860s, she loyally endorsed the founding of the Woman's Medical College of Pennsylvania on the pages of her magazine and participated in coordinating a training program for missionaries at the school. Over the next decades she dutifully reported developments at the institution in her editorials, praising its aims and occasionally appealing on its behalf for money.[22]

Similarly, Marie Zakrzewska received both material and moral support from the local Ladies' Physiological Society, under the leadership of Mrs. Caroline Severance, while attending Cleveland Medical College in the 1850s. Later other networks of women, including Ednah Dow Cheney and Caroline Dall of Boston, facili-tated Zakrzewska's work there by helping to establish the New England Hospital for Women and Children. In New York Eliza-beth Blackwell managed to enlist the aid of a group of Quaker women when she set up practice.[23]

While some parents offered support, others discouraged their daughters' efforts to gain a medical degree. The mother of Eliza Mosher, an early graduate of the University of Michigan and later the school's first dean of women, stubbornly opposed her daughter's aspirations, declaring that she would sooner see her shut up in a lunatic asylum. Maternal objections temporarily delayed Mosher's plans for a medical career.[24] Anne Walter Fearn, an 1893 graduate of Woman's Medical College of Pennsylvania who spent a long and successful medical career in China, recalled that she had been raised by her Southern family to live the life of a social butterfly. Her mother threatened to disown her when she disclosed her medical plans.[25] Bertha Van Hoosen's mother was moved to tears every time her studying medicine was mentioned, and her father, who had previously been open to her ambitions, refused to furnish the money for Van Hoosen to train for something that offended her mother so deeply.[26] Such opposition did not prevent Van Hoosen from attend-ing the University of Michigan and having a strikingly successful career as an obstetrician and surgeon in Chicago.

Another successful women surgeon, Rosalie Slaughter Morton (WMCP 1898), literally had to wait for her father to die before she could put her medical plans into effect. Although her two brothers became physicians, she grew up in an aristocratic Virginia family where her father felt scandalized at the idea of his daughter earn-ing money. "It is essential," he told her, "that society's standards be maintained. . . . Your highest duty is to become a good wife and mother." Similarly, Dorothy Reed Mendenhall, a contemporary of Florence Sabin's and among the first women to attend Johns Hopkins, remembered with ironic humor that her mother was "upset" and her great aunts "aghast" at the idea of her studying medicine. "Aunt Tin, in all the years I was in Baltimore, always alluded to my 'being South for the winter' . . . and Cousin Rouel Kimball's wife . . . wrote my mother that she was sorry that she couldn't entertain me . . . intimating that my profession prevented further social relations with me."[27]

Such negative attitudes were common. Mary Bennett Ritter had spent three years teaching and saving before she began medical study in earnest in 1882. But not, she later recalled, before family and friends "brought out afresh" all their arguments against her plans. "Predictions of failure," she remembered, "were universal but varied. . . . There were the usual caustic remarks about feminine unfitness . . . woman's lack of strength, her instability, natural timidity, and all the other hackneyed objections. . . . Beside all of the above reasons . . . there came this blast: . . . you will 'up and marry' and it will all be wasted." A final argument pitted against her was financial: leaving a successful teaching career and incurring heavy debt promised at best an uncertain livelihood. "As to this prediction," Bennett later remarked with a touch of self-righteous irony, "I can only say that in the first month of my practice I earned as much as the principal's salary in the Fresno school, and after that . . . my income soon equalled that of the highest paid university professor." Her entire debt plus interest was retired in a few years.

"Women in any profession were having a hard time in those days," remembered Anne Fearn, "but women physicians seemed particularly obnoxious to the average man and woman of the eighties and nineties. Study of the ills of the human flesh was a disgustingly unladylike occupation. The young woman student of medicine faced the reproaches of a "disgraced" family, social ostracism, and incalculable difficulties in the struggle to build up a practice."[28] Family opposition could be painful. The majority of objecting parents, however, eventually became reconciled to their daughter's choices, usually after a few years of demonstrated success.

Still, economic difficulties and social disapproval hampered some women to the degree that a significant proportion of them came to the study of medicine considerably older than their male counterparts. Before 1880 the average age of graduation among students at the Woman's Medical College of Pennsylvania for whom records are available was thirty-three years. Although among students after 1880 the age level dropped to twenty-seven years, the fact that many women medical students were already quite mature is nevertheless significant.[29] Male medical graduates were usually in their early twenties.

Another factor determining the older ages of some of these women is that a number of them were either married or widowed. Charlotte Blake Brown was by no means the only wife and mother to take up medicine; others did so as well. Hannah Longshore, a member of the first class at the Woman's Medical College of Pennsylvania, attended to her studies with the approval and support of her husband. In 1876 the University of California graduated its first woman, Mrs. Lucy Wanzer, a thirty-three-year-old schoolteacher who had been married for ten years. A year later, Alice Higgins, forty-one years old, the mother of three and the wife of a doctor, became the first woman to matriculate at Stanford Medical School. Higgins even spent a year doing postgraduate work at the Woman's Medical College in Philadelphia before she settled down to a successful practice in Anaheim. For Hannah Jackson (WMCP, 1881), studying medicine was a childhood dream. Instead she married Joseph D. Price, who was a second lieutenant of the Sixth Pennsylvania Cavalry, serving three years and three months in the Civil War. After migrating with her husband to Kansas and bearing him four children, Mrs. Price was widowed in 1872. Six years later she entered the Woman's Medical College in Philadelphia. By 1881 she was in residency under Anna Broomall at the Woman's Hospital and, a few years afterward, had established a flourishing practice in Chester, Pennsylvania. Another widow, Cornelia Kahn Binswanger, entered the college in 1883, partly as a consolation for the loss of her husband and young child.[30]

Women entered medicine in these years out of a variety of personal motives. Some, of course, came from "reform" families. A number of early women physicians, like Emmeline Cleveland, Eliza Mosher (University of Michigan, 1875), Amanda Sanford (University of Michigan, 1873), Cordelia Greene (Cleveland Medical College, 1856), Samantha Nivison (WMCP, 1855), and Angenette Hunt (WMCP, 1852), grew up in west or central New York, the famous "burned over district," where unorthodox ideas pervaded the atmosphere in which they lived. Eliza Mosher's father, for example, regularly kept her abreast of the newspaper accounts of women's accomplishments, often putting down his paper with the remark, "There, now, Eliza, that's what women are doing nowadays."[31]

For many women who pursued medicine in the early period between 1840 and 1870, religious perfectionism and reform ideology meshed into a desire to contribute to the community welfare. Of course the notion that women, like men, had a moral and religious obligation to society could be relatively controversial if interpreted too broadly. Yet historians have long noted that religious piety often afforded the only means by which women could exercise power and autonomy.[32] Although the doctrine of the Inner Light led Quakers to condone the greatest flexibility of all the protestant sects in defining the boundaries of woman's role, women forged religious justifications for reform activity while subscribing to more orthodox Christian faiths as well. Female influence was particularly discernible in the evangelical fervor of the successive religious revivals which periodically swept New England and western New York in the first half of the nineteenth century.[33]

We have already noted the importance of religious perfectionism in the thought of prominent health reformers. Many women physicians, Elizabeth Blackwell being only one of the most prominent, shared this outlook. Emmeline Cleveland, for example, entered medicine originally to become a missionary. The lives of other women physicians as well linked the "religion of health" preached by the health-reform movement with the formal entrance of women into the medical profession. For example, Cordelia Greene's active interest in applied Christianity provides perhaps the most important clue to understanding her subsequent career. The eldest child of parents who were solid New England farmers—former Quakers turned Presbyterians—she grew up along the banks of the Erie Canal. There her father had purchased a farm shortly before her birth in 1831. Jabez Greene's religious piety was matched only by his interest in progressive education, and his active role as a trustee in the local public school no doubt sparked his daughter's life-long concern with self-improvement. Cordelia became a serious student, and her impressive record earned her a teacher's certificate from the county while she was still in her early teens. As a girl she responded enthusiastically to the evangelism that periodically swept through western New York and shortly after her 17th birthday underwent a religious conversion, apparently helped along by the wife of the local Presbyterian pastor.[34]

In 1849 Jabez Greene, who was also an avid health reformer,

gave up farming and founded a health establishment in Castile, New York, known as the "Water Cure." There Cordelia, manifesting both an interest and a penchant for the care of the sick, assisted her father. Lacking formal medical credentials proved no barrier to practice in these years; the originator of the modern water-cure system, Vincent Priessnitz, was himself a Silesian peasant. Hydropathy, in spite of its lowly beginnings, proved remarkably popular in the 1840s and 1850s in America, and water treatments of various kinds were usually combined with strict attention to diet and general regimen. Cordelia Greene's later approach to medical therapeutics would always bear the influence of her early exposure to health-reform ideas.[35]

While aiding her father, Greene read of Elizabeth Blackwell's graduation from Geneva Medical College and decided to become a physician herself. In 1856 she graduated with honors—along with three other women—from the Cleveland Medical College (Western Reserve). The next six years were spent gaining confidence and clinical experience as the assistant of Dr. Henry Foster, also a graduate of Cleveland, who had founded Clifton Springs Water Cure in upstate New York. Although Foster was a serious-minded and professionally oriented regular physician who kept abreast of new developments in medical practice, he shared his assistant's religious orientation and believed along with Greene that "a strong spiritual atmosphere has a mighty power as a curative agent."[36]

Her father's death in 1864 gave Greene the opportunity to manage her own sanitarium. Urged by her brothers to take over the "Water Cure," she eventually consented, but only after much soul searching. In 1864 she was thirty-four years old, and she would remain the medical director of the establishment she renamed Castile Sanitarium until 1905, when she was succeeded by her niece, Dr. Mary T. Greene (Michigan, 1890).

Her memoirs make it clear that she felt her proprietorship was indeed a religious calling. "I have ever felt," she wrote, "that each patient was sent by a providential hand with the injunction 'Take this child and care for her for Me.' " According to her biographer, "hundreds of patients recall vividly Dr. Greene's serene motherly face as she sat in the centre of her sick 'children' leading the evening prayer service." Her message was the healing of both body and soul. "Holiness," she used to say, "is simply wholeness. Righteousness is rightness—right doing. . . . Our first duty is to work the beautiful enginery of body, intellect, and will in such a way as to make the very best of all the powers God has given us."[37]

Typically, Greene's first medical assistant was Dr. Clara Swain, a graduate of the Woman's Medical College of Pennsylvania and the first woman medical missionary to India. Swain had a long and distinguished career in Asia. The two women remained close friends for over thirty years. When she retired, Swain returned to the United States to make her home in Castile.

Financially secure, Greene donated large sums of money to female social reform causes—homes and hospitals for the needy, the home and foreign missionary boards of the Presbyterian Church. Indeed, the Sanitarium had its own Missionary Society, and it supported numerous Christian Chinese girls through medical training at the Peking Union Medical College.[38] Besides her interest in medical missionary work, Greene had strong ties to the Woman's Christian Temperance Union. She attended their national conventions and was outspoken in favor of temperance in her native Castile. Frances Willard and Mary A. Livermore, warm friends and supporters, came often to the Sanitarium to rest or to visit.

Cordelia Greene's religious orientation was typical of many women doctors. Indeed, transcendental religious experiences were not uncommon among them or, for that matter, among other nineteenth-century women reformers who sought broader avenues of professional activity. Jane Addams, Lillian Wald, Elizabeth Blackwell, Frances Willard, Margaret Sanger, and Dr. Ida Richardson, founder of the West Philadelphia Hospital for Women, were only a few of those who experienced mystical episodes. In the process the religious impulse was transformed into a social commitment and the pursuit of a profession. For many women these incidents, in which they viewed themselves as responding to the call of a higher moral power, helped to legitimate their deviance from prescribed female roles and strengthen their efforts to widen the paths of women's work despite familial disapproval and social opposition.[39]

Protestant Christian idealism aided women physicians of Cordelia Greene's generation in their pursuit of self-development in yet another way. Although many of them had to struggle to attend high school or college, it is also true that they managed, despite numerous obstacles, to gain access to education on a scale simply not available to previous generations of women. A central feature of this education was its infusion with Christian perfectionism. Female academies like Mt. Holyoke set the tone, but even coeducational institutions like Oberlin College applied Christian perfectionism to women in a particular and novel way.

Famous as a hotbed of abolitionism, health reform, and women's rights, Oberlin College had been founded in 1833 by the followers of Charles Grandison Finney for training young ministers for a new type of Evangelical Manhood. Its faculty, however, was drawn from that liberal portion of the Presbyterian-Congregationalist clergy that interpreted the concept of Republican Motherhood to include the broadest moral and religious functions for women. Only three years before Emmeline Cleveland's arrival at the school in 1850, the college had graduated with honors both Lucy Stone and her future sister-in-law and fellow woman's-rights advocate, Antoinette Brown.

Oberlin's policymakers defied the conventional wisdom that claimed that females should be educated exclusively for wifehood and motherhood. Instead they recognized women's physical and mental capacity to pursue an academic program successfully. In almost a direct rebuttal of the most conservative interpretation of the "Cult of True Womanhood," Finney's administrative assistant and presidential successor at Oberlin, James Harris Fairchild, declared in 1852 that the "sphere of women is not so different from that of men" and that before young ladies were taught domesticity it might be "better to say, let them first be educated as human beings."[40]

Yet, as one historian has noted, Oberlin's attitude toward women was distinctive "in degree rather than in kind." The school's leaders, like the large majority of nineteenth-century liberal reformers, still subscribed to the doctrine of separate spheres. As a result, the education of young women remained emphatically subordinate to the education of young men, and the presence of females at the institution was sanctioned partly because of the faculty's belief that their companionship in an unconstrained atmosphere created a natural environment in which young male students could find appropriate wives. Thus, Oberlin aimed to prepare women for a life of usefulness, duty, and good works, but always, Oberlin's official historian is quick to remind us, within a context of "intelligent motherhood and properly subservient wifehood."[41]

The education these women received intentionally failed to relate them in any significant way to the larger occupational structure. Instead it trained them to be moral agents in a culture that generally defined women as passive spectators and consumers. Educated women were thus left to themselves to reconcile such contradictions, and for many of them medicine perfectly meshed personal ambition with ideology. They could pursue a career *and* reform society without overstepping too far the bounds of accepted propriety. Thus, for women like Emmeline Cleveland, being a medical missionary while one's husband ministered to lost souls in foreign lands fit the model perfectly.

Indeed, Cleveland was not the only woman that Oberlin College sent to Philadelphia to study medicine. Nor was Oberlin the only school producing and inspiring women like her. Long after explicitly religious motives ceased to motivate them, women from liberal colleges like Oberlin retained a secularized desire to do good. Such institutions engendered a particular type of nineteenth-century womanhood which Cleveland embodied for many of her students and supporters. For example, contemporaries remember her as a "womanly woman" who, despite a heavy load of professional responsibilities, never slighted her domestic duties. Dean Rachel Bodley left an account of her own first meeting with Cleveland, which provided "a key to the charm of Professor Cleveland's character":

> She was descending the stair of the Woman's Hospital, where at the time she was Resident Physician, bearing aloft on her shoulder, her baby boy, less than a year old. Unconscious of the presence of a stranger, they were beaming the brightest smiles each upon the other, and the laughing child and the happy mother constituted a picture fair to look upon.[42]

The frequent references to Cleveland's "womanliness" are particularly pertinent when contrasted with her reputed skill and courage as a pioneer surgeon. She was one of the first professional women ovariotomists in America, and the several abdominal sections completed at the Woman's Hospital in the 1870s were the earliest known instances of major surgery performed by a woman doctor.[43]

Though women physicians with Emmeline Cleveland's and Cordelia Greene's enthusiasm for Christian perfectionism appear less frequently by the turn of the twentieth century, they persist even into the progressive era, numbering among their ranks enthusiastic activists in agencies identified with the Social Hygiene Movement. Yet while one type of woman physician remained deeply religious, others can be found who were stubborn nonbelievers, choosing medicine out of a love of science or a sustained curiosity about people. Mary Putnam Jacobi, immersed in her medical studies in Paris, felt scientific study to be addictive, and wrote her mother enthusiastically that she couldn't get enough of it. Harriet Belcher's attraction was the physician's opportunity for "the study of human nature." Belcher would have loved to go abroad as a missionary, but she confessed that she could not manage "to hold my tongue on the subject of my rather heterodox religious opinions."[44]

Another especially feminine theme that recurs in the motivation of women towards medicine is a childhood or adolescent encounter with illness—either their own or that of a close friend or relative. Elizabeth Blackwell chose medicine after watching a friend die of uterine cancer. For Eliza Mosher, the death of a beloved brother in 1867 from tuberculosis brought on a religious crisis which strengthened her already budding resolve to become a doctor. Harriot Hunt, one of the earliest women physicians, took up medicine after failures by several male doctors in Boston to cure her sister's neurasthenia.[45] Emily Dunning Barringer (Cornell, 1902) believed that it was the near death of her mother in childbirth that prompted in her the "desire . . . to help the sick and suffering, which later was to lead me into medicine."[46] Similarly, Anna Wessel Williams, a graduate of the New York Infirmary in the 1880s, experienced a startling confrontation with medical ignorance when her sister lost her baby and came close to death herself because of puerperal eclampsia and the incompetence of a rural practitioner. This incident catalyzed her decision to study medicine and try to push back the boundaries of ignorance. From then on she longed, she wrote, "to find out about the what, why, when, and where and how of the mysteries of life. This trait had increased with the years, and finally had become a passion."[47]

Josephine Griffith Davis (WMCP, 1877) originally practiced pharmacy. After several miscarriages, she turned in disappointment to medicine, hoping somehow to find a cure for her personal tragedy. She later specialized in cancer of the uterus and practiced in New York City.[48] Finally, Elizabeth Cohen, probably a graduate of the Eclectic Penn Medical University, settled in New Orleans in 1857 and was the first woman physician there. She began medical study, she recalled on her hundredth birthday, "to help mothers keep their little ones well" after she had lost a small son to the measles.[49]

Other women grappled with their own ill health when they were children or adolescents. Mary Wilson Case, who studied first at Vassar and then graduated from the Woman's Medical College of Pennsylvania in 1881, chose medicine because of a delicate and frail physique.[50] Sarah McCarn-Craig's health broke down when she worked her way through Antioch College. Putting herself in the hands of Drs. Rachel Brooks and Silas Gleason, the proprietors of the Elmira Water Cure, she remained their practically bedridden patient for four years. When her health improved, she read medicine with the Gleasons and then entered the Woman's Medical College in Philadelphia in 1863. Upon graduation she worked for a time at the sanitariums at Elmira and Clifton Springs until, in 1866, she established her own practice in Rochester. Another sickly protégé of the Gleasons, Caroline Winslow, spent several months as their patient shortly before her thirtieth birthday. Their lessons in anatomy, part of their health program, so sparked her interest in medical study that in 1851 she entered the Eclectic Medical College of Cincinnati. Winslow subsequently had a successful career as a physician in Washington, D.C., and edited *The Alpha,* a social-purity journal with feminist leanings. Similarly, Mary A. Stinson's pursuit of medicine was prompted by several unhappy years of adolescent invalidism.[51]

But not all women physicians were either sickly as children or religious idealists. Many confessed openly to the power of sheer ambition, whether or not they identified consciously with the nineteenth-century women's-rights movement. Although Bertha Van Hoosen conceded that her choice of medicine may have been a response "to a call of the woman in me—woman, preserver of the race," she listed as her most important motivations the pursuit of "social status," "the opportunity for growth and advancement in an ever-expanding science." Also of consequence to Van Hoosen was the chance to be her "own boss—to say as Father often did, 'I can speak my mind on any subject . . . I am a free man' "[52] Anna Wessel Williams confessed that her interest was enhanced by the fact that "I was starting on a way that had been practically untrod before by a woman. My belief at that time in human individuality, regardless of sex, race, religion or any factor other than ability was at its strongest. I believed, therefore, that females should have equal opportunities with males to develop their powers to the utmost."[53]

Anita Newcomb McGee also felt that she was "different from most girls." She believed that talented women should pursue careers commensurate with their abilities; indeed, if they did not, she warned, "their unused energy" would degenerate into "neurasthenia." She married a man who was willing to support her professional goals and entered Columbian University's medical department soon after she gave birth to her first child. Many women, no less than men, longed at the end of the century for the high status and financial rewards offered by a professional career. In fact, Belva Lockwood's confession in "My Efforts to Become a Lawyer," an article she wrote for *Lippincott*'s in 1888, "I possessed all the ambition of a man," could be easily applied to many women physicians.[54]

Having attained the necessary preliminary education, a young woman was then faced with embarking on her medical studies. In the decades between 1850 and 1880, students often still read medicine with a preceptor before commencing formal study, although the custom was being discarded. Finding a mentor was not an easy task for the first generation of women because male physicians often refused to take them on as assistants. Thus, J. Ida Sheinman gave testimony to women's difficulties when in 1876 she petitioned the faculty of the Woman's Medical College of Pennsylvania for permission to take first-year exams without having attended the lectures. "I began private study in February, 1874," she explained, "soon after graduation in Oberlin College. I studied leisure hours and during vacations from teaching until coming here in October, 1876. But I had no preceptor because in the places in which I found it was necessary to live, I could find no physician willing to give me preceptorship." Accompanying Sheinman's petition was a curious letter from Dr. John Linton of Garriavillos, Iowa, unabashedly confirming the accuracy of her statement by admitting that he had refused to teach her medicine and had tried to discourage her from her plans.[55]

Already by the 1880s, however, networks of successful female pioneers began to clear a path for the younger women. Often beginners were welcomed as assistants to older women physicians already in practice. Bertha Van Hoosen spent the summer before she entered medical school with Dr. Mary McLean, a recent Michigan graduate, who had just settled in St. Louis. "Dr. McLean," Van Hoosen later wrote of her friend and mentor, "was one of the first women to serve in any official capacity in any hospital in St. Louis. Her record was so exceptionally high and so unusual that few men in the profession did not know of her accomplishments as a skillful operator and an exhaustive diagnostician."[56]

In California Mary Bennett Ritter began her medical study by working with Dr. Euthanasia S. Meade (WMCP, 1869), who had been among the first women physicians to settle there and had a flourishing practice in San Jose. Bennett's relationship with Meade was helpful in numerous ways. The younger woman accompanied her mentor in maternity cases and on her home visits, learning as best she could. Meade also took charge of Bennett's health, putting her on an exercise regimen that was intended to strengthen her endurance. Both married and a mother, Meade provided a strong role model for her student. In addition, her support and encouragement were important to Bennett, as were her extensive social and professional ties to other women physicians in the state. Bennett later spoke of Meade with love, respect, and admiration.[57]

Across the country in Boston, Eliza Mosher spent a year as clinical assistant to Lucy Sewall, one of the earliest attending physicians at the New England Hospital for Women and Children. Sewall broadened Mosher both scientifically and culturally. Her father, Judge Samuel E. Sewall, was a prominent member of the reform elite. He was an abolitionist, an advocate of women's rights, and an early supporter of women in medicine. Lucy Sewall had read medicine with Marie Zakrzewska and, after attending the New England Female Medical College, finished her education with a year of successful study in London and Paris hospitals. Upon Sewall's death Mary Putnam Jacobi wrote:

> Lucy Sewall is especially noteworthy, as having been about the first woman of family, and fortune, to study medicine in America. Her great contribution to our cause, is, that in conservative Boston she first caused medicine to be regarded as a respectable, as a dignified profession for women. . . . The New England Hospital was . . . for many years, sustained by her girlish and singlehearted devotion to a cause, which she had learned to love.[58]

Sewall took seriously the education of her young charge. Mosher accompanied her on hospital visits as well as on calls to private patients. The teacher often discussed diagnoses with her young assistant. Mosher learned the uses and dosage of various drugs so efficiently that she was well versed in materia medica even before she arrived at Michigan medical school. "Because of her studies in Paris and London, and the years of experience gained in hospital work," Mosher wrote years later, "Dr. Sewall was one of the best educated physicians in Boston. She quickly acquired a large and very lucrative practice. I feel that I owe a very great debt . . . which I must repay by assisting other students as she assisted me."[59]

Women's hospitals and dispensaries also began to ease young women's transition into medicine. In the 1860s and 1870s both the New York Infirmary and the New England Hospital accepted apprentice-interns before they sought more formal medical training. In fact, the year previous to her preceptorship with Lucy Sewall, Eliza Mosher had joined her friend Amanda Sanford—fresh from a year's study in Philadelphia—as an intern-apprentice at the New England Hospital.

In 1869 Mosher was one of five intern-apprentices in Boston. Her quickness and maturity soon earned her the chance to do dissections in the hospital laboratory. In addition, she assisted Dr. Sewall at the outpatient dispensary, learned to compound prescriptions and attended operations and obstetrical cases. She also sought private obstetrical instruction from Dr. Helen Morton in order to prepare to deliver her sister's fourth baby.[60]

During this year at the New England Hospital Mosher formed lifetime professional and personal relationships with other women doctors and found worthy, if stern and serious, role models. For half a century after her stay, the hospital continued to provide an opportunity for clinical training to many prominent women physicians: Susan Dimock, C. Annette Buckel, Emma Call, Alice Hamilton, Josephine Baker, Bertha Van Hoosen, Lucy Sewall, and many others.

While Mosher apprenticed in Boston, significant opportunities for women to study medicine became available elsewhere. One day, Mosher recalled, while she and her four fellow-apprentices worked in the laboratory, someone read a newspaper article announcing the opening of the University of Michigan to women. The implications of such an event instantly became apparent and the interns spontaneously joined hands and danced around the table.[61] Although Ann Arbor was the first state university to commit itself to the medical education of women, in the next several decades, a number of universities—Ohio State, Iowa State, Stanford, the University of California among others—followed suit. The tide appeared to be turning in favor of coeducation, and the crowning achievement of all came in 1892 when supporters managed to throw open the doors of Johns Hopkins to women.

Of course, the women's medical colleges offered certain advantages not readily available at coeducational schools. Female faculty served as role models, and the significance to younger women of such exposure should not be minimized. Furthermore, the atmosphere appears to have been at once rigorous and supportive. For example, years later, students spoke highly of both the professionalism and the underlying warmth of their teachers. Anna Wessel Williams, while she took note of the impressive medical record of Professor Chevalier, who taught chemistry at the New York Infirmary, also recalled that Chevalier took "a personal interest" in her, giving her hints as to the way she should dress and as to how she should do her hair. Despite Mary Putnam Jacobi's reputation as an energetically brilliant and demanding teacher, she too gave Williams support and advice and helped her through several crucial decisions. She often "exposed our ignorance," remembered Williams, "but in such a way that we were not so much depressed as encouraged to make it less."[62]

Similar memories abound of the Woman's Medical College of Pennsylvania faculty. Ann Preston, for example, concerned about broadening her students in all ways, often took them to lectures by Lucy Stone and Ralph Waldo Emerson.[63] Emmeline Cleveland combined calm, dignity, warmth, and femininity with undeniable professional competence to create a figure of quiet charisma for those students who knew her. Cleveland's successor in the chair of obstetrics, Anna Broomall, a particularly "busy professor and practitioner," also was remembered by her students for her compassion and her "loyalty to family relationships." "This loyalty," wrote Mary Griscom, "was consistently applied when the families of her assistants needed them. Work never pressed so hard, that we could not go to our families if illness or trouble came to our homes."[64]

Such personal concern carried over into the twentieth century. Rita Finkler, a 1915 graduate who had come to the college as a recent Jewish refugee from Russion pogroms, remembered much kindness from Dean Martha Tracy. Her mentor arranged a special course for her in chemistry in the first year to help Finkler make the transition to a new country and a new language. Before long, Tracy "noticed that I was near-sighted and could not see the formulas on the black-board. I knew that I had defective vision right along, but resisted wearing glasses out of vanity. I was marched off to Dr. Mary Buchanan and in a few days the world appeared clearer and brighter to me." Similarly, Katherine Boucot Sturgis, who in 1935 was burdened with a recent divorce and two young children, remembers that Tracy's main concern in her preliminary interview was what Sturgis fed her children, fearing that they were not getting enough protein.[65]

Thus, the nurturing atmosphere at the women's institutions contributed to easing women students over a difficult transition. On the other hand, female solidarity could be on occasion pitted unfairly against the fulfillment of individual goals. Anna Wessel Williams recalled an incident in her own career when she was pressured by the New York Infirmary faculty to give up a coveted internship. Standing first in her class, she had been offered a position at Babies Hospital in New York, subject to the approval of its founder and director Dr. Ernest Holt, the prestigious pediatrician. When Holt met Williams, he was pleased and sent word to her that she could have the position. "Then I had a shock!," Williams wrote in her autobiography. Emily Blackwell and another member of the faculty, Dr. Davis, "a snip of a consequential woman whom I had tried to ignore," called her in for an interview. Telling Williams that they had talked the matter over with Holt, they revealed that "they had come to the conclusion that perhaps Dr. Parry, the second candidate for the position, might fit in better because of her age (over 30), experience (social work), 'presence' (tall, dignified, assured) . . . and . . . I forgot other reasons, but the chief one was 'she might advance the cause of women more.' " "That finished me," recalled Williams. "I felt like throwing something heavy at them." Later that week Dr. Parry herself came to Williams's home to plead her own case. Disgusted but also defeated, Williams consented to stay another year at the Infirmary to work in the outpatient department, while Parry took the position at Babies Hospital.[66] Pressure to preserve female solidarity could thus also be irritating to those not similarly committed to larger feminist goals.

Women who attended coeducational institutions, however, faced special problems of their own. In the beginning there was overt social ostracism. The hostility could be painful in those pioneer decades. Harriet Belcher (WMCP, 1879) felt the mixed clinics she attended while a student at the woman's college in Philadelphia to be an "ordeal." Male students often made a "scene" with "yells, boos and hisses on all sides." In Michigan, as elsewhere, such treatment had to be taken in stride, recalled Eliza Mosher. Townspeople occasionally refused to rent rooms to "hen medics." Often male students either ignored the women or exhibited deliberate animosity. Even faculty members could not hide their disapproval. Mosher vividly remembered the hazing she and other women received at the lectures in organic chemistry—the one subject the faculty "seemed to think would not injure our morals or those of the men to listen to in the same classroom." "We women," she wrote,

> gathered in a body and filed into the lower lecture room where chairs were placed in front of the Professor's platform for us. It was an ordeal for even strong nerves to listen to the stamping the shouting, the cat-calls and general stampede our entrance elicited. The men behaved more like a set of lunatics than would be Doctors. The worst of it was that the Professor in the department seemed rather pleased than otherwise at the demonstration.

Bertha Van Hoosen, who attended Michigan a decade later, found that the greatest prejudice came from the women students. She recoiled at the epithet "hen medic," calling it "dreadful." "I have never felt the stigma as in Ann Arbor," she wrote.[67]

Dorothy Reed Mendenhall's memoirs testify eloquently to the life of women medical students in Baltimore in 1900. One curious incident occurred during her very first day in the city. Anxious to visit the school, she took a streetcar.

There was only one passenger in the car besides myself, and I soon was aware that I was an object of interest to him. Almost opposite my seat on the bench that ran lengthwise of the car, sat a distinguished gentleman dressed in grey oxford morning coat, striped trousers, and wearing a silk hat. He was short, but so finely built and slender that he did not seem small. I noticed immediately the sallow, ivory-colored tone of his skin and the small hands with tapered fingers folded over a cane which he held between his knees. My appearance seemed to interest him for he literally stared me out of countenance—seeming to go over me from head to foot, as if he were cataloguing every detail for future reference. I decided that he was an oriental—this conclusion brought about by his color and the long, thin rattail moustach that he kept pulling as he inventoried my charms. I knew that he was a gentleman, so I was embarrassed but not alarmed. Thinking to avoid him as soon as possible, when the car stopped at Broadway I hopped out first, and walked quickly in the direction of the hospital gates a block away. He soon caught up with me, and walking along side of me, said very casually, "Are you entering the medical school?" I managed to gasp out that I intended to. "Don't," said he, "go home." And to my amazement without another word walked on ahead of me and went up the long flight of steps leading to the hospital door. Well, thought I, he must be crazy. How would he know that I was going into medicine, or why should he advise me not to? I think this incident dampened my interest in the unprepossessing brick buildings of the hospital and the medical school, for after a very short stay, I found a return street car and took myself back to Miss Conway's and my little room. No other incidents of my first day in Baltimore remain in my memory.

The following morning Mendenhall went back to the medical school for her interview. Waiting nervously with other freshmen to be called, she finally heard her name. Cautiously, she entered an impressive room in which several distinguished-looking gentlemen sat around an enormous table. Led by the dean, Dr. William Welch, the doctors began to question her. Suddenly, as she looked up, she noticed to her amazement the man of the streetcar incident.

I mumbled a reply. Dr. Welch rose and bowed and intimated that the interview was over, telling me to be at the medical school the next morning at 9 o'clock. I got up and not knowing what to do—*backed out* of the room, until I reached the door—feeling that this group represented to me—royalty. Once again in the ante-room, I said to a man waiting there—later known to me as my good friend Dr. Rusk—"Who was the gentleman sitting on the left of Dr. Welch?" He answered, "Why, that is the great Dr. Osler."[68]

Yet disapproval from male faculty was not universal. Despite Mendenhall's curious initial encounter with him, she often spoke of William Osler in her memoirs as a friend. His distaste for feminism did not deter him from treating the women students, once they had arrived at Hopkins, with scrupulous integrity. "Of all the men I have ever known, or even met," she wrote, "William Osler has always seemed to me to have the most vivid personality as well as the finest mind and character. He was the greatest teacher I have ever known; an inspiration to his pupils and colleagues, one of the great gentlemen and influences of his age in the profession. . . . To all of us he was an unfailing guide." Mendenhall spoke similarly of William Welch.[69]

At Michigan Corrydon L. Ford, the head of the anatomy department, was a great favorite with the women. "Professor Ford," Eliza Mosher wrote to her family when still a freshmen, "is just as kind as he can be and has done more than any man living to raise my faith in men!" Michigan's President Angell and his wife also did their best to ease the "hen medic's" social adjustment.[70]

Nevertheless, the women at coeducational institutions had their fill of embarrassing situations. Although Michigan managed to preserve a peaceful and chaste atmosphere by conducting separate classes, not all schools could afford such a luxury. Dr. Ida May Wilson, a Columbus, Ohio, physician who attended the Ohio Medical University in the early 1890s recalled her "first experience with seeing a naked man."

One afternoon it was posted on the bulletin board that Dr. McCurdy was to hold a class of the whole college on regional anatomy. . . . So we all met at the amphitheater. As I was waiting in the hall for the classes to be through reciting, Johnson, a colored man who was janitor of the dissecting room, came upstairs and grinning at me said, "You all going to the recitation this afternoon?" I said yes. He just halted a few minutes, then grinned and went on. So we all gathered for the class, and after a very good lecture from Dr. McCurdy, he said, "Bring that man in," and Johnson came in stark naked—a splendid figure, black and well developed. It was my first sight of a naked man; I had seen some operations on men in the operating room but most of them had been well covered. Well, I gave one look, then looked down in my lap. But when the Doctor began to lecture . . . the men in the college thought it was smart to be annoying, so they began to throw beans at Johnson; and of course they stung his flesh. And though Dr. McCurdy tried his best to get them to listen and behave, it was no use; so he dismissed the class. A week after that he tried it again, but the men again threw corn and beans. Once Johnson jumped over the railing and slapped one fellow and choked another. Again Dr. McCurdy dismissed the class; and though he later had the recitation in orthopedic surgery, he never tried again to teach the location of the different organs on the human.[71]

Sometimes keeping one's composure proved extraordinarily difficult. Mendenhall recorded one experience at Hopkins which "nearly sent me out of medicine." As at any medical school there was both a hospital medical society and an opportunity to attend other evening meetings and lectures during the week.

We heard the other students talking about going to the monthly meetings, and I was very eager to grasp every opportunity that would give me a better chance to do well in medicine. . . . I induced Margaret Long [the daughter of a former Massachusetts governor who became McKinley's Secretary of the Navy] to companion me. We arrived before the crowd and took front seats. . . . I think that we were the only women present. The one woman interne and the women upper classmen, few in number, knew better than to attend this meeting. Simon Flexner presided, sitting at a table just in front of us. The speaker of the evening—Dr. Mackenzie of the nose and throat department—was introduced after some preliminary business. He talked an hour on some disease of the nose. But from the start he dragged in the dirtiest stories I have ever heard, read or imagined, and when he couldn't say it in English he quoted Latin from sources not usually open to the public. Unfortunately, I had majored in Latin at Smith, and 7 years study made most of his quotations understandable to me. Nearly 50 years has passed since this night, but much he said is branded in my mind and still comes up like a decomposing body from the bottom of a pool that is disturbed. It seems impossible that on such a harmless subject a specialist could make it so pornographic. . . . Dr. Mackenzie spent most of his hour discussing the cavernous tissue present in the nasal passages and comparing it with the corpus spongiosa of the penis. We sat just opposite the speaker and the chairman, so that the flushed, bestial face of Dr. Mackenzie, his sly pleasure in making his nasty point, and I imagine the added filip of doing his dirt before two young women, was evident. I knew that we could not go out—not only should not, but I doubted that I could make the distance to the door without faltering. . . . I fastened my gaze on Simon Flexner and prayed that he would not laugh. Roars of laughter filled the room behind us at every dragged-in joke of Dr. Mackenzie. . . . Through it all Simon Flexner sat like a graven image, his face absolutely impassive like the profile on an old Roman coin. All my life I have been grateful for this man's decency, which at the time seemed to be an anchor to buoy me through this ordeal. . . . I cried all the way home—hysterically—and Margaret swore. . . . The next few days I stayed at home . . . debating with myself whether or not to leave the medical school . . . I couldn't make up my mind as to whether or not I was strong enough to rise above such defilement. . . . It is characteristic that Margaret Long was untouched—she put it down to the natural bestiality of man and ignored it entirely. Part of my trouble was that I couldn't face my class, many of whom I had seen thoroughly enjoying themselves at the lecture. . . .[72]

Hopkins never allowed Mendenhall to forget that she was a woman. After several years' effort and one or two more unpleasant and vulgar incidents, she finally settled on a behavioral strategy which worked well for the rest of her medical career:

I decided after much thought that as long as I was in medicine I would never object to anything a fellow student or doctor did to me or in my presence if he would act or speak the same way to a man. . . . But if he discriminated against me because I was a woman—tried to push me around, was offensive in a way he wouldn't be to a man, I would crack down on him myself—or take it up with the authorities if he proved too much for me alone. On the whole, this was the right way to take the position of women in medicine in the 19th-century. It made life bearable, allowed me to make friends with some men who were not very pleasant persons . . . and earned me the respect and friendship of many of my associates. It didn't endear me to one or two I fell afoul of, and undoubtedly I developed an independence, even an arrogance, which was foreign to my original nature. I was distinctly not such a "nice" person, but a stronger one, after Johns Hopkins.[73]

Although there is no reason to doubt the accuracy of Mendenhall's description of events like the one with Dr. Mackenzie, it is also true that an exaggerated sense of female propriety occasionally proved to be the problem. One of the things George W. Corner admired most about Florence Sabin, who was Mendenhall's contemporary at Hopkins and Corner's teacher for many years, was that "she was the first woman I ever met who was free from the prudery in matters of sex anatomy and physiology that was still prevalent in my student days. To hear a woman discuss these subjects before a class mostly of men, with professional detachment, was very instructive to me."[74]

Even well into the twentieth-century, female inhibitions could create unexpected embarrassment in the classroom. Writing to her parents in 1915, Ernestine Howard complained:

> I got quite peeved at Dr. Stearns yesterday in Lab. We were studying various pathological lesions of the male reproductive system. He was supposed to instruct eight of us, so he got us together and as my name was the one he knows best he fired all the questions at me. It's absolutely unheard of to quiz a girl on that subject here—I was perfectly amazed. . . . It's perfect nonsense to make us study that subject. Now I've told you all my troubles—next week I'll probably be very enthusiastic over the whole school again. No matter how coldly scientific one tries to be, the girl in me will pop up occasionally.[75]

Some women were simply tougher than others. Mary Ritter loved to tell of an incident in her own student days which proved to her that women, no less than men, could develop thick skins. In her second year of school she attended an operation—"the most sickening one in my clinical experience:"

> It was a case of cancer of the face. The result was a foregone conclusion, but the patient insisted on the attempt at relief. A facial operation of such magnitude is far more repellent than one on any other part of the body. As it proceeded, a student fainted. Soon another; and then a third. The three men were stretched out on the floor and no further attention was paid them. As the gruesome operation proceeded I gritted my teeth, clenched my hands, and held on. Next to me stood a senior woman student. I watched her turn a greenish white and sway a little. Contrary to the ethics of an operating room, where silence is the rule, I hissed in her ear, 'Don't you dare faint.' She jumped, and flushing with anger, turned on me. In turn I flushed with embarrassment. But the return of blood to our heads by blushing saved the situation. The two women students did not faint and thus disgrace the sex. That three men did faint was merely due to a passing circulatory disturbance of no significance; but had the two women medical students fainted, it would have been incontrovertible evidence of the unfitness of the entire sex for the medical profession.[76]

Small triumphs like these, when a woman had the chance to demonstrate her mettle, punctuated the struggle for acceptance. Eliza Mosher often retold an experience with the Dean of the

Medical Department at Michigan, A.R. Palmer, one of the faculty members openly hostile to women in medicine. Palmer enjoyed announcing to his class that he could "not see how right-minded women can *wish* to study medicine with men." One day he received a rare pathological specimen and asked Mosher to demonstrate it to the women's class. Later Palmer met her in the faculty waiting room with the words, "Miss Mosher, you showed this specimen so well to your class, I want you to demonstrate it to the men's class." "Oh, I cannot possibly do it," protested Mosher. "Do it to please me," he responded in a most persuasive tone.

> Like a flash [I remembered] his words "I fail to see how right-minded women can wish to study medicine with men." The psychological moment had arrived to make him retract these words, and I determined to comply with his request. When I found myself before those 500 men, I longed for an abyss to open to save me. My pride, however, carried me through. Professor Palmer said: "Miss Mosher, has just demonstrated this interesting pathological specimen so well to the women's class I have with great difficulty persuaded her to present it to you." The place became still in a moment, and I was able to make myself heard I think by even the top row of students. I'm not sure but I romanced a little to make my story more impressive. When through I hurried out under a rousing clapping of hands—but not a foot was heard. Professor Palmer followed me joyfully exclaiming: "That's all for you."[77]

Although such incidents fostered necessary inner strength and self-esteem and generated faculty respect and support for women like Mosher, one doubts whether the positive achievements of isolated individuals really altered the opposition of the A.R. Palmers of the world to the principle of women in medicine. Medical school simply demanded a seriousness of purpose that only rare, special, and emphatically resolute women could attain. When such women succeeded, they were often considered atypical. Indeed, many observers praised the "gentlemanly" character traits which supposedly distinguished many women students. Indeed, to be called *masculine* was to inspire disapproval, but to manifest *manly* strength of character, in contrast to the frivolity usually identified with women, could generate much admiration.

Dr. Walter B. Hinsdale vividly recalled his own initial opposition to women students which, he later admitted, was at least partially inspired by the fear that "they'd take away our patients." His recollection of Mosher as a student, however, eloquently illustrates that she was able to change his opinion because she successfully managed to walk a tightrope—exhibiting both determination and pluck without tarnishing her femininity:

> Eliza Mosher was a young woman one couldn't resent. She was so sure of her calling, she went right ahead and never bothered anybody. *She was a gentlewoman* never aggressive, never freakish in dress as some were. She was quiet, determined, I should say eager to learn. . . . She didn't show off her knowledge nor flirt with the men and distract their attention, which was one thing that was feared. She worked well with men. I presume you would say the men liked her businesslike manner.[78]

Florence Sabin, probably the most successful woman student at Johns Hopkins at the turn of the century and the first woman to be appointed to their faculty, had a similar reputation for being "thoroughly businesslike," a "hard worker" but also generous and warm. As one of her woman students remembered her,

> Her appearance was not very feminine and she wore what one would think of as rather practical clothes. She said to a friend of mine, rather wistfully, that she wished she knew how to pick out pretty clothes but she guessed she wouldn't look well in them anyway. It was a surprise to know she cared about anything so frivolous.[79]

Similarly, at a memorial service for Dr. Frances Emily White in 1904 William Salter, director of the Chicago Ethical Culture Society, spoke of her "singularly virile intelligence," and paid her what he sincerely believed was the highest compliment of all when he called her "a man among men."[80]

The two qualities that Hinsdale remembered most in Mosher were that she kept her sexuality under wraps and "worked well with men" by dressing conservatively and maintaining an efficient manner and that she felt "so sure of her calling" that she never lost her self-confidence. Unhappily, not all women medical students managed such feats with equal success. Martha May Eliot (Johns Hopkins, 1918) complained of a fellow intern who was "a funny girl when you come to work with her. She hasn't much tact and doesn't know how to get along with men." Similarly, Ernestine Howard wrote of a woman classmate, "I do wish Katherine Merritt would use her brain more in class. She does act so stupid in Dr. Winternitz' class—we are the only two girls in the division, and he almost always makes me correct her mistakes—which is embarrassing."[81]

Not only appropriate demeanor, but appropriate dress was important. Women remained ambivalent about the kind of image they should project. In 1913, Ernestine Howard wrote to her parents,

> Katherine Merritt and I don't approve of the frivolous clothes the fourth year girls and internes wear around the hospital. So Mary Wright and we two have decided to buy clothes alike next spring for wear in class rooms, etc. Don't you think that a good scheme? We intend to wear white and avoid fluffy ruffles.[82]

In fact, proper clothes remained an issue even after medical school. Emily Dunning Barringer, New York's first woman ambulance surgeon who interned at Gouverneur Hospital in 1902, agonized for days until she found suitable attire for ambulance duty— a suit that "would attract as little attention as possible."[83] Similarly, Josephine Baker (New York Infirmary, 1898), New York City's first head of the Bureau of Child Hygiene, confessed to be loyally grateful to the Gibson Girl for the introduction of shirt-waists and tailored suits into the conventional feminine costume. For her, she wrote, they provided "protective coloring." "As it was," she continued in her autobiography, "I could so dress that, when a masculine colleague of mine looked around the office in a rather critical state of mind, no feminine furbelows would catch his eye and give him an excuse to become irritated by the presence of a woman where, according to him, no woman had a right to be."[84]

A few women failed miserably to strike the delicate balance. While at Ohio, Ida Wilson learned quickly, but she recorded in her memoirs an experience with a woman who unhappily overstepped the bounds of appropriate dress:

> A Miss Belau entered the class in the second year. She was a full German blond, hair of gold and very fair, and was quite loudly dressed the first day she came to class, she was in a vivid scarlet dress . . . sleeveless of course . . . the men could not keep their thoughts or eyes on the doings of the class. I remember [Andrew] Bonnett . . . leaned over and said, "There comes a gay one," and I felt sure a man of his age and place in life knew more than I did. So I never palled around with Miss Belau.

Maintaining one's self-confidence was another nagging problem. Ida Wilson remembered another classmate at Ohio, Mrs. Jesse Smith, who was such a "perfect student" that "she took all the prizes that were offered" and "knew her lessons by heart." Yet, years later, Mrs. Smith confessed to Wilson that "she could never make a living in medicine. She had no confidence in herself and the people seemed to know it."[85] Bertha Van Hoosen, later a successful surgeon and the founder and first president of the Medical Women's National Association, painfully wrote to her parents during her first year at Michigan, "I am so afraid I will not be smart enough and not do well. I am worried all most to death."[86] Ida Wilson herself, discouraged by several lean years after graduating from medical school, considered retraining as a nurse, until her brother, also a physician, made her promise to "stick to it."[87] Happily both Van Hoosen and Wilson overcame their doubts, but other women did not.

Self-doubt may have plagued the women attending coeducational institutions more often than it did those who matriculated at the all women's schools. After Alice Hamilton graduated from Michigan in the early 1890s, she spent several months interning at the Northwestern Hospital for Women and Children in Minneapolis. This institution, founded in 1882 by a graduate of the Woman's Medical College of Pennsylvania, Mary G. Hood, modeled itself after the Philadelphia school's Woman's Hospital and staffed its clinics with so many Philadelphia graduates that its founders looked on it "as literally a younger sister" of the older institution.[88] When Hamilton arrived in Minneapolis, Hood still reigned supreme as senior attending physician, while Ella B. Everitt, a recent gradute of Philadelphia, served as chief of the house staff. Hamilton immediately perceived that "Philadelphia training is very different from Ann Arbor." Although she deplored Everitt's medicine as "desperately unscientific" and her surgery as "slovenly," she admired the Philadelphia woman's self-assurance: "She is so decided," she wrote of Everitt to her cousin Agnes, "has such confidence in herself, such calm authoritarian ways with the nurses and such cheery indifference with the grumbling patients, that I constantly envy her."[89]

Another Michigan graduate, Eveline P. Ballentine, recalled that the Woman's Medical College of Pennsylvania had an allure for women at Ann Arbor. She wrote that when she was a student in the coeducational university, a great deal was heard about the woman's school. Some had already attended there for a year, while others eventually left Michigan to take their senior year in Philadelphia. "There seemed to be a tradition," Ballentine wrote, "that the medical education of a woman was not complete unless at least one of these terms was spent at the Woman's Medical College." When she herself graduated and visited the school for the first time in 1888 she was inspired by the atmosphere: "There was something in the spirit of the place . . . that impressed me that there was a foundation for the tradition. . . . I confess that what I saw filled me with a feeling of loss and regret for some of the good things that had been left out of my student experience." One surmises that Ballentine is here referring to the sense of fellowship and mutual support from both women faculty and students which remained the primary attraction of the woman's school.[90]

When the number of women students was large enough, students at coeducational institutions fought their isolation by coming together in support networks. Eliza Mosher's letters home report a closeness among the women students which seemed essential to her sense of well-being. "We are all very fond of each other," she wrote in 1872.[91]

At Johns Hopkins, the women students created a cohesive and flourishing social and intellectual life of their own. No doubt this was due in part to the influence of M. Carey Thomas and the Baltimore Women's Committee, which continued a watchful scrutiny over the Hopkins women and obsessively monitored their successes. Of course not everyone was grateful for such attention. Dorothy Reed Mendenhall remembered that she and other women came to "know and dread invitations of Miss Garrett to her huge house on Vernon Place."[92] Yet Florence Sabin, a more unflappable personality than her friend, left no such record of annoyance. Indeed, in 1902, when Sabin had already begun to show promise as a researcher with the publication of two remarkable papers, the feminist network in Baltimore lobbied successfully to support her work with an award of $1,000 from the Naples Table Association, an organization dedicated to promoting scientific research by women.

Nor did Martha May Eliot find contact with the women's committee unpleasant a little over a decade later. In 1916 she reported to her mother,

> Yesterday there was a tea at the house at "104" for the Women's Committee of the Medical school and all the dignitaries were there—among them Miss Thomas from Bryn Mawr. . . . She was quite sociable and apparently much interested in us and our welfare. . . . Ethel tried to impress Miss Thomas with the necessity for better living quarters for the girls and she seemed favorably impressed with the idea of a house large enough to hold a good many and with arrangements to provide good meals. . . . Several doctors wives came and it was very pleasant.[93]

In the early 1900s the women at Hopkins founded a secret "fraternity," Zeta Phi. All women students were invited to join. They met often and frequently prestigious older women physicians came to speak. They discussed journal articles together, joined in social activities and occasionally invited men students to teas. Martha May Eliot amusedly wrote home of one such meeting:

> Friday night we had a meeting of the Fraternity and a wild one it was. Such a crowd as the "hens" are when they get together—and such scrappers! The birds don't agree in their nest there are too many odd sticks among us.[94]

From the very beginning women tended to room together, and by the second decade of the twentieth century they had their own house, equipped with housekeeper. Most women students gathered there for meals. "At that time," remembered Marie N. Wherry, "our boarding house, called the Hen House, on Jackson place was notorious." The women also had a "charming sitting room in the hospital and a comfortable rest and lunch room in the Physiological Building, the gift of Mary Garrett," recalled Minerva Herrinton, who entered Hopkins in 1902.[95]

Dr. Alice Ballou Eliot recollected more work than play. "We women kept pretty much to ourselves," she wrote decades later. "We were so busy we had little time for anything outside our work."[96] But occasional letters home contradict Eliot's austere picture. Equally typical was this description by Martha May Eliot of a Friday evening's activity:

> Friday night all thirty hen medics went up the bay in a boat for supper and didn't get back until nearly eleven. We had a fine time and fairly quiet for such a crowd of girls. I guess they were all pretty tired.

Dorothy Reed Mendenhall remembered examination time with particular amusement. "For the big examinations," she wrote in her memoirs,

> Florence Sabin, Rose Fairbank, Mabel Austin and I would get together the night before, coming prepared with a list of questions we had found most difficult to answer and posing them in turn to a jaded audience. Such an evening was very helpful, clearing up many hard knots and usually left us in a hilarious mood.[97]

And yet Johns Hopkins did bring together many diverse personalities among the women—"odd sticks," as Martha May Eliot had put it—and their forced intimacy, often as much a product of necessity as desire, occasionally created friction and resentment. Some of these ambivalent feelings are expressed in Dorothy Reed Mendenhall's memoirs, especially in her description of the women of her class. Mendenhall entered Hopkins in 1900. There were twelve women in a class of forty-three, and Mendenhall, not a person to mince words, passed judgment on them all. Her memoirs, however caustic, give us an insight into the variety of ways women accommodated themselves to the coeducational situation.

For example, she recalled two Vassar graduates, "fine students, and well bred good-looking women" who were both "embittered and supersensitive from association with the men of their classes who made them feel they were not wanted." Another "frump" by the name of Delia Wykoff "represented all that is undesirable in a professional woman." Though she was bright and became an intern at the hospital—an honor extended only to the most promising—she let the men make fun of her and, as Mendenhall saw it, expected special treatment for being a woman. The men "told with glee how she took a day off every month to stay in bed when she menstruated, leaving them to do the work." Such behavior infuriated Mendenhall, who was heckled with Wykoff's failings when she herself appeared on the wards for a clinical rotation. "I determined, at least," she recorded years later, "to ask no favors because of being a woman."[98] Thus, occasional tension in the atmosphere could pit women against other women.

Most of the other "girls" Mendenhall described as "plain." Only Mabel Austin, "a graduate of the University of Minnesota," and a "typical co-education product," was "beautiful" and a "good student." Mendenhall felt Austin knew how to handle men through her experience at a large midwestern university, but was also disappointed at Austin's willingness "to get favors by boot-licking." She was "hail-fellow-well-met" with everyone. With Mabel Austin's help Mendenhall finally relaxed and found her niche. But it was clearly not easy. She later summarized her first year with the observation:

> Both of us being good looking, well dressed, and evidently used to things socially were unusual in a crowd of plain women, introverted types, shy or self-effacing students, or freak personalities. . . . We drew on ourselves much attention, especially from upper classmen— our own class, largely gentlemen, paid very little attention to us. Apparently the older students and some of the staff were dumbfounded to see attractive women in Medical School.[99]

The underlying sexual tension in Mendenhall's memoirs speaks to another difficulty women at coeducational institutions faced. Eliza Mosher's quiet self-assurance gave her an advantage matched only by her asexuality. The same was true for Florence Sabin, of whom an acquaintance wrote, "She was more interested in a career than she was in having beaux."[100] But other women achieved the acceptable affective posture with great difficulty. Women with Mosher's or Sabin's singleminded dedication to work, who refused to be seduced by romantic yearnings for husband, home, and family, managed to escape many of the conflicts that others, perhaps more easily responsive on an emotional level to the opposite sex, could not always avoid. Coeducational institutions could occasionally exacerbate the dilemmas of such women.

Again, Dorothy Reed Mendenhall is a good example. During her last year at Johns Hopkins she was drawn into an unhappy love affair that brought her enormous emotional strain and led to her decision to leave Baltimore and take residency training in New York.[101] Moreover, Mabel S. Glover, a promising Wellesley graduate and one of the three women to enter the first class at Hopkins, fell in love with the school's new young anatomy professor, Dr. Franklin P. Mall, and gave up medicine to become his wife. Years later she wrote, "Dr. Mall always insisted that he made up his mind that first day that he was going to marry me as soon as possible."[102] A bit younger than Glover, Edith Houghton became engaged in the middle of her senior year at Hopkins to Donald Hooker, a fellow classmate and later professor of physiology at the school.[103] She too abandoned medicine. In 1916 Ernestine Howard wrote in some distress about a favorite fellow classmate, Irma Goldman, who had recently become engaged to a man she had known only for a very short time. The psychological stress had become unbearable for Howard's friend and she feared that "Irma . . . is on the way to flunk out." Goldman began to cut classes, and became so worked up over Adolph Meyer's clinics in psychiatry that she began to believe that "she has a psychoneurosis." "All that in addition to getting engaged . . . is too much for her. If she'd attend to business, I think she'd be all right, but the little idiot hasn't got sense enough to do that."[104]

Finally, the tortured letters of Dr. Dorothea Rhodes Lummis Moore to her first husband reveal in rare candor the emotional tightrope walked by women who wanted marriage *and* a career. Dorothea Rhodes had met and secretly married Charles Lummis, later founder of the Los Angeles Southwest Museum and a journalist with the *Los Angeles Times,* when they were both medical students at Boston University in the early 1880s. For several years subsequently the couple lived apart as she completed her medical education and he pursued journalism while living with her parents in Chillicothe, Illinois. Although Dorothea's letters were full of ambition and the determination to succeed in her chosen profession, they also make clear that she was a passionate woman who loved her husband deeply, often felt unsure of his reciprocal affection, and depended on his reassurances. Although she eventually achieved notable success in medicine and was elected president of the Los Angeles County Homeopathic Medical Society, her letters written between 1883–1884 reveal another, more private, side to her personality, suggesting that these years were trying ones, when she occasionally and tearfully regretted their decision to separate:

> I wish I could say Hello to ye today. I am incomplete without you always. (20 September 1883).
>
> Dear Carl Boy! I wish you were here tonight, my mind wants ye, my heart wants ye, and my body wants ye. (5–7 November 1883).
>
> What a horrid world this is, anyhow. Everybody incomplete, except at a few moments of bliss. Here we be, sort o'loving and with young passionate bodies separated by a full thousand of hard real miles. (16–18 November 1883).[105]

Although Moore handled her romantic longings by surrendering to them, other women fought against allowing their emotions to become engaged. Elizabeth Blackwell confessed in her autobiography to the "disturbing influence" exercised upon her by the opposite sex. She chose medicine, she admitted, in order to keep herself permanently distracted from the temptation to marry. Similarly, Anna Wessel Williams wrote of working hard to develop the quality of "detachment—detachment from all disturbing longings," a quality she believed essential to the good physician. "I certainly had longings galore," she recorded. Her diary suggests that dealing with them was for her a lifetime struggle.[106]

Two decades after Mendenhall's time at Johns Hopkins the atmosphere surrounding male-female relationships seems to have become more relaxed. The letters of Ernestine Howard and Martha May Eliot describe a situation of reserved camaraderie. Occasionally the girls who lived at "104," the unofficial women's residence, would have "a 'man' party" and invite their fellow classmates to tea or supper. Often the men and women would see each other in groups. In 1914 Ernestine Howard confessed to her mother that "I think I've learned almost as much about boys this year as I have about anatomy—they certainly look at a great many things in an entirely different way from what girls do."[107] And yet both Howard and Eliot hung back from anything more than friendly, superficial involvement, so much so that Howard was teasingly dubbed "Aunt Sarah" by some of her male classmates. She accepted the sobriquet good-naturedly, but there were times when having to monitor her own and others's behavior caused her to lose her patience. "I'm mad at one of the men who will not keep his hands off me," she wrote home in 1915. "I've sat on him several times slightly—I guess I've got to squelch him good and hard. Sometimes I wish I weren't a girl—I think medical work would be simpler for a man."[108]

While some women struggled, others were simply not much touched by the question of romance. One suspects that Eliza Mosher remained single less out of dedicated conviction, then out of a lack of real interest in marriage. Her intimate letters never reveal a romantic attraction to men, although she got along quite well with them, and she once confessed that she did not marry because she never found a man "who was to me the *only* man." If such a person should ever come along, she claimed, she would have been glad to marry.[109] The fact that such an individual never managed to spark Mosher's interest probably reveals as much about her own indifference as it does about the quality of her male acquaintances.

Still other women found the exposure to men at coeducational schools positively beneficial. Emily Dunning Barringer, who married a classmate, attended Cornell University for her premedical preparation and returned to Cornell Medical School in the last two years of her training when her own medical college—the New York Infirmary—merged with Cornell in 1900. "I learned," she wrote in her autobiography, "to work side by side with men on an equal intellectual level; impersonally, if you will."

> I probably would have never made it through the next ten years of my life, if I hadn't had that day to day contact. It seems extraordinary, in the light of today's mores, to have to labor that point, but women doctors in operating rooms, hospitals, laboratories, dissecting rooms were all but unheard of in those days; and breaking in with a group of men, who were also classmates in elementary biology, dissecting pickled embryonic pigs, was at least the most humane way of conditioning that young women could have had at the time for the later more difficult problems of a medical career.[110]

Eliza Mosher agreed. Long after she graduated from Michigan she wrote: "My acquaintance with men both as Professors and students gave me a conception of the workings of men's minds which has been most helpful in my dealings with them later in my life."[111]

And what of marriage? The decision to marry was not always an easy one to make. Certainly when a woman decided to study medicine in the nineteenth century, she was well aware that in many ways she challenged conventional definitions of woman's role, even if she believed, as many did, that medicine was naturally suited to female talents and abilities. Conventional Victorian marriage neither promoted nor condoned a woman's freedom to pursue personal goals. Often feminists pictured marriage as a dangerous impediment to underdeveloped women who ought instead to seek to live and think independently.[112]

Many women physicians strived for creative means to overcome the fears and psychological strains inherent in the choice of a life of independence. Mary Wright, for example, a student at the Eclectic Medical College in Cincinnati in 1854, explained to a friend how she had arrived at her decision:

> Judging from my own feelings I thought it would be somewhat interesting to you to know what I have been engaged in since you heard from me. Well, I have not turned to be a woman's right's woman in the sense in which that term is generally received but have come to the conclusion that notwithstanding parts of the human family are women, that they and every member of this great family have a right to follow any occupation their tastes and feelings dictate, provided it does not interfere with the rights and happiness of others, and furthermore that no single member of this great body if he is a *man* and no set of men or women have a right to prescribe limits for the occupation of another. I have acted in accordance with this conclusion, and have stepped out of the beaten track marked out for woman to walk in, and have chosen an occupation which heretofore has been followed only by men, I speak of the study and practice of medicine. For nearly two years the most of my attention has been directed to that subject. On the 16th of October I commenced attending a course of medical lectures in Cincinnatti [sic] I like them very much indeed, there are sixteen ladies and about one hundred and eighty gentlemen attending the college I would like to be employed in something that will benefit the parts of the human family that has been oppressed and suffered wrongfully, to wit women. For I do think that they have had their feelings outraged, and suffered wrongs that are derogatory to the customs of an enlightened nation like our own. And I think the practice of medicine is just as much her sphere as it is man's.

Wright concluded her letter by raising the question of marriage. "I am still enjoying a life of single blessedness," she wrote, "and expect to during my whole earthly pilgrimage." Staying single did not "grieve" her in the least. "I think," she explained, "that the great object of this life is to prepare for another state of existence, and to do good to our fellow creatures, and enjoy as much pleasure as we can consistent with goodness. It appears to me that all of these ends can be accomplished as well without being married as to be."[113] Five years later Wright was married, but she continued to practice her profession.

Examining the question of marriage for women physicians on the pages of the *Woman's Medical Journal* in 1894, Dr. Gertrude Baillie rejected the arguments of alarmists who claimed that educated professional women were ruined for wifehood and motherhood. On the contrary, she claimed "it is an undisputed fact, among those in a position to know, that her intelligence, her familiarity with the laws of hygeine [*sic*] and physiology, enable her to do her part . . . with much more efficacy, than her less fortunate sister." Nor did Baillie agree that professional women preferred to remain single because of a "lack of physical impulse" as some critics claimed. Yet Baillie believed that the majority still chose not to marry, because they knew that "no woman can serve two masters" and had learned "to make their bodies subservient to their wills." For every married professional woman with a family, she argued, the conflict between the two roles would eventually prove too grueling: "Either her work or her family will feel the neglect." Women physicians, she concluded, who live "by and for the people" could "least of all" afford to take the risk.[114]

Large numbers of medical women implicitly or explicitly made Baillie's choice, devoting themselves to their work with singular passion. Emily Pope insightfully labeled the New England Hospital the object of Marie Zakrzewska's "most intense affection, the child of her prime and of her old age." Others viewed their relationship to their work as a kind of marriage. Harriot Hunt, who often spoke of herself as being wedded to medicine, celebrated her silver anniversary after twenty-five years of practice in the summer of 1860. Similarly, Harriet Belcher eagerly wrote to her intimate friend Eliza Johnson how much she wished the latter could be present at her graduation, which she termed "my 'wedding day.' " Yet for many the decision to remain single exacted its price. In 1916 Ernestine Howard wrote home to her parents a bit sheepishly, "When you receive this I'll be 27 years old! And not even engaged! I seem to be following in the foot steps of my Aunts pretty well—but there are folks who like me even in Baltimore."[115] Despite Howard's discomfort at deviating from the norm, she cherished warm friendships with both men and women. Others experienced more painful degrees of emotional isolation. Anna Wessel Williams thought a great deal about marriage. When she rejected it for herself it was not without a tinge of sadness. "Marriage!" she once wrote in her notebook. "Of course I want it with the *right* one—but the *right* one?—that is the question."

> How can I be sure? Is there ever a single right one? I can't believe it. Already I have had thrills and longings several times at different stages in my development which have been interfered with, diverted, stopped—or marriage would surely have resulted—and how happy I am that nothing came of them. . . . Rather a divine discontent than happiness through lack of knowledge. . . . I want—more than anything to *know,* not necessarily through actual personal physical knowledge, but through intellectual perception and realization. The actual experience might dim the perception.

Intimate friendships also came hard to Williams. In 1908 she recorded in her diary, "I was told today (by A.) that it was quite pathetic to think that I had no one particular friend. It's too true and tho its probably largely my own fault, yet I do not know that I wholly regret it—considering the life I must lead."[116]

Clelia Mosher, a Hopkins graduate who became resident physician for women at Stanford University, was also plagued by loneliness for most of her professional life. Her notes and unpublished fiction suggest that she felt intensely the conflict between the needs and wants of the independent-minded professional woman, society's prescriptions, and her own romantic longings. In the notes for one story about a beautiful and accomplished woman she wrote:

> Bring out the struggle in the woman's own soul of:
> 1. the right to her intellectual development
> 2. the overwhelming passionate love for a man who is her ideal
> 3. the claims of her motherhood
> 4. the intense religious element in the struggle—her vow to help the cause of woman's intellectual freedom and the recourse of having technically broken that vow. The irresistable force of the affection for the man who is her husband, whose character and mind compel her absolute admiration: The power of his strong personality and his respect and yielding to her wishes; his loyalty; his firmness; his respect for her point of view in which he does not believe. His willingness to give her intellectual freedom even in marriage.
> 6. the yielding to her love loses some of her fineness; irreconcilable in her soul and therefore makes her less fine.[117]

The pursuit of self-development could also engender guilt. Aware that the conventional role for women was to live for others, Harriet Belcher self-consciously caught herself after a lengthy and enthusiastic letter to a friend describing life at medical college. "This letter is 'ego' from first to last," she apologized. "Well, I can't help it, in these days I am wrapped up in myself to a most ignoble extent, but you who are living so *in and for others* write soon to tell me all the news." A year later she commented revealingly to the same friend: "What a family you and Mary have on your hands, my dear! And yet you write as if you do not consider that you are doing much. Why, it seems to me a very heavy charge. . . . Thus far my professional life . . . has been far less onerous to me than my old housekeeping days."[118]

Very often women physicians like Mosher who chose not to marry satisfied their desires for intimacy by establishing relationships with other women, adopting children, or both. Elizabeth Blackwell, Emily Blackwell, Cordelia Greene, Eliza Mosher, Lucy Sewall, and numerous other single women physicians adopted one or more youngsters and raised them to productive adulthood. Greene's six "offspring" called her "mother," and when they married she continued to involve herself in their lives and in the lives of her grandchildren.[119] Although not much is known about Eliza Mosher's relationship with her daughter, whom she adopted from among the prisoners when she was the superintendent of the Massachusetts Reformatory for Women at Sherbon, we do know that she looked to the accomplishments of "my girl" with pride. Regarding the adoption, Mosher once wrote to her sister that if she were never permitted to achieve anything more, "I shall feel as if my life has not been in vain."[120]

Helen Morton, for many years an attending physician at the New England Hospital for Women and Children, retained a close relationship with Mary Elizabeth Watson, even after her friend became Mrs. John Prentiss Hopkinson. Morton's letters to Mrs. Hopkinson are full of expressions of love and emotion, and it is clear that she felt herself able to share through her friend in some significant "female" events. She often wrote of her patients who were babies: "I've got a beauty of a baby on my list. . . . The daintiest piece of perfection I ever saw. She's etherial [*sic*] but she won't fly away. . . . I wouldn't miss seeing her for anything." Morton delivered both Mrs. Hopkinson's daughters, and sent her a long poem on the occasion of the birth of a son. "I wonder if you ever could know how I envy you your beautiful children. . . . You know I'm glad to hear all you tell me about your babies," she wrote.[121]

Women physicians frequently formed lifetime relationships with other women. Often two women doctors lived together, practiced together, and shared work, leisure, and various degrees of emotional commitment. Some of these relationships resembled marriages in the degree of closeness and mutual obligation, like that of Lillian Welsh and Mary Sherwood in Baltimore, or Elizabeth Cushier and Emily Blackwell in New York. Many were undoubtedly homosexual. Others, like that of Eliza Mosher and her partner Lucy Hall, were less intense, and took on a configuration which might be best categorized as that of mentor and novitiate. Nevertheless, in their various forms such creatively diverse solutions to the problem of loneliness and the hunger for connection once again illustrate the presence of a wide spectrum of emotional options for women described so perceptively in recent years by historians.

The correspondence between Elizabeth Clark, an intern at the Woman's Hospital of the Woman's Medical College of Pennsylvania in 1910, and her friend Ada Pierce, reveals the rich intimacy achieved by many women physicians who lived together. Clark shared the home of an older physician on the faculty, Dr. Emma Musson, and letters to their mutual friend Pierce, written between 1910 and 1913, are strikingly descriptive of a world in which men were generally absent and hardly missed. Clark's newsy missives evoke vivid pictures of her medical work as they recount everyday experiences, revealing a satisfying life filled with work, love, play, and occasional disappointment. These women clearly knew how to enjoy themselves: the letters bristle with self-mocking irony, gentle humor, good-natured loyalty, and good times. Musson, for example, who was nicknamed "St. Juliana" by her friends, wrote to Pierce in 1910 that "E is a joy to one's soul and a constant source of delight." Dr. Musson, in turn, called Clark "Izzie." Several other women physicians completed this lively circle of friends, but the primary central relationship remained that between Musson and Clark. When Musson died of pneumonia in 1913, Clark wrote to her friend Ada, "my old heart is clean gone out of me forever & forever."[122]

Many women thus found ways to reject conventional marriage without truncating their emotional lives. For them, the freedom could be exhilarating. They shared the exuberance of Marie Zakrzewska when she confided in her last public message to students and friends, "During my whole life I have had my own way as much as any human being can have it without entirely neglecting social rules or trespassing upon the comfort of others more than is necessary for self-preservation."[123] Such freedom, for women who could tolerate it, was not easily exchanged for a wedding ring.

Others paid dearly in professional terms for the sense of connectedness they felt only a husband and children could bring. Dorothy Reed Mendenhall's recollection of her own decision to marry suggests that she did so out of a desire to share her life with a congenial mate whom she could respect and with whom she could have a family. Although she never abandoned her medical career and, indeed, accomplished much working for the Children's Bureau in the area of public health and preventive medicine, she clearly subordinated her medicine to her familial role. Her brilliant promise as a student in William Welch's laboratory at Johns Hopkins, when she identified and isolated the "Reed cell," important in the diagnosis of Hodgkin's disease, seemed to her teachers to have been betrayed by her subsequent choices. For men like Welch, and singularly dedicated women like Florence Sabin, teaching ignorant mothers diet and hygiene could not compare favorably to the monumental task of moving medical science into the twentieth century. Nor did her significant achievements deter the hostile faculty members opposed to the admission of women to Harvard medical school in the 1940s from citing Mendenhall as an example of "an able woman who had married and failed to use her expensive medical education."[124] Mendenhall herself considered such an accusation a "damned lie," but she nevertheless harbored feelings of bitterness.

Other women physicians did choose to give up medicine entirely or were forced to do so by their husbands. Many of them argued that they had benefited from their medical educations, and quite a few from this group became active in charity and volunteer work. Elizabeth Bollins-Jones (WMCP, 1856), for example, married soon after graduation and had five children, one a daughter who became a physician. Although she surrendered her formal practice, she remained active in charitable work. Another important philanthropic worker was Frances Linton Sharpless (WMCP, 1886), who practiced medicine for four years until her marriage. She stayed active as a lay person in medical charity, remaining for a long time a member of the board of the Chester County Hospital and Training School for Nurses. Frances B. Tyson (WMCP, 1901) practiced for eight years after working her way through medical school until she was ordered to quit by her husband. In 1918, when doctors were desperately needed to handle the influenza epidemic, she went back to work, and refused thereafter to return to retirement. Other women practiced from two to ten years before marriage and children.[125]

Less pessimistic about the possibility of combining marriage with a career, perhaps because she succeeded so brilliantly at the task herself, Mary Putnam Jacobi managed to give the most balanced assessment of the problem. Ultimately, she argued, it was a matter of individual struggle and adjustment. "The question of marriage again," she told her students in 1880,

> which complicates everything else in the life of women, cannot fail to complicate their professional life. It does so, whether the marriage exists or does not exist, that is, as much for unmarried as for married women. . . . Many married women will lose all interest in medicine as soon as they have children, as many now fail to develop the full needed interest precisely because they have no other, and are dispirited by isolation from family ties. Many will interrupt their practice during the first few years after marriage to resume it later. Whatever is done, either with or without marriage, can evidently be well done only in proportion as more complete intellectual development and more perfect training enables the woman to cope with the peculiar difficulties in her destiny.

For all the obvious problems that Jacobi so eloquently delineated in 1880, she herself never regretted her decision to marry, despite the fact that the union was punctuated by occasional stormy interludes.[126]

What is more, married women who ceased to practice medicine remained distinctly in the minority. Contrary to the assumptions of historians and women physicians themselves, available data suggests that the marriage rate for women physcans was disproportionately high in the nineteenth and twentieth centuries, until other professionals caught up in the 1940s. Between one-fifth and one-third of women physicians married in the nineteenth century, and by 1900 their marriage rate was twice that of all employed women and four times the rate among professional women. A significant number of them married men who were themselves doctors. Although most practiced in the United States, a nucleus of these women actually managed to carry out Emmeline Cleveland's youthful dream and became medical missionaries together with their husbands in India, China, Korea, and Japan. While some studied medicine in order to assist or to share in their husband's work, others met and married physicians after they themselves had graduated from medical school. As we have seen, a smaller number of women, like Hannah Longshore and Charlotte Blake Brown, left their families with the permission of their husbands in order to attend medical school. However most women physicians who married in the nineteenth and early twentieth centuries did so after they completed their educations and, judging from impressionistic evidence, were noticeably older than their female counterparts in the general population.[127]

Why did women physicians have such a comparatively high marriage rate? One obvious answer was the nature of the work itself. Medicine, unlike most other professions, still offered the opportunity for self-employment and allowed one to work out of one's home, perhaps combining practice with a physician-husband. Such a situation provided greater flexibility for the woman who wished to pursue marriage and a career. Furthermore, there were neither social nor legal proscriptions against the married woman physician as there were, for example, for teachers.

Another factor which is indicated by the age of women in medicine compared to other occupations seems to be that women physicians were much less likely to abandon their work once they married. Age patterns for all employed women in 1900, for example, suggest that nearly half of them were twenty-four years of age or younger. Professional women follow the same pattern, one which signifies that most women worked only until they married. Hence, the percentages of working women grow smaller in each succeeding age cohort after age 15–24. If we consider that most women classified as "professional" by the census in 1900 were teachers, this pattern makes much sense, since married teachers were usually forced to leave their posts.

Medicine is the only profession in 1900 with an exceptional pattern. Whereas the numbers grow smaller in the successive age cohorts after ages 15–24 for other working women, including professionals, the last three age cohorts—25–34, 35–44, and 45+—remain equal for women physicians. This situation remained stable until after World War II, when professional women began to catch up (see TABLES 5-1 and 5-2)

Information on marriage patterns suggests that women physicians were a small and exceptional group, highly motivated and willing to lead unconventional personal lives. The fact that between 25 and 35 percent in the nineteenth, and 30 and 40 percent in the first half of the twentieth century married suggests that for such women medicine was not an insurmountable barrier to family life. This data is not necessarily incompatible with the conventional

TABLE 5-1   Women's Marriage Rate in Selected Occupations 1900 to 1950 (Percent Married)

	1900	1910	1920	1930	1940[5]	1950[5]
All Occupations	16.0%	24.7%	23.0%	28.9%	37.5%	52.2%
All Professionals	7.4	10.4	12.2	19.3	24.7	43.9
Physicians[1]	31.9	35.6	32.9	32.6	37.2	46.2
Teachers		6.4	9.7	17.9	24.6	47.4
College Professors	4.5[2]	10.0	11.3	14.5	16.5	31.5
Nurses	12.7[3]	7.1	7.5	12.5	19.2	40.0[6]
Social Workers	no data	16.3	11.1[4]	21.8	34.0	43.7
Lawyers	no data	28.7	34.2	33.1	38.6	44.2

[1]Category "Physicians" includes Osteopaths for years 1900 and 1910. Beginning in 1920, "osteopath" is a separate category with a comparable marriage rate—around 35 percent.

[2]Teachers and College Professors are combined in one category for 1900.

[3]The category "Nurses" includes midwives in 1900 which explains the higher marriage rate.

[4]The lower marriage rate for social workers in 1920 probably reflects the rapid growth of the field and the corresponding entry of large numbers of young women in this decade.

[5]The 1940 and 1950 data include among the married a group called "Married, husband absent." In all occupations here, they represented about 10 percent of all the married women.

[6]In 1950 nurses are listed in two categories: "trained nurses" and "student nurses." These categories were combined for consistency.

wisdom that medicine was an unusually difficult field to combine with marriage. Census figures for working women, after all, concern only those women who are actually working at their occupations. Thus, though the percentage of nurses who married, for example, was low relative to that of women physicians, such a figure does not mean that nurses were less likely to get married. On the contrary, it suggests that nurses were less likely to marry *and* to continue their work. Indeed, the age structure of working women in general indicates that women who worked in other areas of employment were more likely to get married than women who entered medicine. However, once married, most abandoned their work. In contrast, medical women seemed exceptionally committed to their profession—so committed, in fact, that even marriage and family could not deter them from it.[128]

But were these marriages happy? Evidence suggests that many were quite successful. Some couples, indeed, managed to create models of egalitarian relationships which their modern day counterparts still struggle to attain. In 1945 Frances Ancell (WMCP, 1896) said of her own marriage: "TEAM WORK! . . . Twenty-three years of happy life and work together!" Her classmate Mary Mellowdew Loog felt equally blessed. "I have loved my work and also my married life," she wrote.[129]

TABLE 5-2   Women Ever Married in Selected Occupations 1900 and 1930

	% Single	% Married, Widowed, Divorced	(% Married)	(% Widowed, Divorced)
All Occupations				
1900	65.0%	35.0%	16.0	19.0%
1930	53.9	46.1	28.9	17.2
1900	87.4	12.6	7.4	5.2
1930	73.1	26.9	19.3	7.6
Physicians				
1900	45.3	54.7	31.9	22.8
1930	51.2	48.8	32.6	16.2
Teachers[1]				
1900	92.2	7.8	4.5	3.3
1930	77.3	22.7	17.9	4.8
Nurses[2]				
1900	58.7	41.3	12.7	28.6
1930	79.5	20.5	12.5	8.0
Social Workers				
1900	no data	—	—	—
1930	58.9	41.2	21.8	19.4
Lawyers				
1900	no data	—	—	—
1930	56.6	43.4	33.1	10.3

[1]In 1900 the category "Teachers" includes college professors. In 1930 the two are separate, but they have similar rates.

[2]In 1900 the category "Nurses" is a semiprofessional category which includes midwives. The inclusion of midwives explains the high percentage of widows. In 1930 "Nurses" means only trained nurses and is listed as a professional category.

Sources
Statistics of Women at Work, Based on unpublished information derived from the schedules of the Twelfth Census, 1900 (Washington: Government Printing Office, 1907); *Fourteenth Census of the United States,* vol. 4: "Population, 1920: Occupations" (Washington, GPO, 1923); *Fifteenth Census of the United States,* vol. 5: "Population, 1930: General Reports on Occupations" (Washington: GPO, 1933); *Sixteenth Census of the United States,* vol. 3: "Population, 1940: The Labor Force," part 1 (Washington: GPO, 1943); *U.S. Census of Population, 1950,* Special Reports: "Occupational Characteristics" (Washington: GPO, 1956).

The success of such marriages certainly depended at least in part on the husbands, who deviated in a number of ways from the classic partriarchal Victorian ideal. Interested not only in their wives' work, but in their ability to develop their full range of talents, they took pride in their spouses' achievements and showed a willingness to aid both materially and practically in their unorthodox aspirations. Thomas Longshore, a teacher and philosopher of religion, whose zeal for social reform, abolition, and women's rights was well known, was one such man. When he married Hannah E. Myers in 1841 she had already expressed a desire to study medicine. Although financial considerations forced her to postpone her plans for several years, even the birth of two children did not deter her enrollment in 1850 in the first class of the Woman's Medical College of Pennsylvania at the age of thirty-one. Longshore encouraged his wife throughout her long medical career. Hannah attended classes with her sister-in-law Anna, who came to live with the Longshores and helped them with household chores. Their daughter remembered that "Aunt Anna studied medicine at night and father helped." He, in fact, was "very instrumental in urging them on. He hunted all the notes for Dr. Longshore's lectures and wrote them for her." Later on, "when Dr. Longshore got busy," Mr. Longshore kept the books and compounded her medicines for her. Similarly, the son of Sarah Cohen (WMCP, 1879) remembered that his father "was quite proud of my mother. When she was teaching in medical school, she would dictate her lectures and he would copy them down in longhand for her."[130]

Other women physicians had husbands who were equally supportive. A niece of Dean Ann Preston studied medicine at the Woman's Medical College five years after she married her physician husband. After taking her degree in 1881 Florence Preston Stubbes joined her husband's practice, concentrating on the diseases of women. For years she balanced work and family life, offering to some observers "an excellent example of what a medical married woman may do, at least in special practice, without neglecting husband or child." When she died, her husband, Dr. H.J. Stubbes, paid her high tribute by pronouncing her a "true woman, a loving mother, a perfect wife," whose professional competence was "ever a source of strength and inspiration to her husband."[131] Dr. Esther Hawkes, an 1857 graduate of the New England Female Medical College had the full backing of her own physician husband, whom she had married when she was still a teacher. A friend wrote of their union: "Marriage to most women means an end to their individual careers. With our friend . . . marriage was simply an entrance to wider usefulness and greater opportunities."[132]

In 1891, four years after Mary Bennett had begun to practice medicine in Berkeley, California, she married William Emerson Ritter, with whom she had fallen in love five years earlier while still a medical student. Ritter was studying biology at the university and, although they became engaged, it was not until he was well along toward the completion of a Ph.D. from Harvard and had received an appointment in the newly created Zoology Department at the University of California that the couple married.

At the end of her life Mary Ritter confessed in her autobiography, "My husband's scientific enterprises have determined the course of our lives."[133] Yet she managed to practice medicine for twenty-two years with his wholehearted support. By her account, the relationship, though childless, was a deeply satisfying one. The two shared many common interests and Mr. Ritter, who founded the Scripps Institution of Oceanography, had an accomplished career. The couple enjoyed friendships with several "medical marriages," and moved in circles where professional activity for married women was not frowned upon.[134]

A generation later Emily Dunning Barringer, who attended the Women's Medical College of the New York Infirmary and was graduated from Cornell when the two schools merged in 1899, wrote of the encouragement she received from her husband, a surgeon whom she met when they were both medical students. Speaking of their initial encounter she mused:

> Fate was certainly very kind to me. I have often wondered what would have happened if I had met an average man . . . [instead of] the extraordinary one I had found. . . . I found him the aggressor in interest in my career. He was the one who crossed the boundaries, discussed, evaluated, and encouraged. And he did it, I found, not to please and flatter me, but because he was genuinely thrilled that the woman he wanted to be his wife was capable of that type of mental development. My life both medical and personal took on a perspective and depth, color and meaning from that day. . . . Ben's love, pride and enthusiasm was the delicate adjustment needed to bring the machine into perfect timing and I settled down with a deep sense of power that brooked no opposition.[135]

Similarly, the pioneer social hygienist and associate of Hull House, Dr. Rachelle Yarros (WMCP, 1893) had complimentary things to say about her own mate, Victor. At the end of a long and full career she wrote to the dean of her alma mater, "I am glad and happy to say that my name is still Slobodinsky-Yarros. . . . I am very fortunate to have such a wonderful companion and inspiring and exacting partner during these long years. He helped me study medicine and in all my subsequent undertakings."[136]

Supportive husbands were not drawn solely from the ranks of professionals and reformers. Maria Minnis Homet graduated with the first class at the Woman's Medical College of Pennsylvania. She deliberately chose a rural practice because, as she later explained, "I thought Alma Mater would be glad to have this obstacle removed." Settling in a small Pennsylvania village she soon met and became engaged to Edward Homet, a farmer and surveyor in the area. Something of the flavor of their courtship has been preserved in a single letter written by Maria to her fiancé on 23 October 1856, one month before the wedding. The note, simple and straightforward, suggests the degree to which these "bold" women tempered their medical concerns with the mundane cares of a more conventional femininity:

Dear Edward:

I want to come see you on Saturday next. Can I come? I thought I would ask you to come down but when crossing the river yesterday, I saw you on the top of the house or on nothing, for I could not see what supported you, and I thought how tired you would be so I said to myself I will not ask him to come down. Then I thought I would like to know, at the close of the week, whether you had escaped all danger, and then at the risk of being called simple I thought I would ask to visit you. If it is not convenient send me a line. I have some business that way so it will not seem like going on purpose.

Miss Slatery sits at one end of the table making my dress. I think it looks quite well.

Tomorrow I calculate to make some fruit cake. It is better when made some time. Oh dear, I wonder if I can make it good enough for Aunt Milly and Aunt Amandy.

I have my hands full—if nobody would get sick for a week or two— but the sick must be attended to and as for other things I will do the best I can and if it does not suit everybody I will try not to cry about it. If you only keep well and no accident happens to you, I will put up with all the rest. But doesn't your head get dizzy when up so high? Then it must make you lame, too. I think I will bring a little of the "medicine" you spoke of but you must take it at night or you might not be able to climb so well.

I am glad you are not afraid. If you were, there would be more danger of falling. Then everybody praises you, and then I feel proud of you and hope "all will be well." But I must confess it made me tremble a little to see you up so high. But you are doing your duty and I trust no harm will come to you.

"Wal" I will not trouble you farther now and close with wishing you very pleasant dreams.

> Yours as ever,
> Maria[137]

Maria and Edward Homet were married on 13 November 1856 and resided near Homet's Ferry, Pennsylvania, for nearly forty years. In 1892 Maria wrote about her practice and her marriage to her friends at the Alumnae Association:

> When I married . . . it was much easier; my husband never allowed me to harness my horse, and if I had a call in the night he always drove for me. Eighteen months after my marriage my only child, a daughter, was born. . . . After practicing thirteen years, my family thought they needed me at home, and that I needed rest. I therefore gave up practice. I now go out occasionally but my visits are gratuitous.[138]

William Osler was once reputed to remark that "human kind might be divided into three groups—men, women and women physicians."[139] Though Osler was known to be scrupulously fair to his women students, his comments reveal that for the most part women physicians were not easily welcomed into the medical profession, and, when not rejected entirely, they were at best tolerated as "different." Their role marginality and role ambivalence, primarily imposed by male physicians, was both resisted *and* internalized by women doctors themselves. They wanted to be accepted into the professional fold, while they struggled to remain both women and physicians. They suffered from male discrimination in their role as Victorian women as well as in their role as Victorian women doctors. In this examination of the ways in which women physicians' professional lives impinged on their womanhood, we have seen that they struggled valiantly to become creditable practitioners without either surrendering or denigrating their femininity. They sought as best they could to mesh the commonplace events of their lives as women with the demands of a professional life hitherto based solely on the male model. It was not an easy task at all, and many of them good-naturedly understood that society would continue to view them as a class apart, no matter what they accomplished. The next chapter will inquire about the ways in which their womanhood affected their adjustment as professionals. We will see that in spite of their unique handicaps, women physicians managed to accomplish a great deal.

Lillian Welsh loved to argue that "out of the mouths of babes and defectives come often current social opinions." In support of her contention, she was fond of telling of an encounter she had with an inmate one Sunday morning when she worked in the Norristown Hospital for the Insane. Suddenly, while doing rounds with her friend Dr. Mary Sherwood, she was confronted with a female patient who "planted herself firmly in our way," and, looking at Dr. Sherwood, asked, "Say are you a doctor or a lady?" "You look so young and pleasant," the woman continued, "I thought you might be a lady." Though public opinion might stubbornly question women physicians' choices, evidence suggests that they managed often quite successfully to balance two identities with sensitivity and grace.[140]

CHAPTER 6

The Woman Professional:
The Lady as a Doctor

> Women Doctors must be as quiet and inconspicuous as possible, so that when they are dead, no one will know that they have lived.
> Attributed to Pliny by Jane E. Robbins, M.D.,
> "Memories of Student Days," 1942.

Women physicians came of age professionally at a time when the organization of medical education and the delivery of medical care was undergoing significant transformation. In the last third of the nineteenth century, in response to bacteriological discoveries and technological innovations that ushered in dramatic advances, the practice of medicine became a science.[1]

In the years between 1850 and 1880, the chaotic conditions produced by urbanization and the growth of a profession which had lost the stability of preindustrial smallness, face-to-face personal relationships and an apprenticeship system that reinforced social elitism as it provided access to a generally respectable clientele had worked in favor of women. The profession's loss of cohesiveness and the intense economic competition of the antebellum period, engendered by the proliferation of low-grade medical schools, the appearance of medical sects, and the abandonment of licensing legislation, eased access to a medical degree for would-be medical practitioners of both sexes. With the erosion of traditional informal mechanisms for controlling who became a physician, the narrow and comparatively homogeneous professional life of the early century was disturbed by the appearance both of men from more diverse family backgrounds and of women.[2]

Paradoxically, the temporary lowering of standards served to maintain a professional identity for most healers by conferring on them the title of "doctor." Such unsettled conditions made it easier for women who wished it to achieve professional status before definitions of professionalism and tracking systems crystallized once more. But as the century closed, and the emergence of scientific medicine boosted physicians' opportunities to improve their financial and occupational status, a successful medical career came to depend more and more on a network of new or revitalized medical institutions: the medical school, the hospital, the dispensary, and professional societies. Such changes would affect the lives and careers of female medical professionals in numerous ways, and this chapter will attempt to describe the various professional paths that women physicians pursued in a changing medical environment.

In the case of the medical schools, we have already seen that women founded their own schools—a few that were generally of high caliber—while at the same time pressing their right to coeducation. These schools successfully trained women physicians until the increasing costs of medical education forced them to close at the end of the nineteenth century. Although few women physicians had actually preferred separate education, the evidence in the last chapter suggests that women students struggled with the problem of becoming female professionals wherever they went to medical school. Both the women's schools and the coeducational schools offered them distinct advantages and disadvantages.

Women's choice of private practice told a similar story. Although conditions changed gradually in the late nineteenth century, it was still possible for the enterprising medical graduate to begin practice directly upon graduation from medical school. But women lacked the needed medical connections and often had a harder time than men. Alida C. Avery, for example, settled in Brooklyn shortly after she completed her studies at the New England Female Medical College. In 1862 she wrote to Caroline Dall of the "discouraging time" she had had office-hunting. "But for the kindness of two friends . . ." she confessed, "I should have given up the idea of locating here in utter despair." And yet, despite Avery's misgivings, she remained excited at the prospect of private practice. "Tomorrow," she continued to Dall, "my shingle will appear beside the door, in all its shining glory of black tin & gilt letters. I must own to a little dread of the publicity that involves. I am not quite callous to doing things that people sneer at & say hateful words about; but I shall not think of that if I have work. *That* is all I ask or pray for at present." Two months later Avery wrote to Dall, "I have little to tell of myself—am waiting with as little impatience as I can. . . . The little . . . I have had to do have been mostly among friends I knew before coming."[3]

Accepted wisdom affirmed that it took women between two and five years to make a private practice self-supporting. The stern and forbidding Marie Zakrzewska, perhaps a bit jaded by the difficulties she experienced as a member of the first generation, warned of "five years of waiting and starvation." But Emily and Augusta Pope found in their survey of women physicians that most managed modest achievement after only two.[4] The *Alumnae Transactions* of the Woman's Medical College of Pennsylvania recount many success stories. However, one must not minimize the psychological and pecuniary difficulties these women endured. Some even gave up dreams of a medical career entirely. Amy Ames, a 1901 graduate of Philadelphia, practiced for a short time in Camden, New Jersey. When her family suffered financial reverses, however, she could no longer afford the luxury of waiting for patients. She finished her career as a clerk typist in St. Louis, where she was at least guaranteed an income. Anna Angell became the first woman to hold a residency at a New York City Hospital—Mt. Sinai—after graduating from the New York Infirmary in 1874. Then she studied pathology for a year and a half in Germany. Yet her superior training couldn't protect her from "self distrust and lack of 'push'." She never established a successful private practice, and eventually found her place in institutional medicine as a resident at the New York Infant Asylum.[5]

Anita Newcomb McGee enjoyed the advantage of prominent family connections when she graduated from the Columbian University medical department in Washington, D.C. Nevertheless, she spent four disappointing years as a struggling practitioner before she gave it up. Although she continued to be involved in medical and women's organizations and served as an acting assistant surgeon general of the United States army in charge of screening nurses during the Spanish-American War, McGee never again returned to practice. On the other hand, Rosalie Slaughter Morton, the daughter of an upper-class Southern family and an 1897 graduate of the Woman's Medical College of Pennsylvania, had little difficulty beginning a flourishing gynecological and surgical practice in the nation's capital.

Still, Morton understood that her good fortune had in some sense been atypical. Musing several decades later on her financial battle to put herself through medical school she wrote:

> Often I have been asked whether I would advise a girl with no income to study medicine. If she is being educated for missionary work, yes. If after proper scholastic education she can borrow enough to see her through four years at medical college, two years of hospital experience and one year of getting established, with the

understanding that she will not be expected to pay interest until she has been in practice for three years, nor begin to repay capital for five years, yes. Otherwise, no. Had I not had a small income and been impelled by a hereditary urge, I should not have ignored the inevitable difficulties. Still I wonder that I accomplished it on schedule.[6]

Women who chose to practice in urban areas particularly needed patience, courage, and grit. The experience of Bertha Van Hoosen was characteristic. After graduating from the University of Michigan in 1888, she spent four additional years in clinical residencies to gain confidence. During this apprenticeship she had recurring nightmares about failing in private practice. In 1890, after one such episode, she wrote to her sister, "Do you know going into practice is worse than getting married there are so many who make failures of it that you stand hesitating and would give up all plans but for the few glorious examples who stand at the front. One begins to want a new backbone. . . . I wish I could know right now that I wouldn't make a failure of it . . . I would start without delay."

Patients came slowly when she finally settled in Chicago, and Van Hoosen was forced to keep "abreast and alive" by teaching anatomy at the Woman's Medical College of Northwestern University and by giving public health lectures to such groups as the Kindergarten Association. In October of 1892 she wrote to her sister, "I am so anxious to get just one patient in this neighborhood"; and a week later, discouraged, she confessed, "It is such a long hard pull I often wonder if it will not end in failure."

But by the spring, her spirits had lifted. "Patients do not bother me much," she confessed to her parents, "but as long as my money holds out my courage does not flag. . . . I think I will get some confinement cases next fall and they will help me a good deal." By the summer Van Hoosen had acquired several new patients, including a female singer from Cincinnati who "always employed a lady physician." "I think I am getting ahead . . ." she ventured, "but it is such slow hard digging." Gradually her practice grew; by the end of the decade it was an indisputable success. In 1899 she reported proudly, "I am feeling very well and my practice is booming."[7]

Harriet Belcher's letters describing her own struggle to survive professionally are a particularly rich source of information. She began to think about setting up practice while she was still in medical school. She first contemplated moving to Cohoes, New Jersey, then Burlington, Vermont, where there was no woman physician and "it is thought a very good opening for one." She also briefly considered becoming a medical missionary. Finally in 1879, she chose Pawtucket, Rhode Island, three miles from Providence. A fellow student for whom Pawtucket was home had also decided to return there. The student's preceptress, Dr. Anita Tyng, was doing splendidly in Providence and would help the women get started. Dr. Tyng promised Belcher social and professional introductions, a State Medical Society well disposed to women physicians, and referrals to some of her own patients.[8]

Belcher arrived in Pawtucket in July 1879, with high hopes. Her male colleagues—"far from looking askance at me and my pretentions—welcomed me, spoke of my joining their societies at once, told me to use their names as references." The following December she was elected to the State Medical Society and the Rhode Island Women's Club. Everyone expected her to succeed. Belcher particularly enjoyed the community of professional women: she assisted Dr. Tyng several times in surgery, and took over the latter's practice, often for extended periods of time, when the older woman was away. But her own patients appeared at her door only infrequently, and staying financially afloat became a problem. A year after she arrived she wrote a friend:

> I am mercenary as possible and growing no better very fast. I am beginning to look at every one who comes to consult with me with a single eye as to how much (in cash) they are good for. And the sick ones get well so disgustingly fast that I want to poison them mildly, just to keep them hanging on my hands. And the poor ones have such a hard time in the struggle for existence that I can't find it possible to make it any harder for them so I have to charge them very little, if anything.

To defray some of her expenses Belcher began giving lectures on health and hygiene. She was enormously proud of her success as a public speaker and believed strongly in the work. "It is a very good idea," she wrote, "and I hope may be only the starting point of a great deal more. Women can do far more than any one else to help other women if they only go the right way."[9]

In the end Belcher had to leave Pawtucket in order to establish herself to her own satisfaction. In 1882 she moved to Santa Barbara, California, to take over the practice of another female physician who was getting married. In the first month she was already doing better than she had done in Rhode Island. By the end of the year she wrote that her "success" was "assured," and letters written in the next several years reveal a large and busy practice and a very satisfying social life.[10]

Many women chose to open rural practices or, like Belcher, to pioneer in the Midwest and West. Though the majority of women physicians by the end of the century were concentrated in the urban East and old Northwest, a significant minority pursued less conventional paths. Indeed, their geographical mobility was quite typical of the age. They went everywhere: to the West Coast, to cities and small towns in the Midwest, to rural areas in western Pennsylvania and New York, even to the South. Most often they went alone.

For example, Ida V. Reel, the youngest of eleven children, found a favorite uncle to finance her medical education. After graduating from the Woman's Medical College in Philadelphia in 1882, she hung out her shingle in Coatesville, Pennsylvania, the only woman physician in the town. She remembered her male colleagues vowing to "run her out of town in three months." But she stuck it out and eventually learned to take "ribbing" from her fellow professionals and to be a "good sport." She practiced in Coatesville for sixty-six years, specializing in obstetrics and bone and plastic surgery. At the close of her career she boasted of having delivered three thousand babies, some under the most primitive rural conditions. She never lost a mother. Similarly, Frances A. Rutherford wrote her fellow alumnae in Philadelphia of her arrival in Grand Rapids, Michigan, in 1868: "I was the pioneer. It was a strong thing for a woman to demand recognition as the peer of the old practitioners, but it has been granted."[11]

Anna Jackson Ferris (WMCP, 1874) met with initial opposition as well when she settled in Meriden, Connecticut. Yet fifteen years of successful practice there prompted her to boast in 1894, "I . . . have proved to a very conservative people that a woman can practice medicine." Nannie A. Stevens, a graduate of the Woman's Medical College in Chicago, left in 1878 to settle in Kansas. First locating in Wichita, she later moved to Kansas City where she engaged in both surgery and general practice. Soon she was joined by a Philadelphia graduate, Helen T. Graves, whose pastor wrote of her that "she had the confidence of the entire community, and her cheery, sunny face was familiar everywhere in Southwest Kansas City." Carrie Leiber-Marvin, an 1881 graduate of Chicago, settled in Hope, Idaho. Marvin became a contract-surgeon for the railroad and attended patients within a 200-mile radius. She reported an "ordinary general practice in a mountainous and unsettled country." Despite the small income, she professed real contentment with her work. So too did Margaret Holland (Chicago, 1873), who wrote from Houston, Texas, that her general practice among women and children earned her a comfortable income and the "respect of the profession," who consulted with her without complaint.[12]

A decade later, Elizabeth B. Ball, who graduated from the University of Illinois medical department in 1907 and interned at the New England Hospital in Boston for three months thereafter, wrote her mentor there, Sarah M. Taylor, of her successful practice in her home town of Quincy, Illinois. "We have two hospitals, one of which does not admit lady physicians, consequently I am dependent on the other one." Nevertheless, she explained, "I really felt honored when the directors notified me that my name had been added to the staff. My work is principally in the obstetrical ward. I have been asked to lecture to the nurses in bacteriology and expect to do so in a short time."[13]

Colorful letters like these from determined women who struck out on their own abound in the alumnae records of the women's medical colleges in Philadelphia, Chicago, and New York. But perhaps Helen T. Graves's report to her alma mater written a few years after she left Kansas City to relocate forty-five miles further west in Lawrence best catches the flavor of these women's experience. "Dear Friends and Fellow-Workers," she wrote in 1886,

> Regretting that I cannot be present in person at this time, I wish to send greeting from this Western country, and to wish you all Godspeed in the profession. I have been located in Lawrence, Kansas, since August, 1883, and after the "waiting" which is to every one of us harder than the "working," have begun to realize a few of my anticipations. It has been with me a very slowly-growing practice, in chronic diseases, and disorders of no particular moment or significance. My predecessor was a Homeopathic physician, who won golden laurels and an excellent lucrative practice, and then retired (?) to married life. Since then, a period of four years, there has been no other woman physician here. I have not met with any opposition, but the utmost indifference from the other physicians, which is about as much as one can expect in some places. Women are eligible to all the Medical Societies of the State, and have been so for some years.
>
> Lawrence is a delightful place to live in. . . . Every one finds in embarking in any career or profession that they must be "weighed in the balance," their qualities tested, their knowledge and skill tried.
>
> I find a great deal of tonsilitis here during the winter months; sometimes the diagnosis between it and diptheria is quite difficult,

and sometimes there are frequent relapses, which make it a serious disease. There is a peculiar skin disease prevalent here, not confined to any particular locality or season, and, like most skin diseases, is very obstinate in some patients. In common parlance it is known as "Prairie Itch." . . . It is contagious in some degree, and is generally of short duration, but chronic in a few cases.[14]

Women physicians new to private practice often utilized public health lecturing as a means of self-support in lean times and as a method of attracting patients. Teaching hygiene courses proved a significant professional activity for women physicians in the nineteenth and early twentieth century, beginning with Elizabeth Blackwell, who offered one of the first such courses on the physical education of girls in the spring of 1852. Blackwell admitted years later that the lectures gave her "my first start in practical medical life." And so it was with hundreds of women physicians in cities and towns throughout the country who not only took seriously Blackwell's dictum that they should be the "connecting link" between science and the everyday life of women, but also understood the practical benefits of such public exposure. While they lacked both the professional connections and the easy tolerance from male peers that facilitated hospital appointments leading directly to public acceptance and professional recognition, and until the 1870s were denied membership in most professional societies which were increasingly essential to success as the century came to a close, women physicians found the means to be resourceful in other ways.[15]

Early success in private practice was sometimes assured because with some social groups women physicians were in demand. Indeed, while public disapproval often proved discouraging, some women found ready acceptance, especially, but not exclusively, among the expanding immigrant populations of the cities. Sara Josephine Baker and a friend graduated from the New York Infirmary in 1898 and, with the usual misgivings and doubts, opened a practice together on New York City's Upper West Side. Several well-established women doctors that Baker consulted had advised her to go to a small town, predicting five years of real financial hardship and another five years of tenuous existence. But the predictions proved false. "Paradoxically," Baker recalled, "our only asset was that we were women doctors. . . . For many years women came to us because we were women and the competition in that line was small." Like many male physicians, women doctors usually became established with a family first through a successful childbirth. So it was with Baker. "Obstetrics," she wrote, "have been a godsend to many a young doctor just starting his career. . . . It is an opening wedge of considerable importance . . . when in the natural order of events the father or mother comes down with a cold or some other minor ailment . . . you are consulted and have other patients. It was in this way that my practice was built up and became a truly family affair."[16]

In similar fashion, Eliza Mosher and Elizabeth Gerow, graduates of the University of Michigan, enjoyed almost instant success among women and girls when they opened their practice in Poughkeepsie in 1875. Later Mosher moved to Brooklyn and again she and her new partner, Lucy Hall, found themselves being consulted by prominent male physicians wishing to refer patients who preferred to be treated by a woman. In 1887 Mosher wrote proudly to her family:

> I am getting quite a practice among young girls who are over doing and under eating. and need a good overhauling—life, habits & all. It pleases the mothers, evidently, to have me make a careful examination, and note the condition of the various organs and parts. and sum up regarding the needs. I really am able to put a hand on such a girl which she does not resent yet which is firm enough to hold her to right living and I do not *want* better work to do.

In Baltimore Amanda Taylor (WMCP, 1880), reported that although she had been in practice only two months, "ladies" came to her, "glad to be treated by one of their own sex." Similarly, Dr. Jessie F. Shane confessed that her own large country practice had gotten off to a slow start until "one and then another woman came to me, suffering from some 'inward trouble,' as they almost invariably stated it, obtained relief, told others."[17]

In some communities, being the "woman's doctor" carried a considerable amount of informal authority. Pauline Stitt, a physician interviewed in connection with the Women in Medicine Oral History Project, grew up in western New York in a tiny town, Frewsburg, in the 1910s. She remembered that Dr. Jane Lincoln Greeley, rumored to be a cousin of Horace Greeley's, "practiced regularly and was the most esteemed physician for women." Greeley did general medicine and gynecology. "It was an era when a lady found it easier to go to a woman," Stitt recalled. Greeley was "called the doyenne, the dean, of physicians in Chatauqua County."

> I recall . . . that Grandma Stitt went a few times to Dr. Jane Greeley when she had what she regarded as "female problems." . . .

As long as Dr. Jane Greeley was at their sides, matrons who were careful of propriety could access other care, too, because Dr. Greeley's recommendation conferred respectability on referral. She could send a patient to another doctor and he would be acceptable. If a referral was needed Dr. Greeley was alert to arrange it, and she stood by her patients literally and symbolically. Her patients proclaimed, "There's nothing wrong in going to Dr. Whosit; Dr. Jane Lincoln Greeley sent me there." She not only wrote referral notes, she even accompanied patients on some visits. Everything was done with dignity, and a woman patient could make that clear to her husband, too.[18]

Besides private practice, a career option that opened to women in the last third of the nineteenth century was institutional work. Not surprisingly, women were particularly happy to take such positions, though the work carried low professional status and was often scorned by the more ambitious male physicians favoring private practice. D. W. Cathell, M.D., in his widely read book *The Physician Himself, And Things That Concern His Reputation and Success,* warned the enterprising that offices such as "vaccine physician, coroner, city dispensary physician, sanitary inspector, etc." tended to "dwarf one's ultimate progress" by creating a "low grade reputation" that was hard to outlive. Even "permanent physician or assistant physician to hospitals, infirmaries, lunatic asylums, dispensaries, almshouses, reformatory or penal institutions" should be avoided, according to Cathell, since they looked to many people "like a confession of impecuniosity or inferiority."[19] Uncertain of the rewards of private practice, women were often attracted by the security of such appointments, and the opportunities they afforded to gain expertise.

One of the earliest types of institutional work was employment in a water-cure establishment, something akin to today's spa. Although many of these health resorts were originally founded by sectarian physicians, regular physicians too understood the practical and therapeutic benefits of sanitarium work. Cordelia Greene, we remember, attended regular institutions—the Woman's Medical College of Pennsylvania and Cleveland Medical College (Western Reserve). Greene's interest in sanitarium work was shared by many women physicians of her generation. Samantha Nivison (WMCP, 1855), Angenette Hunt (WMCP, 1852), Fanny Hurd Brown (University of Michigan, 1891), Rachel Brooks Gleason (Central Medical College, Syracuse, 1850), and several others preferred practicing medicine in this setting. Because sectarian institutions had proved initially far more receptive both to hydropathic precepts and to the idea of women in medicine, some of the earliest female water-cure physicians were irregulars. As the century wore on, however, new opportunities for study appeared with the founding of the regular women's medical schools and the admission of women to some of the regular state schools. By the end of the century, a far smaller proportion of women physicians practiced sectarian medicine, and most water-cure physicians had a regular degree.

The relationship between middle-class women and the female water-cure physician had significant cultural dimensions, implying a great deal about social relations and gender in Victorian America. Chapter 2 chronicled the rise of female health as a feminist issue in the nineteenth century, and described how the rituals of female invalidism and its treatment bound women together through companionship, mutual concern, and consolation.[20] The water cure provided one locus in which such bonds between women could be acted out. Women suffering from the physical and psychological debilities of nineteenth century marriage, sexuality, and child rearing flocked to these sanitariums to share their troubles with other women. Here they cared for each other's illnesses, expressed affection for one another, established and renewed ties of friendship and intimacy. Superintending the entire process was the woman physician—strong, wise, motherly, sympathetic. Compassionate yet firm, she had listened to the "heart-histories" of hundreds of women, and she offered the wisdom of science as a panacea.[21] Her prescriptions included physiological knowledge, healthy diet and dress, sensible exercise and, almost as often, meaningful and interesting work. She preached an end to the frivolity and ornamentalism which haunted the lives of nineteenth-century middle-class women and made them sick, and the feminist implications of her entreaties were often not far below the surface. It is no wonder that many water-cure establishments were run by husband-and-wife or father-daughter teams, or that male proprietors eagerly sought women physicians to handle their female clientele. The names of well-known nineteenth-century feminists appeared often on the patient rolls of such institutions.[22]

A more modern type of institutional work became available to women for the first time in the 1880s: resident positions at many state reformatories and asylums. Nearly two hundred women physicians served in this capacity in the last three decades of the nineteenth century.[23] In the beginning, a handful of progressive hospital superintendents discovered that women doctors' services were extremely beneficial to insane women patients, who often were likely to respond sexually to male physicians. Doctors like Merrick Bemis of the Worcester Asylum in Massachusetts, the man who first hired Dr. Mary Stinson in 1869 as assistant physician in the department for women, understood that because women doctors' professional options were limited, they were easy to hire and easy to retain. To be sure, most hospital administrators remained staunchly opposed to the innovation, but after a brief struggle and significant pressure from feminists, the employment of women doctors in public institutions eventually came to be required by statute in several states. In 1900 Calista V. Luther, herself a psychiatrist, reported to the alumnae of the Woman's Medical College of Pennsylvania that out of 133 public institutions for the insane, thirty-eight—a little over one-fourth—employed women physicians. These positions were distributed among seventeen states in the East and the Midwest.[24]

Asylum work was attractive for the female medical neophyte because it offered an opportunity to treat a variety of physical and mental ailments, provided economic security in the form of room and board, and even presented a chance to make contacts or to build a reputation in the neighboring community which would later on ease the transition to private practice. Upon leaving institutional service, men and women established practices in nearby areas. The occasion for social intercourse with other physicians was perhaps a less anticipated by-product for these institutionally-employed women doctors: but, according to Constance McGovern, at least two dozen of them married men who served with them on medical staffs.[25]

Women physicians pressed enthusiastically for the chance to do asylum work, both for the clinical experience it provided and because of their increasing interest in psychiatry. Characteristically, many of them believed that women had a unique contribution to make to the care of the insane. "The field of psychiatric work calls loudly for an invasion by the woman physician," Louise G. Rabinovitch told the alumnae association of the Philadelphia Woman's Medical College in 1903. "I doubt whether there is any other branch of medicine that can less afford to dispense with her services. Those of you who are acquainted with the history of the insane asylums previous to the advent of the woman physician into them . . . probably appreciate but too well the crying necessity for women's more active participation in this work."[26]

Though they did provide some women with invaluable clinical

experience, institutional appointments in psychiatric hospitals did not fulfill their promise as an avenue of professional advancement. A strong undercurrent of skepticism about women physicians pervaded the fledgling psychiatric profession and thus blocked avenues to achievement. Women were not welcomed at the meetings of the American Psychiatric Association until the turn of the century. Although by that time the percentage of women physicians choosing to specialize in psychiatry was on the increase and would continue to rise in the twentieth century, most found the unequal treatment they received at state institutions less desirable than private practice. Regularly passed over for promotion, systematically paid lower salaries, and frequently forced to confront an unsupportive superintendent, women in psychiatric hospitals often found the plethora of dead-end positions a real limitation on their success in this new speciality.[27]

Women's schools and colleges, and later on, the large coeducational universities, also provided institutional employment for women physicians in the last third of the nineteenth century. When E. H. Clarke argued that higher education impaired the health of adolescent girls, he may have unwittingly helped to create more jobs for women doctors. The response of many educators to Clarke's dire predictions was not to bar women from college, but to hire female resident physicians to monitor the physical well-being of women students and teach hygiene and physical culture. As Dr. Grace Wolcott explained to the Woman's Medical College of Pennsylvania alumnae in 1892, "We constantly receive application for young women graduates in medicine who would be capable of taking charge intelligently of the course on physical culture in girls schools or colleges. Such a position usually involves also instruction in elementary physiology."[28] School positions, like asylum work, offered varied advantages in terms of security and income for those not willing to risk the hardships of private practice.

By the end of the nineteenth century, the more progressive coeducational universities had joined in the clamor for a resident physician for women students. And yet here, too, professional advancement was both shaped and constrained by gender.

The story of Eliza Mosher's tenure at the University of Michigan is illustrative of women physicians' experience. Because she lived a full and busy life in private practice in Brooklyn, Mosher felt only cautiously receptive in 1895 when President James B. Angell of the University of Michigan asked her to Ann Arbor to become the school's first dean of women. Although most coeducational institutions strictly supervised the comings and goings of their women students, Michigan until the 1890s had boasted of a relatively permissive atmosphere that implicitly trusted much to the women themselves. Pressures from parents, alumnae, and faculty, and the desire of the women students for their own gymnasium finally led Angell in 1895 to conclude that the ideal solution would be to hire a woman physician who could supervise health, direct physical education, and offer counsel and guidance on personal problems. Angell had been impressed with Mosher when she studied at Michigan's medical school, and he wanted her for the job.[29]

But negotiations dragged on for over a year. Mosher, justly proud of her medical degree, assumed as a matter of course that she would have an appointment in the medical school, where she could teach gynecology. The reluctance of the dean of the medical department, Dr. Victor Vaughan, to appoint a woman to the medical faculty, despite Michigan's liberal record on women students, proved typical of the disadvantages to women of medical coeducation. Even where women gained admittance to schools as students, female faculty consistently despaired of prestigious medical appointments. The position of resident physician all too frequently became the only one available to women doctors in universities. Such appointments carried neither the status nor the power of a regular place in the medical school.[30]

In the end, the title Dean of Women and Professor of Hygiene in the Literary Department was agreed upon, still making Mosher the first woman faculty member at Michigan. She also served as resident physician to women and director of physical education. Feminists hailed the appointment as a breakthrough, despite Mosher's inability to get her way with the medical school.[31]

Mosher considered the professorship of hygiene an important part of her job. She taught not only personal hygiene and home economics to young men and women, but sanitation, preventive medicine, and public health. Her courses anticipated much of the thinking in public health and preventive medicine which became standard fare in the progressive era. They also were the precursors of later courses in euthenics and home economics designed specifically to professionalize homemaking and make it a science.[32] Indeed, women physicians with positions like Mosher's are not given the credit they deserve for being pioneers in the field of public health education and home economics.

Lilian Welsh, a graduate of the Woman's Medical College of Pennsylvania who became Professor of physiology and physical

training at Goucher College in 1894, accurately described the status of preventive medicine at the time:

> A woman who accepted a position in a woman's college in 1890 to
> develop a department of hygiene entered an unworked field and
> could practically make of it what she pleased. She could expect little
> or no help from her colleagues in trying to give her department
> academic rank because the subject of hygiene as a dignified subject
> for department standing in a college of liberal arts was unheard of
> and a professor of physical training was given scant
> consideration. . . . Indeed doctors of medicine themselves looked
> with doubtful eyes on teachers of college hygiene who supposedly
> gave their time to teaching gymnastics.[33]

The disdain of male colleagues' doubled, Welsh pointed out, when
teachers of college hygiene were women doctors. Hygiene was still
considered women's work.

Undaunted, Mosher established a rigid system of preventive
medicine and physical education for Michigan's coeds. She personally examined all the girls, measured and advised them as to cor-
rective exercises, reviving an elaborate system of record-keeping
which she and her partner Lucy Hall had developed in the 1880s
when they had worked part-time at Vassar. One of her most dramatic accomplishments was the vaccination of over three hundred
girls for smallpox early in the first year.[34]

Ironically, Mosher never received more than a lukewarm recep-
tion from the women students. Contemporary reports indicate that
males took to her much more easily. An imposing physical presence—nearly six feet tall, large-boned and straight-backed with a
crown of white hair and steel rimmed spectacles—her missionary
zeal seemed too dictatorial to some. She had strong opinions about
proper posture, healthful dress, and physical education for women.
Remembered one student: "She marched us around like a regi-
ment of soldiers. It was useless to say one word against physical
education. Dr. Mosher called anyone who didn't like it 'just plain
lazy.' "[35]

Lilian Welsh faced similar opposition at Goucher and dryly attributed it to the desire to preserve personal liberty—"that is the
liberty of the individual to enjoy poor health unmolested." But
other students were offended by Mosher's no-nonsense approach
to physiological instruction and her connection of such instruction
with an "old-fashioned" brand of militant feminism. She had
sewed for herself out of brightly colored silk a whole set of models
of internal organs, and these she made use of constantly in her

classes, draping them over her body for visual effect. Commented one student, "Her lectures on anatomy and physiology were horrible to us. She'd try on her silk organs like a dress and talk about them freely. It made us shudder."[36]

Another area where Mosher occasionally trod on toes was in her belief that the University should act "in loco parentis" by closely supervising the coeds. Rules for social conduct appeared suddenly, and the new dean enforced them without mercy. Girls who traveled to and from Ann Arbor were for the first time required to do so by day or by pullman sleeper overnight. One freshman who sat up in a coach all night on a trip home was promptly suspended despite protests from her mother. When on appeal Angell upheld the dean's decision, the angry young lady left Ann Arbor for more liberal quarters. Surely many of these Old Guard women physicians harbored behavioral expectations that inevitably clashed with those of their charges—a new generation of women with less puritanical inclinations.[37]

The women's medical schools also provided teaching positions for outstanding medical women. Especially in Chicago, Philadelphia, and New York, female faculty became respected members of the medical community, enjoying because of their position a unique and cordial relationship with the more liberal male members of the profession. Hospital work connected with these schools afforded an opportunity to do clinical research. But, most important, these separate female institutions provided a visible professional platform from which women physicians could do creative medical work while giving them the power to strengthen networks among medical women—networks that contributed so much to the viability of the movement to train women in medicine. Historians of women are just beginning to describe and assess the importance of the connection between strong, separate female institutions and the success of feminist goals more generally.[38] The women's schools became a training ground for faculty as well as for students, and their diminished number in the twentieth century severely handicapped women's advances in medical academia.

When the New York Infirmary closed its doors in 1900 to merge with Cornell, for example, a competent faculty of women was displaced, for Cornell refused to hire women. In her closing address to students and faculty, Dean Emily Blackwell acknowledged the situation with sadness, admitting that the women's schools had been the only institutions willing to "offer advanced positions to women who will work for them." There was nothing the friends of the Infirmary college regretted more in closing the school, she admitted, "than the fact that it cut short, temporarily at least, the teaching career of a group of capable and rising young women teachers."[39] Unfortunately, Blackwell's hope that the situation would be only temporary proved to be merely wishful thinking.

The reluctance of coeducational medical schools to hire women faculty also hampered women's careers in research. In the 1880s and 1890s, a life of full-time research at a medical school or a research institute was still primarily a thing of the future, but women, of course, endured the additional disadvantage of gender. There were dozens of women attracted to bacteriology at the end of the century, and many managed to train abroad. Edith Cadwallader (WMCP, 1900) studied in Vienna with Wechselbaum and Landsteiner. Mary Sherwood, a graduate of the University of Zurich, spent several years working in Kleb's laboratory there, where her close friend Lilian Welsh (WMCP, 1889), also hoping to do research, had joined her. But when the two women returned to the United States after a year of studying pathology together they were forced by circumstances to change their direction. Although they maintained informal connections with William Welch's laboratory at Johns Hopkins, there could be no position there for either of them, and both became resident physicians, at Bryn Mawr School and Goucher College, respectively.

Only a handful of women had more success in achieving their research goals. Martha Wollstein did private work in pathology for several hospitals in New York after her graduation from the New York Infirmary, and she ultimately won an appointment at the Rockefeller Institute of Medical Research, founded in 1904. With Mary Putnam Jacobi's help, Anna Wessel Williams managed to obtain a position as a full-time staff member working with William Hallock Park, an early exponent of applied biology, at the newly established diagnostic laboratory of the New York City Department of Health. It was Williams who isolated a strain of the diptheria baccillus in 1894 that subsequently became known throughout the world as Park-Williams #8, or the Park strain. William's discovery significantly facilitated antitoxin production and allowed the city to launch its first successful antidiptheria campaign. Although Park was on vacation at the time of the isolation, much of the credit for the discovery characteristically fell to him because of his position as laboratory director.[40]

The most prominent of the early women physicians in research, however, was Florence Sabin. A classmate of Dorothy Reed Mendenhall's at Johns Hopkins in the 1890s, Sabin attracted the attention of the great anatomist Franklin P. Mall, probably the most outstanding scientist on the Hopkins faculty. She became his protégé, and under his guidance constructed the first three-dimensional model of the brain stem of a newborn. This early work, completed while she was still a medical student, was soon published as *An Atlas of the Medulla and Midbrain.*[41]

Although her early promise made her a likely candidate for a teaching position, the medical school proved reluctant to welcome a woman to its faculty. A glance at the Johns Hopkins faculty in the next decades indicates that, despite its commitment to the acceptance of women as students, the school remained as recalcitrant on the question of female faculty as institutions elsewhere in the country. Such stubborn discrimination rankled many women physicians, who understood that it would prove a major stumbling block to their professional advancement in the twentieth century.[42] In Chicago Alice Hamilton, for example, remembered with irony her early association at the Memorial Institute for Infectious Diseases with the brilliant bacteriologist Ruth Tunnicliffe. At the turn of the century, Tunnicliffe had already achieved distinction, but the limitations imposed on her career opportunities because of her gender did not escape Hamilton's notice:

> She could be a member of any scientific society she chose, could read papers and publish them and win the respect of her colleagues quite as well as if she were a man, but she could not hope to gain a position of any importance in a medical school. I remember taking her to see the head of a department of pathology in a medical school where the chair of bacteriology was vacant. The pathologist received her with cordiality and respect and together they discussed their work for some time, then he spoke of the vacancy in the medical school and went over with her the qualifications of the different candidates who were being considered. Had she been a man she would almost certainly have been chosen, but it never occurred to him even to consider her.[43]

More fortunate, perhaps, than Tunnicliffe, Florence Sabin did not have to brook sex barriers for long. When the reluctance of the Hopkins faculty to hire her became known to the Baltimore feminist community, they secured her a fellowship to continue her laboratory work. A year later her outstanding ability could no longer be overlooked, and she became the first woman to teach at Hopkins, as an assistant in the Department of Anatomy.

For the next twenty-three years, Sabin distinguished herself there both as a scientific investigator in embryology and histology and as an inspiring mentor. Throughout her career she emphasized a philosophy of self-education and student research that she had learned from Mall. "Books," she often told her students, "are merely records of what other people have thought and observed. The material is a far safer guide."[44] Like Mall, Sabin developed a keen eye for the gifted student, and she inspired many to careers in research. Although she was always supportive in her contacts with other women physicians, the young scientists she worked with most closely were all men. She never managed to attract directly a woman to become her protégé.[45]

Sabin's lack of female followers remains one indication that the branch of medicine she chose proved particularly resistant to women. But perhaps another more subtle impediment lay in the image of herself which she projected. One young male protégé remembered her in a histology class in 1909: "Dressed very plainly, usually with a plain brown skirt of tweed," he recalled. "No cosmetics. Neat but not ostentatious. After all, business was business."[46]

It was not that Sabin was unfeminine. Most descriptions of her take note of her qualities of sympathetic understanding, maternal gentleness, and humanity. Yet one wonders what kind of role model she presented to a younger generation of women physicians whom she herself regretted were no longer "serious minded" enough, but were just "nice girls." For an increasing number of educated women in the twentieth century seeking to balance marriage and a career, Sabin, who essentially had chosen work over marriage, may have been able to provide little in the way of encouragement or advice. Indeed, when the daughter of a friend expressed interest in becoming a doctor, Sabin advised against it, arguing that the girl was too pretty and would drop out of school after a few years to get married.[47]

Though Sabin was in a position to notice the disappointing effects of sex bias, she remained reluctant to recognize discrimination, even when it affected her own career. In 1917 the death of Franklin Mall forced Hopkins to seek a new chairperson for the anatomy department. To the shock of almost everyone, Sabin was passed over for promotion in favor of Lewis Weed, one of her own former students. Friends immediately joined with Baltimore feminists to protest. Hastily Sabin was appointed professor of histology, the first full-time woman professor on the faculty. Although her biographer suggests that she reacted to the incident with dismay and disappointment, she lodged no public complaint and loyally remained at Hopkins for another seven years. Only when Simon Flexner enticed her to join the Rockefeller Institute as its first woman fellow in 1925, did she leave her beloved alma mater.[48]

Although she remained unwilling to make herself an "issue," Sabin practiced her own brand of quiet feminism. Living among Baltimore's strong and militant feminist network, which included several women linked to the medical community, kept her aware of women's concerns. There was, of course, the original Woman's Committee under the leadership of M. Carey Thomas. In addition, Sabin developed warm and lasting friendships with two "faculty wives"—Mabel Mall and Edith Hooker. Both women had met their husbands while attending the medical school. While each abandoned medicine and settled down to raise large families, neither of them surrendered their intellectual acuity or their active interest in social issues. Both ardently supported suffrage for women; indeed, Edith Hooker rose to prominence as chairwoman of the Woman's Party. Her affluent and genteel home became a gathering place for feminists. Mall and Hooker, along with Sabin's occasional good-natured aid addressing envelopes, published the Maryland *Suffrage News,* a local feminist bulletin.[49]

Sabin also cultivated an enduring friendship with Lilian Welsh and Mary Sherwood. The three physicians often met for lunch on Saturday afternoons to discuss medical research and women's issues. Sabin knew that Welsh's original desire had been to do medical research, and remarked with admiration that Welsh "got the most intense enjoyment out of seeing younger women get the opportunities she had lacked." Sabin admired Welsh's lack of bitterness. Such an attitude tells much about Sabin herself. Despite her quiet devotion to women's rights, Sabin often expressed the belief that "it matters little whether men or women have the more brains: all we women need to do to exert our proper influence is use all the brains we have."[50]

Sabin's career suggests that she persistently followed her own advice. Her brilliance, combined with a compliant and reserved personality marked by personal dignity and maternal generosity, won her an honored position in the male world of twentieth-century scientific medicine. But her success was not typical of the majority of her medical sisters, who found pathways to influential places in the medical elite closed to them.

By the end of the nineteenth century a successful medical career came to depend increasingly on connection with medical institutions—hospitals, dispensaries, schools, professional societies. The hospital had already emerged both as a central institution for the care of the sick and a major center for the education of physicians. Clinical training there became more and more important for the young doctor wishing to become well established, especially as advances in surgery and medical technology rendered therapeutic skills more complex and more important. Such changes in the delivery of medical care presented a dilemma for the woman physician. She too must move with the times, all the while attempting to do so in a professional and social atmosphere often unwilling to extend to her equality of opportunity.

Hospital appointments, for example, were an early goal of female medical educators. Male students often studied with preceptors who had clinical positions in various hospitals throughout the city, but such contacts were difficult for women to obtain. Efforts were first directed at securing for them the opportunity to attend clinical lectures and surgical operations performed regularly in hospital amphitheaters. The right merely to observe was not always won easily. Although authorities at Blockley Hospital in Philadelphia agreed readily in 1868 to admit students from the Philadelphia woman's medical college to the general clinics, and Dr. Alfred Stillé, the prominent Philadelphia physician who taught there, welcomed the ladies "cordially" a year later when they presented themselves for Saturday morning clinic at Pennsylvania Hospital, a near riot ensued. In spite of the permission granted to the women by the hospital managers, the male students at the Pennsylvania would tolerate no women.[51]

In New York Anna Manning Comfort, a student at the homeopathic New York Medical College for Women, recalled similar rude treatment when she and other women students first began attending clinics at Bellevue Hospital in the late 1860s. Yet in other cities, women were accepted without fanfare: Boston City Hospital and Cook County in Chicago both welcomed them quietly in the 1880s.[52]

Female medical educators who well understood the new trends in scientific medicine, however, rightly viewed these large clinics as a poor substitute for ward work. Most agreed with Mary Putnam Jacobi's observation, "To students habituated to the daily visits in the wards of the best European hospitals, this form of clinical instruction, where the patient studied is seen but once, and then at a distance, must be seen as ludicrously inadequate."[53] Of course male and female students suffered such defects indiscriminately, except that men could more easily remedy their situation by securing clinical residencies at city hospitals or dispensaries. Consequently, female leaders strove to open these competitive appointments to women as well.

Such opportunities came slowly, and remained woefully deficient well through the first half of the twentieth century.[54] Emily Dunning Barringer recalled in her autobiography the disappointment and anger she felt in 1901, when her four years of medical study were drawing to a close and she contemplated the next step after graduation. She felt, she wrote, like a pianist who had practiced long and hard to perfect his technique, only to be told at the last minute that he could not try his skill on the Steinway. "Surely it was illogical," she complained, "for the medical school to train women physicians equally with men, and then make no adequate arrangements for them to obtain internships."[55] Clinical appointments for women at large city hospitals, when they were available at all, were scattered and irregular. In New York City, for example, Dr. Annie Angell and Dr. Josephine Walter, both graduates of the New York Infirmary, won three-year appointments as resident physicians at Mt. Sinai hospital after severe competitive examinations. Yet when Dr. Walter finished her term in 1887, New York City went without a female resident at any of its major hospitals until Barringer, spunky and determined, and backed from behind the scenes by the powerful Mary Putnam Jacobi, wrested an internship at Bellevue Hospital's downtown branch despite the almost successful efforts of the Commissioner of Hospitals to block the appointment of a woman.[56]

Similarly, Boston's regular hospitals barred women from clinical positions until World War I. That even then hospital internships remained a problem is clear from the correspondence from 1916 and 1920 between two Johns Hopkins students, Ernestine Howard and Martha May Eliot, and their prominent Boston parents. Internships for women were frequently the subject of discussion. In 1916 Eliot burst out to her mother after witnessing her first surgical operation:

> It was terribly interesting and made me wish that there were chances in the big hospitals for women to go into surgery. That is the great trouble now. This hospital here and Bellevue in N.Y. are the only two which will even let women compete, that is among the big hospitals. I can't see why M.G.H. & the P.B.B. can't be broad enough to admit us or at least let us try. . . . It is all very well for Dr. Cabot to say that he admits that there should be a few good women physi-

cians—but how is he going to get them if he doesn't give them an
equal chance to get good experience in hospitals with men?[57]

In Philadelphia women competed for internships at Blockley
after 1883 and received twelve such appointments in the next decade. Chicago proved the most liberal in this regard, however.
Cook County opened its examinations to women in 1877, and by
1889 four hospitals in the city were willing to accept women interns
and residents.[58]

Securing an appointment, of course, did not necessarily imply
acceptance by colleagues or staff. Emily Dunning Barringer weathered only with heroic determination the most malicious hazing from
four "headstrong" and "ruthless" male interns who were willing to
stage a "battle royal" to "get me off the staff."[59] And even at Johns
Hopkins, whose charter bound the administration to a nondiscrimi-
natory policy, women occasionally had trouble. One memorable
incident regarded the appointment of Florence Sabin and Dorothy
Reed Mendenhall as interns in 1900. Because of Hopkins's commitment to equal treatment, outstanding women had won hospital internships from the beginning, but there had never been more than
one woman on a service at a time. When the matter of hospital
appointments arose that year, however, Sabin stood third in the
class, while Mendenhall ranked fourth. Although there were four
internships each in surgery, medicine, and gynecology, the most
coveted positions were those under Dr. Osler in medicine. Because
the top ranking student's health barred him from vigorous work and
the second in the class chose surgery, nothing stood in the way of
both Sabin and Mendenhall's right to choose medicine.

Faced with the possibility of two women interns on the medical
service, William Welch, who had been a warm and generous
mentor to Mendenhall, summoned her to his office to explain
"that there was a serious embarrassment over the fact that Florence Sabin and I were both honor students and of course there
could never be more than one woman interne and would I like to
take surgery or gynecology as he thought there could not possibly
be two women in medicine. This would necessitate one of us
working the colored wards—men and women—and this seemed
unwise." "He was kindness itself," recalled Mendenhall, "really
solicitous of my future and desirous of helping me to make the
decision."

But Mendenhall stood firm. She wanted medicine. Although
Sabin wavered, Mendenhall refused to let her friend buckle under.

In the end, Welch and Osler, honorable men both, reluctantly backed two women.

Mendenhall's private victory was not won without cost, however. She later incurred the wrath of several men near the top of the class who felt cheated out of their "rightful" positions. And when she and Sabin arrived that September to take up their duties, they were harassed by the hospital superintendant, Dr. Henry M. Hurd, who made an ugly scene and accused them of "abnormal sex interests," for their willingness to work on the male colored ward.[60]

More numerous and slightly less competitive, dispensary appointments were easier for women to secure than hospital residencies. Mary Putnam Jacobi listed fourteen New York City dispensary positions held by women in the year 1891 alone. But dispensaries were a relatively short-lived institution for the delivery of health care. Appearing in the 1880s and 1890s, they were already in decline by the 1920s, and with their demise women lost a significant source of clinical experience.[61]

Besides pressing persistently for equal treatment at established institutions, women physicians moved unilaterally to solve their problems of inadequate postgraduate training in two additional ways. For those who could afford it, work in Europe became extremely common, just as it was for the male medical elite. Ironically, the great medical centers in France, Germany, Switzerland, and Great Britain proved quite cordial to women in the last third of the nineteenth century. Hundreds of women physicians took advantage of European opportunities. Most of the attending staff at the New England Hospital for Women and Children—including Susan Dimock, Lucy Sewall, Helen Morton, Elizabeth Keller, Fanny Berlin, Emma Call, and Mary A. Smith—spent at least a year abroad. Mary Putnam Jacobi sought an additional medical degree from the prestigious École de Médicine in Paris. At the Woman's Medical College of Pennsylvania, Emmeline Cleveland, Anna Broomall, and Frances Emily White were only a few of the female faculty members who finished their clinical training outside of the United States. Others, like Lillian Welsh (WMCP, 1889), Anna Wessel Williams (New York Infirmary, 1891), and Anna A. Angell (New York Infirmary, 1871) were drawn to the great pathological laboratories in Germany, although opportunities in laboratory research did not open up for women until the very end of the century.[62]

Women physicians partially solved their need for clinical experience by founding their own hospitals and dispensaries. Although the dispensary as a medical institution was relatively short-lived, many of the hospitals proved remarkably hardy in the transition from nineteenth-century to twentieth-century scientific medicine: the New York Infirmary on Manhattan's Lower East Side, Boston's New England Hospital for Women and Children, Children's Hospital in San Francisco, the Mary H. Thompson Hospital in Chicago, Northwestern Hospital for Women and Children in Minneapolis, the Sara Mayo Hospital in New Orleans. More transient, but equally important to their professional success, dispensaries run by groups of women physicians, like Baltimore's Evening Dispensary for Working Women and Girls, appeared and disappeared in rhythmic succession on the medical landscape in almost every city where there were more than a handful of women doctors. Together these institutions brought several generations of women physicians to professional maturity. Here was an opportunity to work with women physicians often trained in Europe; here were women physicians and surgeons providing competent and thoroughly professional role models to young women still deprived of a clear sense of their place in medicine.

A young intern at the New England Hospital in the 1880s recalled decades later that the atmosphere there was one of commitment and competence. Women were "well aware" she remembered, "that they were under the critical eye of contemporary men, and, therefore, must excel in whatever they do." Consequently, life was "indeed serious" for the unseasoned women who came under the "watchful" eye of these early pioneers. "If in an unguarded moment," recalled Dr. Kate Campbell Hurd-Mead,

> the interne was heard humming a little air or whistling softly at her work, or even if her shoes squeaked a trifle she was taken to task by one of these dignified censors and questioned as to her reasons for studying medicine and for her unseemly deportment. To a very earnest but immature interne the tall and serious bearing of Dr. Zakrzewska was especially awe-inspiring, but by her contemporaries she was very much beloved. Her own early struggles for independence led her to watch even the spare time of the young doctors.[63]

At the New York Infirmary, one of the great attractions was the opportunity to work with Mary Putnam Jacobi. "Dr. Jacobi," recalled one of her favorite students, "had an amazing fund of general medical knowledge and was said to be the most widely read medical person in New York City at that time." Although her prolific medical writings were well known and admired, she also excelled as a clinician. "Her knowledge of diagnosis and differential diagnosis was profound," remembered Emily Dunning Barringer, "and based on fundamental understanding of the basic sciences back of medicine. She was a hard taskmaster; there were no short cuts in establishing a diagnosis. . . . What could have been more valuable for an impressionable young doctor just starting out, than to find herself in this atmosphere of truly great scientific accomplishment and to have all her standards of medical procedure crystallized day by day?"[64]

The female clinicians in these hospitals excelled particularly in obstetrics and gynecological surgery. Young women interns who came of age professionally at the end of the nineteenth century and had the opportunity to observe the changes wrought by scientific medicine, believed that women doctors trained in obstetrics in this period received instruction superior to most men. Of her apprenticeship to Helen Morton at the New England Hospital Eliza Mosher wrote:

> Dr. Morton was by far the finest obstetrician in Boston at that time, having spent four years in the great Lying-In Hospital of Paris. . . . Never afterward did I receive such teaching as she gave us that winter. We were permitted to examine as carefully as we wished, all the confinement patients in the different stages of labor. During those months there were over fifty confinements in the hospital. We were expected to make a diagnosis of position and condition and watch every delivery.[65]

In Philadelphia Anna E. Broomall, who spent several years studying in Germany, dominated the wards of the Woman's Hospital when she succeeded Emmeline Cleveland in the chair of obstetrics upon the latter's death in 1879. Here she made several innovations, establishing a separate maternity hospital connected with the college and emphasizing prenatal and postnatal care well before it became accepted by the majority of physicians. Always the bold clinician, Broomall was one of the first physicians to recommend routine episiotomy in obstetrical cases.

Though she was an expert surgeon as well, the Board of Directors of the Woman's Hospital had typically decreed that a male surgeon must attend Broomall in the amphitheater for all laporatomies. After a few such instances of monitoring, her male colleagues refused to continue the humiliation on the grounds that she was more skillful than most of them. Of Broomall's striking expertise one of her students wrote: "Of one thing I am confident, Dr.

Broomall was far ahead of her time in teaching obstetrics, and her students were greatly superior in mechanical skill to the young men who graduated from the universities during the eighties and nineties."[66]

Some of these women pioneers managed to retain a personal warmth in their dealings with younger women, despite the crustiness that their hard-won accomplishments had demanded of them. Though students remembered Anna Broomall as imposing, colleagues also recalled her commitment to family relationships as quite "astonishing." Similarly, Mary Bennett Ritter, a graduate of Stanford's Cooper Medical College in California in 1886, discovered Charlotte Blake Brown, the founder and dominant figure at San Francisco's Children's Hospital, to be warm, "beautiful," and "always like a mother to me." Ritter interned at Children's in 1887. Brown's personable style, Ritter remembered, did not deter her mentor from developing a reputation as a remarkably innovative and highly respected professional. It was she, for example, who diagnosed Ritter's chronic ill health as septaecemia, and in a bold and still-rare surgical move, cured her by removing an intestinal abcess which the younger woman had endured unknowingly since the age of twelve. Brown performed the first ovariotomy by a woman in the West, and was particularly popular among San Francisco's Chinese population, who preferred that their women be treated by women.[67]

Indeed, the unique atmosphere of the women's hospitals often elicited genuine enthusiasm from open-minded men. Professor James Chadwick of Harvard Medical School publicly praised the New England Hospital for its special atmosphere in an article published in the Boston *Evening Transcript* in 1882: "There are probably few hospitals in the country," he wrote,

> where patients feel the rigors of institution life less than in the New England Hospital. Not only is "the interior sunny and cheerful," but the physicians and surgeons in attendance are, as a rule, sunny and cheerful too, as well as careful and skillful; and taken all in all, it may be justly described as a model hospital.
>
> I once had the pleasure of making the round of its surgical wards with the lady surgeon in attendance, on her semi-weekly visit, and though I have visited the best hospitals in this country and have also had some opportunity for observation abroad, I have never seen neater wards, brighter faces, nor more prompt assistants than I saw there. There seemed to be the best possible understanding between

the surgeon and her patients—gentleness and sympathy as well as skill on the one hand, with confidence, cheerfulness and hope on the other. In short, the *atmosphere* (figuratively as well as literally), was just what it should be in such a place . . . there was nothing forbidding or disagreeable in any of the appointments. . . . When the dressings were removed in the case of amputation . . . I was almost compelled to admit that even the wound itself was devoid of the repulsiveness which generally belongs to such a condition.[68]

While taking into account Chadwick's hyperbole, it seems likely that the women's institutions strove to create a nurturing atmosphere, and in many cases they succeeded.

Like the hospitals, the dispensaries founded by women physicians in the late nineteenth century also had a peculiar flavor of their own. As did all dispensaries, they catered to the working class, but treated primarily the women and children of the immigrant and native-born poor. The first such dispensary was that connected with the New York Infirmary, which ran an extensive outpractice on the Lower East Side. The work included home visits by nurses or interns. Although insufficient funding and sparse personnel cramped the dispensary's operations between 1853 and 1879, work in the outpatient department became a requirement of the medical curriculum in 1889, and funding was then put on a firmer basis. Annie Sturges Daniel took over direction of the Dispensary in 1879 when she graduated from the Infirmary and for the next sixty years charted its course. Daniel was an impressive figure, well respected by students and beloved by the immigrant poor. Her radical outspokenness on prison reform and on the elimination of tenement houses and sweatshops, for example, earned her the nickname "The Angel of the Lower East Side."[69]

Dispensary work often shocked and dismayed young women physicians who, despite their own courageous willingness to stray from prescribed paths, generally viewed life from the solid perspective of the middle class. As Daniel herself admitted, "The degree of wretchedness, filth, of utter degradation in the abodes of many of the poor would be inconceivable to the majority of women in comfortable circumstances." While working in the outpatient dispensary of the New England Hospital, Harriet Belcher wrote of being called to a case of criminal abortion in a brothel. "I did not want to be mixed up in any such affair," she wrote her friend Eliza. "After getting her out of immediate danger you may imagine I informed them that they could call in another physician.

I am learning many lessons besides professional ones, and not the least is to be more thankful each day I live for the happy protected life I have had."[70]

Some women physicians never got used to the squalor. "The work was often thrilling," wrote Anna Wessel Williams of her year as Daniel's assistant at the Infirmary's dispensary, "but mostly disappointing and depressing. Such a mass of dirty, irresponsible, non-responding people I met that I came to the conclusion that they were not ready for what we were able to give them. Crowded back tenements, dark broken stairs, no fire, with mother and children in bed to keep warm, street beggars with plenty in their tenement homes—these and more were the impossible situations I was constantly meeting. How dissatisfied it all made me."[71]

For others, however, work in the slums could be radicalizing. Women physicians clearly performed a form of social work years before it became fashionable or professionalized. Daniels has often been cited for her innovative and groundbreaking programs. "The medical problems which present themselves to the physicians are so closely connected with the social problems," she wrote in 1891, "that it is impossible to study one alone. The people are sick because of insufficient food and clothing and unsanitary surroundings, and these conditions exist because the people are poor. They are often poor because they have no work." Consequently, the dispensary often provided food, fuel, clothing, and rent, made loans, aided in securing work, and even helped some of its patients to emigrate west. For children Christmas trees and Thanksgiving dinners were the rule, and many young people were sent to the country in the summer for two-week outings.[72]

In Philadelphia four alumnae of the Woman's Medical College—Marie B. Werner, Ida Richardson, Marie K. Formad, and Calista V. Luther—founded another type of outpractice, "The Medical Aid Society for Self-Supporting Women," an evening dispensary located "in the central part of the city, so as to make it possible for those employed during the day to obtain advice and treatment." Most dispensaries of this type charged a nominal fee "to avoid the pauperizing effect" of outright charity.[73]

In Boston the Trinity Dispensary grew in 1885 out of the Girls Industrial Club of the Church of the Trinity, which had invited several of the city's women doctors to lecture on hygiene and advise on health problems. Before long Drs. Grace Wolcott and Lena V. Ingraham had expanded the staff to include six physicians, some of them specialists. Weekly lectures on dress and evening classes in calisthenics added diversity to the dispensary's program. Keeping evening hours proved particularly successful with all such clinics. "Then we reach," reported Dr. Ingraham, "a portion of the community that has scarcely been touched before."[74]

From 1891 to 1910 when the Evening Dispensary for Working Women and Girls in Baltimore closed, it remained yet another exemplary women's institution which practiced social medicine with compassionate determination. Founded by two graduates of Philadelphia, Kate Campbell Hurd-Mead and Alice Hall, the dispensary was a mutual social service organization between patient and physician, intending to give free care to the needy while affording supervised postgraduate training to young women doctors. Before long several prominent women physicians in Baltimore joined the staff, including Lilian Welsh and Mary Sherwood, while others, like Florence Sabin and Elizabeth Hurdon, a surgical protégé of Howard Kelly's at Johns Hopkins, donated their time.

The dispensary staff gave hundreds of lectures to women and girls on hygiene. It employed the first visiting nurse in Baltimore, and established the city's first distribution of clean milk to sick babies of the poor. It started the city's first public bath, made a special study of midwives and birth registration, and became the second institution in Baltimore to organize a social service department under a trained social worker. Finally, its careful study of deaths from tuberculosis for the years 1890 to 1900 helped to inspire the founding of the National Tuberculosis Association.[75]

And yet, despite the substantial and innovative contribution these female-run institutions made, both to the training of women physicians and to health care more generally, tough-minded professionals like Mary Putnam Jacobi never deceived themselves regarding their ultimate value. The small women's hospitals, concentrating as they did on obstetrics and gynecology, tended toward "specialism," she wrote, "which, though useful for the patients, is detrimental to the physicians who must find all their training in them." Equally unnerving to Jacobi was a gnawing fear that "isolated groups of women cannot maintain the same intellectual standards as are established and maintained by men."[76]

There is some evidence that Jacobi's worries may have been justified. When the locus of physician education shifted from the medical school to the hospital, the women's hospitals all experienced institutional crises of one sort or another in addition to the unwanted effects of de facto specialization. Gradually the complex technology and treatment that became the hallmark of modern medicine was concentrated within hospital walls. Indeed, a leading spokesman for scientific medicine regarded the hospital as so essential to the medical school curriculum that, in 1900, he declared in the *Journal of the American Medical Association* that "to a large extent, the hospital [with all its facilities] *is* the medical school."[77] Women's hospitals, if they were to serve their purpose as training institutions, needed to be responsive to the professional needs of those who sought to learn clinical medicine on their wards. But some of these institutions were slow to recognize the increasingly crucial role of the hospital in teaching young doctors, and fell behind in their willingness to provide up-to-date clinical experience to women students and interns.

In Philadelphia, for example, disagreements over giving students actual ward responsibilities arose between the Woman's Hospital's Board of Lady Managers, always jealous of the institution's reputation, and the faculty of the Woman's Medical College. The tension led the school in 1904 to sever its half-century old ties with the institution and build a new hospital, one more directly under the control of the teaching faculty.[78] The controversy temporarily hampered the quality of clinical education the school could offer.

In Boston ill-feeling over the kind and quality of clinical experience available mounted between attending staff and interns at the New England Hospital for Women and Children in the 1880s and 1890s. Evidence suggests that old-guard physicians under the leadership of Marie Zakrzewska remained insensitive to the professional needs of newly graduated interns. The younger women complained of being treated with disrespect and asked to be trusted with more direct responsibility for patient care. In several written communications in 1883 Zakrzewska repeatedly patronized her charges, declaring that "the main object of the NEH" was to give young women the chance to see women physicians and surgeons in action so "that thereby they may acquire courage and self-reliance, which can never be so completely gained by seeing *men* acting as physicians and surgeons."[79]

Zakrzewska did not respond adequately to the interns' demands, and although the crisis passed temporarily, tempers flared again in 1891. In that year Dr. Bertha Van Hoosen, fresh from the University of Michigan and an additional year of clinical experience at Kalamazoo State Hospital for the Insane, accepted an appointment as resident physician in Boston. But she resigned after several months' service. Van Hoosen's letter of resignation suggested numerous changes in the organization of responsibility throughout the hospital. Her recurring complaint was that the interns needed more clinical responsibilities. They rightly felt, she observed, that they were "losing ground," because "so many privileges that would be readily acceded to physicians elsewhere" were denied them at the NEH. They did not get what they needed the most—a chance to manage patients by themselves. After all, Van Hoosen reminded the directors, although discrimination still existed, positions for medical women had multiplied over the last years and many of the interns could go elsewhere. "Where there was one opportunity for women 20 years ago there are now twenty. Opportunities for observing the best medical work are now ample in every city. What women want now is opportunities for doing."[80]

Once again, Zakrzewska's response appears in retrospect unsympathetic and inadequate. Though she made vague reference to "important changes in the division of work" in the future, she again reminded her critics that "there is no position in life which does not have its annoyances" and that she expected better from "helpers, in one of the great historical reforms." Unwilling to engage in a productive exchange of views, she invoked the cause of women in medicine, expecting compliance from young women interns merely because they were women at a woman's institution.[81]

Contemporaries remembered Zakrzewska as "serious," "awe-inspiring," not particularly harsh or cruel, and by her female colleagues "very much beloved."[82] And yet the qualities of defiance and determination that helped her to accomplish so much in establishing the New England Hospital on a firm footing worked against her at the end of the century, when flexibility and openness to new medical ideas became imperative. Her reluctance to respond adequately to the changing needs of a new generation of women under her authority, more and more of whom were coming to the NEH from progressive coeducational institutions like Michigan, gradually made the New England Hospital less attractive to women clinically, especially when hospital opportunities opened up elsewhere.

There were others at the NEH who were prepared to acknowledge the problem more readily than Zakrzewska herself. In 1895, for example, Dr. Mary Hobart, who had worked on the attending staff for nine years, bluntly warned her colleagues to change their ways. "It is well known," she observed courageously at a physicians' meeting, "that the staff of the New England Hospital already has the reputation of being narrow and to repulse bright women who might otherwise be valuable as co-workers."[83]

But it was Alice Hamilton, trained at Michigan in the early

1890s, who best summed up the problems the hospital faced, and her message seemed sadly to confirm Mary Putnam Jacobi's worst fears: that separation, when it became isolation, could breed inferiority. Hamilton came to Boston in 1893 full of enthusiasm, but that excitement soon waned as she encountered outdated rules and inadequate opportunities for clinical experience. First, there was not enough work to do: "I have not enough to keep me busy," she wrote her sister. "I feel that I am simply losing a year which I cannot spare." But worse, she found the hospital "narrow, petty, squabbly, idiotic," because of its ancient rules and regulations. "We have an amount of etiquette or red tape that would overstock Bellevue. Most of [the rules] date things years back and were made for interns who were only prospective medical students, but they are still kept up and handed down to us graduates."

Hamilton's most scathing criticism, however, was reserved for the attending physicians themselves: "The visiting physicians," she wrote in disgust in 1893, are "bland and patronizing and so convinced that there is no hospital like the New England and no advantages like ours. They are narrow women *who escape discovering their own inferiority merely by avoiding their superiors.*"[84] Such women, Hamilton lamented, needed to take refuge in extreme authoritarianism. The result was that the sort of girl who succeeded at the New England Hospital was "the one who rides rough-shod over her subordinates and cringes to her superiors." Nor was Hamilton alone in her displeasure. During her internship at the NEH she became close with Rachelle Yarros, a graduate of the Woman's Medical College of Pennsylvania and a woman who eventually became professionally active working for Hull House in Chicago. Together they bemoaned their fate at the hospital, giving each other support and encouragement during the all-too-frequent clashes with their superiors.

Hamilton thought hard about the reasons for the New England's deficiencies. She concluded that its faults could not be blamed on "the fact that they are all women." Indeed, she had a basis for comparison, because she had spent time before coming to Boston at the Northwestern Hospital for Women and Children in Minneapolis, a similar all-women's institution founded in 1883 by a graduate of Philadelphia. The women at the NEH, she believed, were, in contrast to her mentors in Minneapolis, "narrow-women," women "who lived in a state of self-distrustful antagonism to all men doctors," and who "study gynecology and obstetrics and know absolutely nothing else." She regretted leaving an "excellent place" in Minneapolis, she wrote to her cousin, in order to come to an institution that she discovered to her disappointment was "living on the ashes of its former reputation." It rankled her that women physicians still had not enough good internships to choose from, and that a place like the NEH was thus not under enough pressure to change its ways. "It irritates me to think," she burst out, "that there is not a man medical graduate in the country who would accept so inferior a position as this; yet here we are, who know just as much as men students, obliged to accept places where we must divide with six the work that is only enough for two."[85] Hamilton was unable to tolerate the situation. In April 1894 she resigned from the hospital.

It would be a mistake to conclude either that the New England Hospital's difficulties were typical of all women's hospitals, or that all the women who interned there had an unhappy experience. There were those who believed, along with Josephine Baker, that the institution "fitted my needs admirably. It was staffed entirely by women of first-rate calibre. . . . It provided a wide range of medical, surgical and obstetrical work."[86]

Many of the New England's problems had to do with the personality of its founder, Marie Zakrzewska, and the women she gathered around her. The product of an earlier struggle, Zakrzewska advocated a brand of feminism that could potentially divide the loyalties of women seeking to be both women physicians and members of a larger, integrated professional network. While successfully preserving the female character of her institution in the crucial years, her inflexibility rendered her ideas antiquated by the 1890s, and jeopardized the hospital's reputation both among the male profession and among younger women physicians.

The hospital's aura of feminist militancy annoyed some more than others. Alice Hamilton never adjusted to it. Margaret Noyes, on the other hand, took it in stride. Fifty years later, while reminiscing about Dr. Mary Smith, the woman superior Hamilton disliked so intensely, and her partner, Dr. Emma B. Culbertson, Noyes could still describe the pair's idiosyncrasies with good-natured humour:

> I was married in 1916. . . . They were both horrified. They really hated men. Not just as feminists, but just because men were men. They lost no opportunity to expound on the subject. . . . They drove about in a Stanley Steamer and insisted on my going with them at times, I did not enjoy it much as they quarrelled so much. They lived together. . . . In the O.R. they were always having their altercations

too. . . . But with it all I liked them and was grateful to them as they
really helped me get started.

Similarly, Alice Bigelow was ready to forgive Smith her idiosyncrasies. She knew that Smith belonged to "the generation of women
doctors who had to fight for every bit of education" and that the
"long battle" had made her a "trifle belligerent." "If the layout of
instruments in the operating room was not perfect," Bigelow recalled, "the sharp rebukes to nurses and interns was something to
remember." Still, she wrote, Smith had a "heart of gold."[87]
  It would be helpful to know more about how other women's
hospitals faced such dilemmas, but the information is too fragmen-
tary. The New York Infirmary remained a small but respectable
woman's institution through the first half of the twentieth century,
in part because of the devotion of several wealthy female trustees.
It did not develop the reputation for abrasiveness that eventually
warned some women physicians away from Boston. Yet the fate of
women's hospitals elsewhere suggests that Zakrzewska's fear that
too much flexibility could lead to a loss of identity was real.
Neither the Woman's and Children's Hospital in San Francisco,
nor the Northwestern in Minneapolis, for example, remained exclusively female-run institutions for very long into the twentieth
century. San Francisco Children's eventually affiliated with the
University of California, and by 1900, though it still sought only
women interns, there were a number of male physicians on the
attending staff.[88]
  In Minneapolis, Northwestern Hospital eventually merged with
Abbott Hospital, a private institution founded by a male physician,
and became connected with the University of Minnesota. Both
these institutions, and many others like them, weathered the transition from nineteenth- to twentieth-century medicine with foresight
and skill. But in the process their exclusively feminine character first
diminished and then disappeared. No doubt Zakrzewska dreaded
such a fate for the New England, and her fears likely nurtured the
atmosphere of "distrustful antagonism to all men doctors" which so
disgusted Alice Hamilton in the 1890s. But Hamilton represented
the attitudes of a new generation of women physicians, one which
appeared more relaxed in a coeducational professional world, in
part because their own experience with discrimination was more
subtle. Yet this generation, too, cared a great deal about the future
of women in medicine, and it would be incorrect to conclude that
they rejected entirely the benefits of female medical networks. On

the contrary, many younger women would feel more acutely torn than their elders were between separatism and assimilation, and the psychological confusion that accompanied such tension could at times be painful, even confusing.

We must remember that the marginality of women physicians like Zakrzewska was never entirely self-imposed. The pioneer generation had fought tirelessly for entry into male professional societies and for the right to consult with male physicians. But such access came neither easily nor all at once. In some regions, including much of the Midwest, women gained admission to local and state societies quietly and without incident. In other places, such as Massachusetts, Philadelphia, San Francisco, and Washington, D.C., the struggle was bitter and protracted. The Massachusetts Medical Society, for example, one of the most stubborn, first considered the idea of admitting women in 1850 and again in the 1870s. However, it was not until 1884 that the friends of women physicians finally succeeded in winning their goal. Even the American Medical Association preceded Massachusetts, by agreeing in 1876 to seat Dr. Sarah Hackett Stevenson, a female delegate from Chicago—although the acceptance of women in the AMA remained only de facto, and was not formalized until 1915.

Women physicians exposed the hyprocisy of male objections at every opportunity—especially complaints that women were not adequately trained. Wrote the dean of the Woman's Medical College of Pennsylvania in a commencement address in 1879, "An objection sometimes urged by our medical brethren to the admission of women into their organizations is that . . . women like men must show themselves qualified before expecting recognition. But is qualification the invariable standard for men? I think not. Occasionally, at least, it is not competence but the diploma which is made the open sesame of doors still closed to us."[89]

Such difficulties were never easy to overcome. For example, Harriet Belcher wrote of assisting with four other women physicians at a delicate operation to remove several ovarian tumors early in her career. Waiting to see if the patient would recover was "a mental and physical strain," and Belcher confessed to "utter thankfulness" when she "saw her coming through safely." The patient's recovery "meant to us not only a life in which we had a strong personal interest, but success or failure was so much more to us professionally that it would have been to men." In addition to the burden of having to prove themselves continuously, women often disliked being outnumbered even after they gained entrance into the male societies. Feelings of isolation may account for their low professional participation, even where the opportunity to do so was available.[90] In a report published in the *Alumnae Transactions* of the Woman's Medical College of Pennsylvania in 1900, Ida C. Barnes, Class of 1890, wrote from Topeka, Kansas, of women's cordial acceptance by the medical societies in the state: "Their membership in the societies is as eagerly sought as that of their brother practitioners," she reported, and they were often invited to give papers and to hold office. Indeed, she concluded, "Women physicians in the West, at least, could have more positions in the medical societies if they would attend more regularly, and give close attention to the reading of papers and to the business of the session."[91]

Similarly, the editor of the *Colorado Medical Journal* chided women physicians in his state for their poor participation in medical society activities. Conceding that the women were "truly . . . doing nobly by their profession," he nevertheless complained that they gave too much attention to their own organization, the Denver Clinical Society. "That society," he argued, "is properly classed with the special and restricted societies, membership in which should supplement and not supplant that in the general societies."[92]

Ironically it was in the cities in which women had already gained admission to the larger medical associations that local women's medical societies were most likely to appear. These societies apparently evolved to strengthen ties between women professionals where networks of female physicians already existed. Sometimes, as was the case in San Francisco, Boston, Minneapolis, Washington, D.C., and Philadelphia, charter members had already cooperated in founding a hospital or a dispensary. Stressing primarily the importance of female professional companionship, these groups served as clearing houses for the exchange of scientific information, and occasionally as pressure groups for social action. Founders often explained the decision to organize, not by pointing to overt discrimination, but by citing the more subtle effects of their minority status. Mary Stark, for example, a charter member of the Practitioners Society of Rochester, founded in 1887, explained:

> We are members of a learned profession of which the opposite sex are as sands of the sea compared with us in number. . . . The medical societies are under their control; we have been admitted to these after the persistent knocking of the pioneer women of the profession, but we are not at home there as in our own circles. We need

the general societies to broaden our minds and give us lines of thought but our work and growth should be free where we are without embarrassment or restraint.[93]

The situation of women doctors in Iowa was not very different from those in Rochester. In 1901 there were over seventy women physicians.[94] Iowa's male practitioners were praised in the pages of the *Women's Medical Journal* for their justice, courtesy, and liberality toward women colleagues. Not only were women admitted to all medical societies, but they were also accepted in official positions of all kinds and sent as delegates from local to state and from state to national conventions. In 1893, for example, Iowa was represented in the Pan-American Medical Congress by a woman. The state's hospitals for the insane were among the first in the country to include women on the staff, and the majority of general hospitals had one or more women on either the active or consulting staff by the turn of the century. The *Iowa State Medical Reporter* and the *Iowa Medical Journal* had female assistant editors. Finally, the medical, pharmacy, and dental schools in the state were all coeducational.

But a woman's medical society fulfilled a need in the lives of women doctors that even this liberal atmosphere of acceptance could not totally satisfy, and consequently the State Society of Iowa Medical Women was founded in 1898. As Dr. Azuba King explained in her 1901 Presidential Address to the group: "Our professional brothers long ago recognized the truth: In union there is strength . . . let us profit by their example. The woman physician—alone either in city or town has an isolated professional life, the brother practitioner may be courteous, and ethical—she is alone nevertheless."[95]

Those women who did not have families longed for the intimacy that shared goals and shared experience could provide. Others craved social, professional, and psychological support. The women's medical societies gave this sought-after fellowship, while simultaneously training their members in the unwritten "rules" of professionalism. Often, for example, the women's society proposed its members as officers in the regular state society. In 1901 two of their candidates were elected without fanfare to high offices in the Iowa State Medical Society. Local societies also coached younger and timid or reserved women in self-confidence before they went on to grapple with the forbidding world of male colleagues.

For example, though the Iowa Women's Medical Society especially urged its members to submit papers to the regular state medical meetings, it also gave them the chance to deliver their remarks before an all-woman audience first. Here, at the intimate meetings of the women's society, the "less experienced" could "with friendly criticism," cultivate their powers of expression, stimulate growth in their professional life, and develop their capabilities. In 1902 the society's president, Jennie McGowen, explained that the Iowa Women's Society was

> a council chamber where the younger women, embryo practitioners fresh from graduation may freely ask questions and receive advice and help, where ethical questions may be discussed and difficulties of all kinds considered. . . . There must be no haughty self-isolation, no false pride, no patronizing toleration. Each must give the best that is in her for the good of all, and there must be no spirit of clique or exclusiveness. But standing shoulder to shoulder, and holding out hands of sympathy and helpfulness and good cheer to all new comers, the dignity of this aim, and the earnestness with which it is pursued, cannot fail to guarantee to Iowa medical women the sensible widening of their sphere of influence.[96]

One must marvel at this rhetoric of mutual support, with its wholesale rejection of competitive values, for it stands in firm contrast to the harsher ethos of professionalism developing simultaneously in the medical world at large. The women's medical societies founded in these years strove toward cooperation rather than competition, for mutual support and fellowship rather than aggressive individualism. Perhaps no other single fact testifies more eloquently to the psychological importance of separate female organizations, to the persistence of both overt and more subtle forms of discrimination, or to the continued ambivalence of women physicians about their relationship to the male medical world.

The professional work of women physicians, as it developed in the late nineteenth and early twentieth centuries, generally drew them toward "feminine" areas of endeavor—public health and the teaching of social hygiene, work with adolescent girls in schools, gynecology, pediatrics, obstetrics. This was true because cultural and professional sanctions concerning proper behavior for a woman doctor converged with women physicians' sincere desire to make a contribution to the profession that was uniquely their own. With professional lines hardening at the end of the nineteenth century, women continued to be tracked into the less glamorous, lower-paying medical roles. Yet these roles also seemed to be the very positions that put them in touch with what they cared about most in medicine: female health, family life, and the scientific management of child growth. These concerns linked them most closely with the private sphere. Like Mary Putnam Jacobi and Elizabeth Blackwell before them, women physicians continued to criticise the narrow professionalism and crass materialism that they often found characteristic of their male colleagues, offering instead the compassionate dedication to serving others that they themselves considered woman's particular strength. Ida Reel (WMCP, 1882) for example, continually deplored "mercenary physicians . . . those who are only in the profession for the money they can get" and wore her modest means like a badge of honor. "I haven't made much money," she wrote her fellow alumnae at the Woman's Medical College in Philadelphia, "but there is a satisfaction in the gratitude of patients—a satisfaction which money couldn't buy." Similarly, Dr. Mary McKibben-Harper, in a retrospective article on Anna Broomall, found it particularly noteworthy that Broomall kept her fees to the minimum on principle. "She had great fear," remarked Harper admiringly, "lest our profession became commercialized."[97]

Thus, no matter how successful individual and exceptional women physicians would be in integrating themselves into the male professional world in the late nineteenth and early twentieth centuries, as a group women physicians remained poised around the edges of that world, making contributions that were socially useful but otherwise devoid of the flashy éclat which measured success by male professional standards. Marginal to their profession, perhaps, they still made substantial contributions to the community. Beula Sundell, a graduate of the Woman's Medical College of Pennsylvania in 1930, might well have spoken for several earlier generations of medical women when she answered, with a combination of defensiveness, apology, and pride, a questionnaire about her career sent out by her alma mater:

> This information on the first three pages would not make a very glamorous write-up for a Who's Who. However, the mother whose child has a convulsion at midnight does not care about degrees, etc. She wants a doctor who will *come* to see her babe, and make him well. Most of my activity is built around healing the sick."[98]

Science, Morality, and Women Doctors: Mary Putnam Jacobi and Elizabeth Blackwell as Representative Types

The professional career of Dr. Elizabeth Blackwell was distinguished by intense devotion to the interests of the medical education of women . . . and in works of charity. . . . The crowning feature of that life was the demonstration of the value of woman's influence upon men . . . and the wisdom of the fiat of the Council of Creation, "It is not good that the man should be alone."

Dr. Steven Smith, 1911

Such one-sidedness as Elizabeth Blackwell exhibited in some things has always appeared to me to amount almost to a virtue. She was always occupied, her thoughts and feelings ran in the direction of usefulness to the great many. . . . It was not for her . . . to find new roads in science. . . . Hers was its application.

Dr. Abraham Jacobi, 1911

One of the most important lessons I learned as a student . . . was unconsciously taught by Dr. Jacobi. . . . From hearing her . . . I formed a standard of value for testing medical discussion that it has never been necessary to raise. . . . With rare power of keen analysis, and a thorough knowledge born of wide acquaintance with medical literature, she was able to select surely and swiftly what was of value, to reject positively and promptly the false and worthless. In all my experience in medical meetings since then I have known but two other persons who possessed the same quick critical judgment . . . and these were both men. . . . She was not only a woman eminent among women, but she was a physician eminent among physicians.

Dr. Lilian Welsh, 1907

On Christmas Day, 1888, Dr. Mary Putnam Jacobi sat at her desk to write a long, frank, and remarkably revealing letter to Elizabeth Blackwell. Although Blackwell was several years her senior, both women belonged to the pioneer generation of women physicians. Yet the two women never knew each other well. In 1869, shortly after Blackwell established the Woman's Medical College of the

New York Infirmary, she left America and took up permanent residence in England, where she believed she could accomplish more in behalf of women physicians. She consigned the school to the competent administration of her sister Emily and an able faculty, which included Jacobi, a handful of recent graduates, and a few young, sympathetic male physicians.

Both women had fine reputations and were recognized leaders among the rapidly expanding ranks of women physicians. But though they admired each other deeply, it is also clear that their cordiality and mutual respect was enhanced rather than hampered by the geographical distance between them. No two temperaments differed more profoundly. Jacobi had not a trace of sentimentality about her. Her quick and penetrating intellect cut to the core of things with a rapidity which left lesser minds bewildered. No one valued rational thinking more highly; no one remained more frustrated with mushy generalities that could not be grounded in empirical investigation and factual analysis. Jacobi chose medicine out of a love for scientific rationalism. She adored chemistry and pursued medical study with the enthusiasm of a mind comfortably at home with its rigors.

Blackwell, in contrast, was nothing if not sentimental. She entered medicine with a perfectionist conception of morality and her own role in the moral universe. Believing that the realm of medicine and health must be a fundamental area of concern for the reformer, she wrote in 1889, "The progress and welfare of society is more intimately bound up with the prevailing tone and influence of the medical profession than with the status of any other class of men."[1] Indeed, Victor Robinson, a younger physician who knew and admired her, called her a "Swedenborgian-theosophical-theological-Christian-metaphysician, instead of just an unadulterated scientist."[2]

To the amused Robinson, such idiosyncrasies could be tolerated in great pioneers. But, as Jacobi formulated her thoughts on that Christmas morning in 1888, she realized that Blackwell's thinking raised her "antagonistic hairs" particularly because the woman was a pioneer. Sentimentality hurt the cause. Blackwell's preoccupation with the abstract struggle to make a place for women in medicine, Jacobi complained, never allowed her to descend from her vision "into the sphere of practical life within which, that vision if anywhere must be realized. You left that for others to do." What rankled Jacobi most was Blackwell's dominant "mental habit,—principle,—or method, . . . the well known Transcendental method of arriving at conclusions by the force of meditative insight, and then refusing to submit these to tests of verification. "Indeed," Jacobi continued upon further reflection,

> it is the latter omission I really object to: the Transcendental vision probably always comes first in all large generalizations. . . . But whether these are to stand as effective truths or not depends upon how far they can bear the tests of close conflicts with facts, with innumerable details: how they can sustain the onslaught of argument and criticism. Your sex, your age, and your cast of mind render all this difficult. . . . You resemble your sister Anna sufficiently to prefer to remain within the sphere of large, often half mystical assertion.

What mystified and frustrated Jacobi was Blackwell's inattention to clinical medicine. "You have always disliked, ignored and neglected medicine!" she wrote, and the "one real occasion where from your position you should have shown me much, yet failed to show me anything, was when I began to study medicine under your direction in New York." Jacobi could sympathize with the "immense" obstacles in the way of Blackwell's reading and being taught medicine at midcentury, but she confessed she had always suspected that her friend's "greatest real difficulty" was "your own intense indifference to the work."[3]

The differences between the two women were partly temperamental. But in the last third of the nineteenth century, they also reflected tensions within the medical profession created by the new discoveries in immunology and bacteriology. Women physicians, as they came to see themselves more and more as active participants in a changing profession, were not immune to the ethical and scientific debates that took place within its ranks. One of the most important was the question of the role of the physician in specific areas of reform—a debate intensified by the dramatic discoveries concerning the origin of disease which were made in the laboratory in the 1880s and 1890s. Like many male physicians, Jacobi and Blackwell disagreed sharply over the scientific meaning and ethical implications of bacteriology. Intertwined with the different responses to what became a medical issue of considerable consequence, however, were their divergent views on the role of the woman physician. Their lives and their opinions merit further exploration because each of them represents a pole in a wide spectrum delineating the various responses of female medical professionals to these crucial questions. Women physicians, by nature of their being physicians, ranged themselves on different sides of the controversies shared by their medical brethren. By virtue of their being women, they also faced dilemmas from which their male colleagues were spared. Most of these centered on the fact of their womanhood and its meaning with regard to their larger connection with the profession. But even here their solutions, as we shall see when we examine Jacobi and Blackwell's views more closely, could dissent from one another in significant ways.

One of the most bewildering controversies to twentieth-century observers remains the reluctance of many nineteenth-century physicians and public-health advocates—known as sanitarians—to accept the discoveries of the bacteriologists. How could such men and women persist in speaking of "effluvia," "miasma," and "filth" when the precise experimentation of Pasteur, Koch, and their followers had, by reproducing various diseases in the laboratory and indentifying various "germs," ushered in the concept of "specific etiology?"

To make sense of the sanitarians' objections we must remember that bacteriological concepts called into question an older and deeply internalized view of disease that was holistic in its scope, moralistic in its implications, and fundamentally religious in its point of departure. In the minds of many sanitarians, Elizabeth Blackwell included, health was the natural order of things, a gift to be enjoyed by people if they governed their lives wisely and well. Disease was neither the abitrary visitation of an Angry God nor the quixotic outcome of Blind Fate, instead it was the inevitable result of one's violation of the laws of Nature made manifest by a benevolent Deity. Disease, so often equated in their cosmology with sin, was permitted by God to exist, but conscience and revelation on the one hand and reason and science on the other were the tools provided by Him for man to combat these evils. Medicine's task was to reveal and teach the laws by which people could ensure the proper balance between environment and individual behavior. Chapter 2 demonstrated the role of women and the health-reform movement in popularizing such attitudes.

From a modern perspective, nineteenth-century sanitarians and health reformers may have been scientifically naive, but their ideas exhibited an internal consistency which linked together a perfectionist world view with the more personal concerns of men and women interested in active and dramatic social reform. They reasoned that, since disease was always accompanied by ugliness, want, and pollution, health could be achieved by replacing these modern blights with the pure food, air, water, and the pleasant surroundings enjoyed in the preindustrial age.[4]

Louis Pasteur's discovery of germs in the laborabory created a tension between environmentalism and the concept of specific etiology which agitated the medical community at the end of the nineteenth century both in America and abroad. To be sure, the controversy represented different points of view on a continuum rather than a conflict between two opposing camps. As early as the 1840s and 1850s individual physicians spoke of "germs" and used the term to identify a cause of disease that defied mere cleanliness and purity. Some even suggested that conscience and clean living were not always enough to keep people well.[5] Enlightened Americans, like Lemuel Shattuck or Dr. Henry Ingersoll Bowditch, for example, carefully balanced traditional sanitation theory, with its emphasis on filth, against new concepts pointing to a specific microbial invader. Nevertheless, the social implications of the two poles of thought can be usefully contrasted. Blackwell, perhaps because her scientific opinions exhibited none of the subtlety of contemporaries like Shattuck, Bowditch, or Mary Putnam Jacobi, stands as an appropriate representative of an older, more conservative tradition, still unmoved by the startling new discoveries of laboratory experimentation.

One clue to Blackwell's thinking lies in the fact that her interest in moral reform antedated her attraction to medicine. In part this was due to her remarkable family background. The children of the abolitionist Samuel Blackwell immersed themselves in the traditions of Christian perfectionism and reformist activity. Elizabeth's brothers, Henry and Samuel, supported antislavery and women's rights: the former married the feminist Lucy Stone and the latter married Antoinette Brown, the first formally ordained woman minister in the United States. Sister Emily also became a physician, and another, Anna, a poet and translator. Several family members dabbled in spiritualism. Blackwell's approach to medical issues confidently bore the stamp of her family's progressive tendencies.

The idea of studying medicine did not come easily to Blackwell, for she admitted in her autobiography that as a young adult she "hated everything connected with the body" and "the very thought of dwelling on . . . its various physical ailments filled me with disgust." Yet other circumstances pushed her toward her life's work. One was her burning desire for engrossing, ennobling activity. When she finally decided to become a physician, Elizabeth could hardly "put the idea . . . away." She knew even then that the term "female physician" referred primarily at that time to abortionists, the most notorious of whom was New York's Madame Restell. Such misuse of female power directly offended her growing mystical fascination with what she later termed "the spiritual power of maternity." The Madame Restells of the world represented "the gross perversion and destruction" of womanhood and "utter degradation of what might and should become a noble position for women." With determination she concluded to do what she could to " 'redeem the hells' . . . especially the one form of hell thus forced upon my notice."[6]

Blackwell seems to have consciously chosen a life that would protect her from marriage and intimacy with men. Her autobiography reveals that her choice of career came in part from fear of her susceptibility to romantic longings. Although she was constantly "falling in love" she shrank from the implications of those feelings, "repelled" by the idea of intimacy and a "life association." Soon after seizing upon the idea of medical practice, she confided to her journal:

> I felt more determined than ever to become a physician, and thus place a strong barrier between me and all ordinary marriage. I must have something to engross my thoughts, some object in life which will fill this vacuum and prevent this sad wearing away of the heart.[7]

Like Cordelia Greene, and many other women physicians of her generation and the next, Blackwell often used a traditionally religious vocabulary to articulate these goals. She turned for aid "to that Friend with whom I am beginning to hold true communion," and shortly after she began preparing for her future course her fears and doubts were dispelled by a mystical experience which left her confident that her individual work was divinely inspired and "in accordance with the great providential ordering of our race's progress."[8] This conversion of religious impulses into paths of professional activity was characteristic of many sanitarians during the antebellum period, both in America and in England.[9]

Similar themes pervaded Blackwell's writings as she formulated her two major concerns, the role of the physician in society and the place of women in the profession. Because her approach to disease was holistic, she argued that the physician had more to do than merely cure. She constantly spoke of the union of the spiritual and the physical, warning her students frequently against the dangers of materialism. "True science," she wrote, "supports the noblest intuitions of humanity, and its tendency is to furnish proof suited to our age of these intuitions." When "the recognition of the higher facts of consciousness is obscured, and the physician is unable to perceive life more real than the narrow limits of sensation," she warned, the loss to practical medicine was "immense."[10]

The bacteriologists obscured "the higher facts of consciousness," according to Blackwell, because bacteriology *appeared* to develop at the expense of sanitation, hygiene, preventive medicine, and most important, morality itself. By equating disease with a specific microbial invader, laboratory scientists seemed to be challenging the older view of health as equilibrium and threatening the work of those reformers who supported massive sanitary measures to remove the filth, want, and pollution that they believed caused disease. The traditional art of medicine, whose monistic pathologies bid the physician treat only after a careful balance of emotional, environmental, and physio-psychological factors, was rendered obsolete. Not laboratory experimentation, dissented Blackwell, but "pure air, cleanliness, and decent house-room secured to all . . . form the true prophylaxis of small-pox."[11] "The arbitrary distinction," she continued elsewhere, "between the physician of the body and the physician of the soul . . . tends to disappear as science advances."[12]

Blackwell continued to explore these themes when she turned her attention to the role of women in the profession. In 1889 she wrote that the sense of right and wrong must constantly govern medical research and practice, "the Moral must guide the Intellectual, or there is no halting-place in the rapid incline to error." Because she shared with many feminists the belief that women innately exhibited a higher moral sense than did men, she saw the role of medical women as integral to the proper and healthy progress of the profession as a whole. Indeed, a "distinguishing characteristic" of the nineteenth century, she argued, was the "increasing devotion of women to the relief of social suffering" through the "spiritual power of maternity." By this she meant "the subordination of self to the welfare of others; the recognition of the claim which helplessness and ignorance make upon the stronger and more intelligent; the joy of creation and bestowal of life; the pity and sympathy which tend to make every women the born foe of cruelty and injustice." Women were accomplishing great deeds. Such "spiritual mothers of the race," she judged "often more truly incarnations of the grand maternal life, than those who are technically mothers in the lower physical sense."

Women physicians, she argued, must monitor medical progress so that it did not violate moral truth. "Whatever revolts our moral sense as earnest women," she reminded her students, "is not in accordance with steady progress" and "cannot be permanently true." It was through the "moral, guiding the intellectual" that the "beneficial influence of women in any new sphere of activity" would be felt.

Bacteriology and its penchant for vaccination offended Blackwell because its concept of specific etiology undermined her sense of the moral order. A concomitant of modern laboratory science—animal experimentation—represented something much worse: the triumph of the intellect over morality. Blackwell probably opposed vaccination primarily because early in her practice she lost a young child whom she had vaccinated against small pox. Vivisection, however, represented to her an attempt to do good by evil means. Animal experimentation, she felt, hardened the heart, blunted the moral sense and injured the "intelligent sympathy with suffering" which was the mark of a good physician. Ultimately it led to the dangerous habit of treating the poor and helpless with indifference by regarding them merely as "clinical material."[13] Blackwell regretted this tendency particularly among younger physicians, and she felt it the responsibility of women doctors to discourage such inhumane practices. In 1891 she addressed a letter of protest to the Alumnae Association of the Woman's Medical College of the New York Infirmary in which she opposed their endowment of a new experimental laboratory. She reminded her female colleagues of their "duty" as potential mothers to oppose the cruelty and narrow materialism of which, to her mind, the new laboratory was symbolic.

Blackwell even connected the corruption of the moral sense resulting from "unrestrained experiment on the lower animals" to the increase in gynecological surgery at the end of the century. To her, ovariotomy represented "mutilation" and was especially heinous because it rendered women incapable of having children. Again she looked to women physicians to remind the profession that "moral error may engender intellectual error" and talked often of returning to the United States to rally women's attention on these issues.[14]

Fascinated and energized by recent events in laboratory medicine, Mary Putnam Jacobi could muster little enthusiasm for Blackwell's views. In her private life she too confronted the moral dilemmas of the reformer, and she enthusiastically supported numerous meliorist efforts, including the Consumer's League, woman's suffrage, and the reform of primary education in the direction of manual training and physical culture. But though she understood that the pursuit of truth could never be divorced totally from moral life, she approached the acquisition of medical knowledge as something quite independent of morality. Believing in science with an earnestness that was almost extreme, she nevertheless remained uncomfortable with Blackwell's traditional religious vocabulary, and she viewed scientific research as an absolute good because it added to the fund of human knowledge.

As a young medical student Jacobi had written her mother that her vision of Heaven was "simply the Region of Pure Thought" emancipated from "the overwhelming dominion of personal emotion and instinct." Her desire to pursue a scientific career developed early, and she hesitated only when deciding whether to concentrate on medical practice or laboratory research. The oldest daughter of the publisher George Palmer Putnam, Jacobi, like Blackwell, received considerable support from her family. Although the Putnams were not active reformers, they were nevertheless New Englanders who remained sympathetic to many of the progressive causes of the day. Mary's Aunt Elizabeth Peabody, for example, kept her in touch with every new social "ism." Yet Mary· remained too hardheaded and practical to identify herself with trends and fads. She once wrote to her mother, "I detest vulgarity, pretention, . . . inanity, twaddle, insipidity and pretention in velvet. I will have none of either. No homeopaths, no spiritualists, few "female" orators . . ."[15]

The Putnams were not pleased with their daughter's choice of career, but their disappointment did not hinder their providing emotional and material support. Jacobi's father considered medical science to be a "repulsive pursuit" but nevertheless took great pride in Mary's success. He begged only that she shun the company of "strong-minded women," saying, "Your self-will and independence . .·. are strong enough already," and asking that she preserve her "feminine character:" "Be a lady from the dotting of your i's to the color of your ribbons," he wrote to her in 1863, soon after she began her studies at the Woman's Medical College of Pennsylvania, "and if you must be a doctor and a philosopher, be an attractive and agreeable one."[16]

Jacobi appreciated and respected her parents' advice because she understood the significance of their liberalism with regard to her aspirations. "You have always been such a dear good father," she once wrote to George Putnam. Grateful to them particularly for the "liberty" they gave her to make her own decisions and correct her own mistakes, Jacobi felt that she could not have succeeded without her parents's open-minded support."[17]

Their tolerance of her plans was indeed remarkable for Victorian parents. Jacobi was headstrong, and she spent long years stubbornly pursuing her goals—years that the oldest girl of an upper-middle-class New York family might have passed making more of a contribution to home life as daughter, sister, and eventually, a wife. After receiving a degree in 1863 from the New York College of Pharmacy, Jacobi attended the Woman's Medical College in Philadelphia and was graduated a year later, the only student in the history of the school to write her thesis in Latin. She spent the next several months studying clinical medicine with Marie Zakrzewska and Lucy Sewall at the New England Hospital for Women and Children. Yet, neither experience satisfied her thirst for formal medical training, and in 1866 she left the United States for France, where she hoped to be admitted to the École de Médicine in Paris. Looking back on this decision in 1871, she wrote to her mother, "I cannot do a thing half way. When I was in Boston, Lucy Sewall considered me stupid, because I could not do things without having studied them, and could not accept her methods without question. In Paris, I am considered one of the most successful students, because I have been able to 'go the whole horse.' Explain it as you may, I always find the whole of a thing easier to manage than the half."[18]

Jacobi's time in Paris testified to her persistence and determination. Although she immediately began attending hospital clinics, lectures, and laboratories, it took her two years of dogged perseverance to achieve her goal of admission to the École. Characteristically, she passed her examinations with high honors and won a bronze medal for her graduating thesis in 1871.

In Paris Jacobi pursued the most advanced medical science of her day. Soon after her arrival there she wrote enthusiastically to her mother, "I have a fair prospect here of becoming a thoroughly educated physician," adding that "unless I am, I certainly will never undertake to practice medicine." Her commitment to the laboratory made it easy to welcome the discoveries of the bacteriologists and seek to stay abreast of their findings. She perceived early that opportunities for medical study in America did not begin to compare with those abroad. In another letter to her mother she spoke of New York City's inadequacies:

> I have already sufficient terror of the demoralization imminent from the atmosphere of New York, with its very slack interest in medical science or progress, its deficient libraries, badly organized schools and hospitals, etc. I am doing my best to accumulate a sufficient fund of original force to make headway against these adverse influ-

ences, and to subordinate them to my purposes, instead of allowing
them to subordinate me.

Yet at the same time Jacobi shunned opportunities for practicing
medicine that would take her out of the mainstream, as inadequate
as it was. She would not even consider teaching at the Woman's
Medical College in Philadelphia, which she believed to be sincere
but deficient, and when offered the position of resident physician
at one of the women's colleges, she remarked that such isolation
from the medical world would be "suicidal."[19]
In 1871 Jacobi returned to New York to join the faculty of the
Woman's Medical College of the New York Infirmary as professor
of therapeutics and materia medica. She also set up private practice, feeling satisfied that "few young physicians could have a better opening." Family considerations and a sense of duty determined the subordination of chemistry—her first love—to private
practice. As she explained to her mother, "After all the sacrifices
you have made . . . I see more chance of satisfying you if I am a
practical physician than if, without fortune, I try to become a
scientific chemist."[20]
Plunging herself into the world of New York medicine, Jacobi
fulfilled her ambitions to become a first-rate physician and scientist. She was the first woman to be admitted to the New York
Academy of Medicine and later chaired their section on neurology.
She gained admission to numerous other medical societies as well
and sustained her interest in research by publishing nine books and
over 120 medical articles. The respect of her male colleagues was
never in doubt. One younger member of the Pathological Society,
for example, remembered her as a woman "whose knowledge of
pathology was so thorough, whose range of the literature was so
wide and whose criticism was so keen, fearless and just that in our
discussions, we felt it prudent to shun the field of speculation and
to walk strictly in the path of demonstrated fact."[21]
Perhaps Jacobi's successes in the male professional world were
due at least in part to her willingness to accept men as equals.
Certainly Jacobi did not share Blackwell's ambivalence toward romantic attachments to men, and her private correspondence never
reveals the suspicion of marriage characteristic of many accomplished women of her generation. Nevertheless, she sought in a
mate a rare thing in the nineteenth century—an intellectual and
spiritual companion who could fully support her commitment to
her work. Although she was capable of passion, she was prepared

to forgo marriage if she did not find such a man and broke two engagements before she joined the ranks of New York's professional medical elite. While still in Paris she had written on the subject of marriage to her mother:

> I have no particular desire to marry at any time; nevertheless, if at home, I should ever come across a physician, intelligent, refined, more enthusiastic for his science than me, . . . I think I would marry such a person if he asked me, and would leave me full liberty to exercise my profession.[22]

Fortunately, Jacobi did meet such a man. In 1873 she became the wife of Dr. Abraham Jacobi, a German-Jewish refugee from the revolutionary upheavals of 1848. Jacobi was already one of the most distinguished physicians in America and has often been called the father of modern pediatrics.[23] The couple shared common medical interests and collaborated occasionally. Although the marriage was occasionally tempestuous, it remained a relationship of equals, despite Jacobi's assuredly ironic remark to her students that "it is desirable that every woman remain as inferior to her own husband as may be feasible and convenient."[24]

Jacobi's personal and professional history made her understandably impatient with Blackwell's rigid theorizing, and glimpses of irritability appear in her comments concerning Blackwell's proposed trip to America. On Blackwell's antivivisectionism she remarked coolly, "Of course . . . you know . . . I should oppose you," adding with humor and a touch of wistful regret that a campaign among women physicians would be useless because "I am tolerably confident that I am the only woman in the United States who experiments on animals!"

As for the "problem" of gynecological surgery, Jacobi was less polite: "When you shudder at 'mutilation,' " she wrote,

> it seems to me you can never have handled a degenerated ovary or a suppurating Fallopian tube—or you would admit that the mutilation had been effected by disease,—possibly by the ignorance or neglect of a series of physicians, before the surgeon intervened. You always seem so much more impressed with the personalities,—sufficiently faulty,—of doctors, than with the terrific difficulties of the problems they have to face. . . . There has been much reprehensible malpractice. But I do not see that malpractice which may render a woman incapable of bearing children differs . . . from the malpractice which may result in the loss of a limb or of an eye. *There is not such special sanctity about the ovary!*

To Blackwell's suggestion that women physicians ought to avoid performing gynecological surgery she retorted, "And why should not women be delighted if they succeed in achieving a difficult and useful triumph in technical medicine," adding that she did not feel women physicians should be urged to strike out for independent views until they had "demonstrated an equality of achievement in the urgent practical problems,—*not of sociology but of medicine.*"[25] The chief task of women physicians, she believed, was not the fostering of morality ("sociology") but "the creation of a scientific spirit" among them.[26]

In the end, it was on the question of the role of women in medicine that their divergent attractions to the potentialities inherent in medical practice led Blackwell and Jacobi to differ most intensely. Blackwell's thought derived from the ideology of domesticity, which emphasized not the essential identity between men and women but their differences. Women should become physicians because they exhibited unique qualities which would allow them to make a distinct contribution to the profession.

In her writings Blackwell constantly underscored the singular capabilities of women as physicians, which led to a peculiar kind of female chauvinism. The purpose of teaching women medicine was not to convert them into "physicians rather inferior to men," but to occupy "positions which men cannot fully occupy," and exercise "an influence which men cannot wield at all." Those positions had mainly to do with women, children, and the family. Women physicians must bring science to bear on daily life. This could be done best as family physicians, obstetricians, public-health advocates, and teachers of preventive medicine and hygiene, because it was in these areas that women could excel. Other branches of medicine reeked to Blackwell of the tyranny of male authority unmitigated by the dictates of conscience. She cautioned her students against the "blind acceptance of what is called 'authority' in medicine," which she equated with the "male intellect." "It is not blind imitation of men, nor thoughtless acceptance of whatever may be taught by them that is required," she wrote. Women students, she regretted, were as yet too "accustomed to accept the government and instruction of men as final, and it hardly occurs to them to question it." They must be taught that "methods and conclusions formed by one-half of the race only, must necessarily require revision as the other half of humanity rises into conscious responsibility."[27]

In advocating this position Blackwell voluntarily set herself and women physicians apart from the mainstream of professional developments. Rather than assimilate women into the larger group, she preferred to give them special responsibilities in order to achieve what she believed was a higher social and moral purpose. Women physicians were to be "in" the profession, but not "of" it.

This stress on the primacy of the maternal qualities of sympathy and instinct troubled Jacobi because she objected to female-centered, moralistic, and separatist standards for women. Her concern for objective science and the centrality of intellectual endeavor remained fundamentally universalistic and assimilationist. For Jacobi the physician dwelt in two realms, the intellectual and the practical. Although she admitted that moral considerations occasionally entered into the equation, she hailed the liberation of science from the mystic and demonic influences of the past and believed that the physician should deal with rational concepts based on objective knowledge. Ideally his business was to "take conditions which science has abstracted for the purpose of thought and to recombine them for the purpose of life. In the absence of the physician there would be no one to do this." Thus, the physician was the link between theory and practice. Moral issues were often beside the point. The intrinsic difficulty in medicine, she wrote, was not moral, but remained "the great mass of facts which it is necessary to know" and "the variety of sciences which must be understood in order to interpret these facts."

Where Blackwell emphasized sympathy and compassion and identified such qualities with women, Jacobi spoke rarely of exclusively feminine contributions to medical practice. Having a sympathetic nature, she argued, did not necessarily make one a good physician. He or she must be interested primarily in the facts. In the end, she wrote, unless "the interest in the disease be not habitually greater than the interest in the patient," the patient would surely suffer. She saw women participating in the profession, not as a distinct entity unto themselves, but as separate individuals united with men by objective, demonstrable, and professional criteria in the search for truth. "Indeed," she cautioned her students in 1883, "you are liable to be so much and so frequently reminded that you are women physicians, that you are almost liable to forget that you are, first of all, physicians."[28]

Jacobi did not reject entirely the notion that women had special strengths, although it is apparent that she believed such characteristics were acquired rather than innate. She admitted, for example, that "it is impossible to deny that women are intrinsically more suitable than men to take charge of insane women," because of their "superior kindness and conscientiousness." She quarreled little with the common wisdom that "tact, acuteness, and sympathetic insight [were] natural to women." Indeed, while stressing the importance of first-rate training she graciously conceded that "the special capacities of women as a class for dealing with sick persons are so great, that in virtue of them alone hundreds have succeeded in medical practice, though most insufficiently endowed with intellectual or educational qualifications."[29]

Yet despite women's unique skills, Jacobi insisted that they be fully integrated into the profession. She deplored the tendency of women doctors "to nestle within a little circle of personal friends and to accept their dictum as the ultimate law of things." Their role must not be supplementary or distinctive; inevitably skilled women physicians should displace inferior men. There was nothing earth-shattering about women competing with men: "Since society is, numerically speaking, already supplied with quite enough doctors," she wrote, "the only way in which women physicians can possibly gain any footing is by displacing a certain number of men." In order to do so, of course, they needed to be either equal or superior, and this meant receiving a better medical education than had yet been possible.

While Blackwell urged women to specialize, Jacobi continuously cautioned women not to concentrate in obstetrics and gynecology, but to devote themselves to a "liberal study of the whole field." Treating women and children should be used only "as a stepping-stone to general medicine." If women "do not obtain a foothold" there, if they "content themselves with claiming this little corner," she warned, "they will never really gain a high place even there."[30]

Although Jacobi remained suspicious of separatism, she also conceded that the "opposition to women students and practitioners of medicine has been so bitter, so brutal . . . so multiple in its hypocrisy" that women did have common interests as an oppressed class. She repeatedly prescribed grit and hard work in the face of discrimination: "I have always advised you . . . to so saturate and permeate your consciousness with the feeling for medicine," she told the graduating class of the Woman's Medical College of the New York Infirmary in 1883, "that you would entirely forget that public opinion continued to assign you to a special, and on the whole, inferior" position. She even urged students to forget that they "have in any way braved public opinion." "Acclimate," she implored, "as quickly and as thoroughly as possible" to your "new place," and don't "keep dawdling on the threshhold to forever remind yourselves and everyone else that you have just come in." Medicine remained too demanding a profession for conscientious doctors to allow themselves to be concerned with problems of "social status." If you do not find the facts of medicine more interesting than any other facts," she cautioned, "you are not fit to be physicians."

Yet if Jacobi lost patience with those who "dawdled on the threshold," the "monopoly" which excluded "one half of the race [from] the advantages of education and the facilities of increased life which that confers" rankled even more. She was not naive; she knew such opposition could be removed only after "much effort, individual and collective, persistent, patient, far-sighted, indomitable." Thus she devoted considerable time and effort to examining the practical difficulties involved in assimilating women into the male professional world. For her the most obvious problem remained what she knew was "the most delicate:" "actually raising to an equality the class which hitherto has been really inferior."[31]

In acknowledging and working to overcome women's shortcomings Jacobi and Blackwell remained of one mind. Indeed, one suspects that, however substantial were their disagreements on theoretical points, practical issues of strategy continuously drew them together. Both women deplored women's inferior preparatory education, an education that rendered them deficient in intellectual initiative, dependent on authority, and apathetic—all qualities which Jacobi perceptively labeled characteristics of the subordination of "colonial life." In order to rectify such disadvantages, she wrote, medical women must combine as a class to remove the obstacles that have blocked their progress. Their first task was to create among themselves a "scientific spirit," by improving medical education for women and encouraging "free, self-sustained, self-reliant intellectual activity." Jacobi hoped that this "gradual progress in mental culture would improve "mental initiative" in women and hopefully render them equal to men "in every work that both undertake."[32]

Blackwell had no quarrel with these points. She agreed that the barriers to women's equal access to quality medical education must be removed as quickly as possible, and she understood that only thorough scientific training would promote women's success. Both women hoped that the unique opportunities offered by the Woman's Medical College of the New York Infirmary would begin to alleviate some of these difficulties. The two stood united as well in the battle to widen women's opportunities for clinical experience and professional association, and both, for different reasons, enthusiastically welcomed the advance of medical coeducation. But where Jacobi's brand of feminism strived to minimize the differences between men and women and to integrate female physicians into the profession as rapidly as possible, Blackwell adhered to the very end to a vision of the woman doctor's unique contribution. This was true at least in part because her concept of disease was linked to her notions of morality and her belief that authentic moral understanding depended on female intuition. Such assumptions allowed her to equate bacteriology with male science and its triumph with the victory of the male principle over the female. That such a victory would lead inevitably to the denigration of inuition and morality in medicine was deplorable enough, but the final and most egregious consequence would be that women would be deprived of their power, purpose, and unique advantage in the profession—and this at the very moment when civilized society was beginning at long last to afford them a role appropriate to their highest capacities.

Blackwell's suspicions of "ignorant male domination" caused her to worry that women physicians accepted male models uncritically. "The only disappointment which comes to me now, as I draw towards the close of a life full of joy and gratitude," she mused in 1889, "is the surprise with which I recognize that our women physicians do not all and always see the glorious moral mission, which as women physicians they are called on to fulfill. It is not by simply following the lead of male physicians, and imitating their practices, that any new and vitalizing force will be brought into the profession."[33]

Indeed, a central theme in the story of women in medicine has been the tension between "femininity," "feminism" and "morality," on the one hand; and "masculinity," "professionalism" and "science," on the other. In a society that continually emphasized woman's primary maternal role, the stepping out of prescribed avenues of endeavor inevitably involved for its participants some explanation of purpose. Did women have the right to pursue professional goals, usually considered masculine, with the same vigor as their male colleagues and for similar reasons of self-interest and personal fulfillment? Was the goal of equality a legitimate one for women, or need they contribute as well to some higher female mission? What obligations did women professionals have to other women, or to "female values" in general? Must women emulate the professionalism of men, or seek to temper dominant male values by asserting their uniquely feminine characteristics? Women physicians were the first female professionals to grapple with such questions in the nineteenth century, and we shall see that their contemporary descendants in the profession still do. Nor have other women professionals in the twentieth century escaped such conflicts.

Jacobi and Blackwell, as first-generation women physicians, struggled to formulate answers that would ease women physicians' transition into the public and professional world. They shared similar goals as well as the common experience of being pioneers. In retrospect, their differences on the issue of women appear less pronounced than their broad areas of agreement. Each struggled defiantly in her own way with the humiliating effects of discrimination while holding fast to her objective of broadening the sphere of constructive activity for all women. Both saw the role of women in medicine idealistically, in the sense that they rejected its pursuit on the grounds of self-interest and emphasized instead the physician's larger social responsibilities. Jacobi, for example, once declared to her mother that "I look upon a rich physician with as much suspicion as a rich priest." In 1889 Blackwell wrote in the same vein, "I say emphatically that anyone who makes pecuniary gain the chief motive for entering upon a medical career is an unworthy student: he is not fit to become a doctor." Both women believed that the success of women in the profession had immense importance for the general success of women "in every other department of society."[34] On questions of strategy, too, they were usually of one mind: both hoped to widen the access of medical women to superior scientific training and to increase their professional and clinical opportunities. Nevertheless, the two women represented distinct approaches to the problem of women in medicine, and their differences were passed on to succeeding generations of professional women.

Although the fact of their womanhood was central to them both, we must not forget that Jacobi and Blackwell differed in the final analysis on medical issues as well—medical issues that went well beyond questions of gender. The achievements of the bacteriologists and the introduction of the concept of specific etiology unleashed in the late nineteenth century constructive forces that would dominate developments in scientific medicine for the next century. Yet the scientific medicine that would flourish after 1900 would do so increasingly at the expense of a holistic approach to the problem of illness. In many respects the worst fears of Eliza-

beth Blackwell concerning the neglect of psychological, environmental, social, and personal factors would come to pass. Doctors
would begin gradually to overlook treatment of the whole patient,
concentrating instead merely on the disease. The nurturing aspects
of nineteenth-century practice, with its heavy emphasis on intuition, sympathy, and art, would gradually give way to a medical
science becoming aggressively more "masculine." From the perspective of the nineteenth century, Jacobi's enthusiasm for laboratory science, her identification with the most revolutionary and
dramatic achievements of her profession were progressive and refreshing. Blackwell's ideas, heavy with religious overtones and
convoluted personal idiosyncrasies appeared to many to be reac-
tionary, uninformed, and annoyingly short-sighted. But the passage of time would gradually reveal the shocking limitations of
laboratory science. Once again researchers would begin to see the
value in studying factors in disease causation that cannot be measured, recorded, or recreated in an experimental setting.

To be sure, our contemporary interest in holistic approaches to
disease is something very different from the kind of position Elizabeth Blackwell occupied a century ago, and could have come
about, in fact, only after scientific reductionism became institution-
alized in medicine. However, in the midst of such an about-face,
Blackwell's vision seems almost prophetic as she mused to a friend
in 1853:

> I hope some day to arrange a hospital on truer principles than any
> that we have yet seen—but in thinking of this subject, I feel continu-
> ally the want of the *Science* of reform, which I believe is as yet
> unknown—I should want my hospital to be a center of Science, and
> of moral growth—in the scientific department I should be puzzled to
> know how far I ought to unite men and women—In the future I have
> no doubt that the two sexes, in varying proportions, will unite in
> every act of life—but now there are difficulties both in their separa-
> tion and their combination. . . . I should want also in my Hospital to
> cure my patients spiritually as well as physically, and what innumera-
> ble aids that would necessitate! I must have the church, the school,
> the workshop . . . to cure my patients—a whole society, in fact.[35]

Doctors and Patients: Gender and Medical Treatment in Nineteenth-Century America

"Medicine is indeed a science, but its practice is an art."
Professor Henry Hartshorne, M.D.,
Valedictory Address, 1872

Some of the most interesting research to emerge from the confluence of social history, women's history, and the history of medicine has been the investigation of the therapeutical relationship between physicians and their patients. Women accounted for a disproportionately large percentage of the nineteenth-century physician's clientele, and some historians have claimed that the medicine practiced in this century reflected a belief system that encouraged male doctors to oppress their female patients. Physicians' cultural prejudices, it has been argued, biased both treatment and the doctor-patient relationship. Physicians have been accused of administering harsh and painful therapies to punish and control females who were unresponsive to the dictates of "true womanhood." Clinicians' treatment allegedly attempted to reinforce childlike dependency in women, defined females as inherently weak and sickly, and discouraged excessive mental or physical exertion that might have turned a woman's attention to pursuits beyond her sphere.

Even those scholars who do not believe that male physicians were consciously hostile to women admit that the traditional patriarchal verities that informed nineteenth-century American culture guided doctors' treatment, leaving practitioners all too often oblivious to women patients' real needs. For example, physicians presumably tortured women pitilessly with heroic therapy. They harassed discontented housewives with "rest cures" and labeled them as hysterical when their behavior deviated only slightly from accepted norms. In addition, doctors warned women that higher education and the autonomy it could provide would cause the degeneration of their reproductive organs and the ultimate decline of civilization and the family.[1]

Even worse, doctors took the management of childbirth out of women's hands, drawing into professional auspices a process that had been hitherto defined as natural, and limiting women's right to handle—with other women—a traditionally female event. The result was the increased incidence of mechanical intervention, which actually endangered the lives of those who might otherwise have done better under the more cautious supervision of a midwife content to "wait on nature." Male doctors allegedly resorted to forceps out of impatience, thereby increasing the possibility of infection and tearing, while remaining stubbornly unresponsive to growing evidence that the obstetrician himself often spread puerperal fever because of improper sanitary precautions.[2]

While male physicians have been criticized, women doctors have been depicted as leaders in a struggle against the medical oppression of their sex. Indeed, a few scholars have argued that women physicians founded a "woman's medical movement" to combat erroneous and self-fulfilling concepts of female health that pictured women as innately weak and sickly. They have assumed, for example, that women were more sensitive to the natural birthing process, that they were less likely than men to hurry a patient through labor by resorting to forceps or drugs, and that they remained eager to minimize the risks of infection. Outraged at the ravages of puerperal fever, female practitioners seemed to some historians more willing to entertain the idea that the physician might be a source of infection.

Others have claimed that women physicians universally and consistently shunned heroic dosing and were much more reluctant than their male colleagues to use the physician's arsenal for questionable diagnoses. Women physicians are credited with the organized rebellion against the medical wisdom that held females to be prisoners of their reproductive systems, and are described as seeking to redefine female health and disease in a manner more commensurate with autonomy and independence. "The women doctors who began to appear on the American scene in the 1850s," wrote Ann Douglas in 1974, "saw women's diseases as a *result* of submission, and promoted independence from masculine domination, whether professional or sexual, as their cure for feminine ailments." Though such intentions might have led them to unscientific conclusions on occasion, women doctors could be excused, Douglas observed, because "these women bypassed science in large part because they had a goal quite distinct from its advancement: namely, the advancement of their sex."[3]

No historian of women physicians can fail to address the important issues—issues of crucial significance to our understanding of the relationship between nineteenth-century culture and nineteenth-century medicine—raised by these scholars. In addition, the motivations and purposes attributed to women physicians—especially the assumption that they were rebellious reformers rather than authentic medical professionals—invite further investigation, especially in the light of our comparison of the differing approaches of leading women physicians like Mary Putnam Jacobi and Elizabeth Blackwell to the problem of women in medicine. This chapter, then, will speak to two important questions that underlie the historical debate. The first is whether, how, and in what ways either medical theory or practice was used as an instrument of power over women. The second asks if women physicians were aware of the use of medicine for conservative cultural ends and, if so, how they coped with this perception without jeopardizing their role as medical professionals.

An answer to the first question about medical theory must begin with the acknowledgment that many, though not all, male physicians in the nineteenth century played a central and conservative role in the debate over woman's nature. Especially in the latter half of the century, when ministerial authority declined and increasing secularization enshrined science as a new touchstone for truth, physicians, who wrote much of the prescriptive literature regarding health, sexuality, and gender roles, gave voice to traditional definitions of femininity which limited women's social role to domesticity. We have already examined most of the objections to an expanded role for women raised by these doctors, for their suppositions were used as well to oppose the entrance of women into the medical profession. After the Civil War, the spiritual arguments developed in the antebellum period gave way to more rigid biological sanctions promoting an increasingly inflexible conception of woman's nature and capacity.

Indeed, the last third of the nineteenth century was an era of extreme somaticism in which physiological explanations for character, class, race, and gender traits became accepted as a matter of course. The optimistic environmentalism of the antebellum period gave way to the social Darwinism of Herbert Spencer and William Graham Sumner.[4] According to Spencer, the human body was a closed energy system in which any abnormal demands made on one part would inevitably deplete the healthy development of some other part. This theory was often applied to men, particularly when physicians discussed sexuality, but historians have discovered an even greater willingness among medical thinkers to appeal to variations of the closed energy theory when discussing women. It formed, for example, the basis for the contention of E. H. Clarke and his medical disciples that the mental strain of a college education would have dire effects on the natural development of women's reproductive organs.[5]

Historians have carefully investigated and exposed the medical and biological views regarding women that saw them both as prisoners and products of their reproductive systems. The modern reader may find nineteenth-century medical theories at best peculiar, but such theories could also be blatantly oppressive. To many physicians woman's diseases—indeed woman herself—were defined primarily by her uterus. It was, wrote one commentator in 1870 "as if the Almighty, in creating the female sex, had taken the uterus and built up a woman around it." Most female complaints, argued another, "will be found, on due investigation, to be in reality no disease at all, but merely the sympathetic reaction or the symptoms of one disease, namely a disease of the womb." As late as 1900 the president of the American Gynecological Society could state about female health:

> Many a young life is battered and forever crippled in the breakers of puberty; if it crosses these unharmed and is not dashed to pieces on the rock of childbirth, it may still ground on the ever-recurring shallow of menstruation, and lastly, upon the final bar of the menopause ere protection is found in the unruffled waters of the harbor beyond the reach of sexual storms.[6]

There was nothing particularly novel about the idea that woman's capacity was limited by and connected to her reproductive organs. Indeed, the theory was as old as antiquity, and it was the Greeks who coined the term "hysteria," meaning "wandering womb." But in the latter half of the nineteenth century, the social need to muster indisputable justification for keeping women in the home became particularly urgent, and historians have rightly seen a connection between social needs and doctors' medical theories, even if a few scholars have tended to overstate the case.[7]

What caused this growing tension and social anxiety in the latter half of the nineteenth century? The ideology of separate spheres had provided a measure of emotional sustenance to men and women who needed to come to terms with change. On the simplest level it explained and justified visible changes in individual's lives, offering to them a social explanation for economic alterations which threatened traditional assumptions about how they were supposed to behave. Industrialization separated home and work. Just as it was characterized by differentiation and specialization, so, too, the identification of home and work with contrasting women's and men's spheres linked changes taking place in the economic realm with more specialized conceptions of gender roles and called it progress. Herbert Spencer himself believed the divergence of male and female roles to be the inevitable result of higher civilization.

But as we have seen in chapters 2 and 3, however comforting was the sexual division of labor, the new domesticity also endowed woman's role with social and political meaning by invoking her central obligation to regenerate family life and social morality. The result was that women threatened to achieve new forms of power and influence in the nineteenth century, first in the family and then in the public sphere. Mothers gained more power over child-rearing and implicitly over the rearing of sons; wives asserted the right to control their own bodies in matters of sex and reproduction and thus presumably gained a degree of power over husbands. Female moral reformers and temperance advocates occasionally wielded the power of public exposure over men.[8] Meanwhile industrial expansion tempted farm girls to leave their families for work in the factory. Middle-class women participated in health reform, abolitionism, and benevolent work of all kinds. By the middle of the nineteenth century women were taking over the teaching profession. Some demanded the right to higher education and a few asserted their intention to practice medicine and law. The closer some women's activities came to blurring the lines between the home and the world—even if it was often done in the name of a higher domesticity—the more anxious were conservative social commentators to reassert the boundaries between men's and women's spheres.

With the growing American respect for science, doctors found themselves the spokespersons for the affirmation of traditional cultural verities. Many of them relished the opportunity to wield such authority and were particularly assiduous in giving attention to problems regarding women's role. Physicians like S. Weir Mitchell, J. Marion Sims, E. H. Clarke, Augustus K. Gardner, and C. W. Meigs have come under particular attack in the last decade for their denigration of women only superficially veiled by medical theory. And yet the pronouncements of these conservative male physicians regarding female nature tell us less about male physicians in general—or even about the conspiratorial hostility toward women of particular individuals—than about the cultural component of scientific assumptions and the power that those who are recognized interpreters of scientific theory began to exert in the social realm.

Scientific discovery and scientific explanation, Tristam Englehardt has so cogently argued, always depend on the researcher's prior evaluation of reality. In the nineteenth century evaluations of female health were informed not by empirical evidence tested carefully in the laboratory, but by cultural assumptions that had a particular non-medical use in ordering social and power relationships. "Moral values influence the search for goals in nature and direct attention," Englehardt writes, "to what will be considered natural, normal and non-deviant." Englehardt's observations concerning the "disease of masturbation" in the nineteenth century can easily be applied to physicians' pronouncements regarding women's health:

> Medicine turns to what has been judged to be naturally ugly or deviant, and then develops etiological accounts in order to explain and treat in a coherent fashion a manifold of displeasing signs and symptoms. The notion of the "deviant" structures the concept of disease providing a purpose and direction for explanation and for action, that is, for diagnosis and prognosis, and for therapy. A "disease entity" operates as a conceptual form organizing phenomena in a fashion deemed useful for certain goals. The goals, though, involve choice by man and are not objective facts, data "given" by nature.[9]

Little wonder, then, that doctors warned women who violated the "goals" of "Nature" that they would inevitably suffer disease. The majority of physicians could not be expected to notice scientific "facts" which stood in contradistinction to traditional assumptions about women's proper role.

Although it is possible to argue convincingly, as many historians have, that women unreasonably bore the brunt of the late nineteenth-century emphasis on somatic justifications for social roles, they were not the only group to experience this form of social constriction. Blacks, immigrants, and the poor were also subjected to scientific labeling when the aim was to define broadly the accepted cultural parameters of the normal. Furthermore, the control of sexuality that was one goal of medical practice subjected men as well as women to intrusive therapeutical treatments which tortured their bodies and troubled their souls. The unfortunate young man who was treated with doses of quinine, strychnine, calomel, and podophyllin, and whose penis and scrotum were on alternate days given such strong quantities of faradic and galvanic shock that he fainted after the meatus was cut in order to tolerate an even larger sized electric sound—all because he was plagued by seminal emissions "accompanied by lascivious dreams" assumed to be induced by early masturbation—believed, as surely as did his doctor, that he had a serious disease. Though doctors did not use medical theory to control men's activity in the public world, they did use science to control male sexuality as well as female, believing that they did so in the interests of general cultural stability.[10]

Indeed, we are witnessing in all these examples of the social usage of diagnosis and treatment the beginnings of what Christopher Lasch has labeled the "medicalization of society." In the period after 1900 the helping professions gained increasing leave to intrude on the family in various ways, disseminating the principles of efficiency of function, expertise, and science, and rationalizing emotional life. Educators, psychiatrists, social workers, penologists, and public-health advocates would all increasingly use the metaphor of a sick society in order to best define their own newly developed social role: as agents of a more scientific, more humane, and more rationalized social order. Doctors, too, would participate in these changes, while their medical theorizing reflected the gradual equation of deviance not with crime or sin, but with illness.[11]

Women physicians, by virtue of their being professionals, could not help but be influenced by the growing use of the medical profession as an instrument of social control. They, too, naturally turned to science to buttress their cultural theory. It is important that we keep this in mind as we address the second question raised at the beginning of this chapter. How aware were women physicians of the use of medical practice for conservative cultural definitions of woman's role, and how did they cope with their perceptions while continuing to maintain their self-respect as qualified medical professionals? Did they indeed offer a coherent critique of male medical procedure, either in theory or in practice, as some historians have claimed?

To begin with, many women physicians seem to have expected their medical practice to differ in a number of important ways from that of their male teachers and colleagues. Since they based their arguments in favor of women's role in medicine on their difference from men, it is hardly surprising that such would have been the case. Nor did the assumption that women and children would be their primary constituency trouble them, because they sincerely believed that women usually were more effective than men in treating women.[12] Ella Ridgeway wrote in her 1873 thesis at the Woman's Medical College of Pennsylvania that women had been called upon to "supply a deficiency" in medicine "in regard to the diseases of women." There were many questions about the subject that "no doubt" have arisen in the "mind of every woman student which are not answered either by our professors or the books. One of these is why do women generally suffer so much more from ill health than men?" Anna Longshore-Potts also displayed pique at her male colleagues when she wrote that their opinions about women were "cut and dried" and if women had pursued medicine earlier, "today women would have had more healthy bodies." A generation later, Rosalie Slaughter Morton agreed that even well-intentioned male physicians misdiagnosed women. "Diagnoses made by men often indicated," she wrote, "they they either did not, or could not, fully understand the diseases classified as those of women. Their analyses lacked clarity through insufficent differentiation from male disorders." Consequently, Mary E. Bates chided those few women physicians who "have cherished the ambition to be consulted solely because of medical attainment," preaching the doctrine "that there should be 'no sex in medicine.' " "So long as there are men and women patients there will be sex in medical problems," she warned, and women needed women physicians to understand their ailments best.[13]

In addition, women physicians readily acknowledge that they practiced a more nurturing, milder, and a more holistic brand of therapeutics. Sarah Adamson Dolley urged her students to meet patients "as something more than a static entity or dynamic quantity whose muscles, nerves, and joints are not simply a bundle of levers, pulleys and hinges, but are the instruments of that mysterious something which we call life." Similarly, Dean Clara Marshall emphasized this point to her graduating classes in Philadelphia. Study people as well as diseases, she warned. "A distinguished physician has said 'there are no diseases, only patients,' " she told a group of students in 1879, "and you will often reach patients and cure them too, by a scientific use of your humanity." Susan Dimock, the brilliant young surgeon at the New England Hospital, frequently commented that if she were asked "to do without sympathy or medicine, I should say do without medicine." "A woman physician sees life without its mask," observed the surgeon Rosalie Slaughter Morton. "[She] gets closer to the inner thought of other women in understanding the many domestic and social factors in illness . . . because her mother heart has scientific facts to support intuition and sympathy."[14]

So pervasive was the belief that women had more patience and insight, that even the greater physician Oliver Wendell Holmes, Sr., admitted to a suspicion that male physicians all too often resorted to drugs when empathy was all that was in order. "I have often wished," he mused,

> that disease could be hunted by its professional antagonists in couples—a doctor and a doctor's quick witted wife—with their united capacities. For I am quite sure there is a natural clairvoyance in a woman which would make her . . . much the superior of man in some particulars of diagnosis. . . . Many a suicide would have been prevented if the doctor's wife had visited the day before it happened. She would have seen in the merchant's face his impending bankruptcy while her stupid husband was prescribing for his dyspepsia and endorsing his note.[15]

Implicit in such sentiments, of course, was a critique not unlike Elizabeth Blackwell's, of the male style. Men were presumably neglectful of important but subtle aspects of medical practice and could not be expected to change because such deficiencies were a reflection of both the strengths and weaknesses of the male character. Not inherently altruistic like women, men lacked the "spirit of self-sacrifice" and thus could not do as well with children because they had "neither enough love or patience." Male physicians were apt to reject the insane "pitilessly," whereas women took the time to communicate with them. The interests of men lay in pure science, not in its sympathetic application. In obstetrics, argued Effa Davis, this meant that it had always been "the mechanical side" that had "appealed to men from the beginning." Preparing the patient for childbirth through instruction and advice has been less "alluring." Indeed, male physicians' most serious deficiency was found to be in the area of prevention.[16]

Evidence to support these assumptions about male and female differences is intriguing but inconclusive. The Philadelphia physician Arthur Ames Bliss offered some indirect verification for the "male" medical style when he noted in his memoirs about his early days at Blockley that:

It must be confessed that the young medical man was too often disposed to be sarcastic, cynical, suspicious and anxious to drive away every applicant who did not bear in his or her body the symptoms of being an interesting medical or surgical case.[17]

In contrast, Harriet Belcher reported her own internship at the New England Hospital as a "ceaseless round of care, work, and anxiety." "The Maternity is the saddest of places to me," she told a friend. "Most of the women are unmarried, and except for the respectability of the thing, by far the greater number had better not be—the Husbands being brutal wretches who abuse them in every way." Proud of the efforts of the hospital's lady managers to help such unfortunate women find work and a home, Belcher concluded, "I have always been interested in such work . . . and I am very glad, as you may imagine, to take any part in it."[18]

As far as criticizing actual practice is concerned, many of the published case studies of women physicians are specifically concerned with alternative therapies to "scientifically applied therapeutics." In 1884 Dr. Sarah R. Munro argued that women physicians were better at curing dysmenorrhea in young girls first because "they will not be contented with giving morphia month by month as the main remedy," and, second, because they would put greater emphasis on preventive hygiene. Three years later Lena V. Ingraham reminded her listeners at the Woman's Medical College of Pennsylvania in a paper on "Preventive Medicine" that drugs, pledgets of cotton, and pessaries should not be resorted to in cases of prolapsed or retroverted uterus until proper attention had been paid to healthful dress. Finally, Dr. Bertha R. Lewis spoke in a paper on correcting spinal curvature, of her sense of male doctors' reluctance to use exercise therapy as a cure. "It is so much easier to put on a stiff brace," she observed. "I think the few men physicians who do approve of giving exercises for lateral curvature, are unwilling or unable to find time to give the necessary personal supervision," she concluded.[19]

It is clear from their published work that women physicians admired a therapeutic style that reflected sensitivity to the patient's feelings. In remembering her mentors at the New England Hospital at the end of the nineteenth century, Dr. Alice Bigelow emphasized Dr. Sarah Bond's gentle speech. "I never heard it harsh. . . . Her patients adored her, and she went through the old medical building like sunshine." Likewise, Dr. Elsie Brown was a woman full of "kindliness." Attending a seminar on gynecological surgery, Mary E. Bates was particularly offended by the fact that the speakers "limited their attacks to the offending . . . uterus," while "practically ignoring the patient." Harriet Belcher believed that women even handled dissection differently in their medical schools. In a letter in 1875, she noted her own surprise at finding dissection less difficult to endure than she had expected. "I find that when the spirit of scientific research and inquiry is roused, you soon lose sight of all the rest," she explained. Nevertheless, she concluded, "from what I hear of it in other colleges I have no doubt that a dissection as managed by women is a very different matter from one under the charge of male attendants. Every possible precaution is taken to spare the sense and feelings of those engaged in it."[20]

A fascinating first-hand description of one highly respected woman physician's empathic style has been left to us by the feminist writer Charlotte Perkins Gilman. Gilman's account is particularly noteworthy, because in 1885, soon after the birth of her daughter, she experienced a nervous breakdown and was for a short time placed under the care of S. Weir Mitchell, the eminent Philadelphia neurologist who was renowned for his treatment of hysteria. Though Mitchell's paternalistic "rest cure"—placing the patient in an isolated room under the care of a nurse for complete bed rest and total inactivity—worked with scores of women in the late nineteenth century, he failed miserably with independent-minded individuals like Gilman whose very lives stood as indictments of Victorian traditionalism. Gilman's meeting with Mitchell was so unsatisfactory that she wrote a brilliantly critical caricature of him and the "rest cure" in her gripping short story "The Yellow Wall-Paper."[21]

Unable to find complete relief for her ill health, Gilman suffered from nervousness the rest of her life. She was helped in 1902, however, by the treatment of Mary Putnam Jacobi, and left the following account of their relationship:

When I met her I found we were more or less interested in the same things. She became most kindly interested in my variety of neurasthenia and made a proposition to me. She said she had originated a system of treatment which she desired to try for that ailment, and nobody would allow her to do so. I said I was perfectly willing to let her try it on me, and we formed a compact. She proceeded to develop with me the original system, and the result was admirable. I worked under her for some months, going to her office every day, and she put me through a course of most remarkable performances and gave me this compliment—that I was the most *patient* patient she ever had. I found her the most patient physician I had ever known, and the most perceptive. She seemed to enter into the mind of the sufferer and know what was going on there, and I have carried with me, and always shall, the deepest . . . feelings for that broad mind. . . . I have heard it said that women physicians are, if anything, *more* given to respect authority than men physicians. Dr. Jacobi seemed to me an example of a free and original mind, thinking for itself and working out its own methods, not only taking accepted knowledge on a subject, but adding to it.[22]

One wishes that Gilman had left us a more detailed record of Jacobi's actual course of treatment. But Jacobi's willingness to engage Gilman as an equal partner in effecting her cure stood in direct contrast to S. Weir Mitchell's authoritarian approach, so disdainfully described in "The Yellow Wallpaper."

Besides the question of variations in style, there was also the contention that women physicians used drugs differently. Many argued that women physicians would reject heroic dosing and that some women doctors actually preferred milder therapies. Certainly this may have been partially true. In a letter to Elizabeth Blackwell, for example, Marie Zakrzewska confessed her dislike for drugs, admitting that her "whole success in practice" was based upon viewing medicines as "secondary," often using drugs as placebos. "I have the reputation among my large clientele, men, women & children as giving hardly any medicine but teaching people how to keep well without it . . . I can assure you," she concluded, "it is far harder, requiring more strength, and more endurance & more patience to practise Hygiene then [*sic*] what is called medicine."[23]

Yet we cannot generalize about women physicians and heroic therapy. Scores of male physicians rejected harsh dosing, while one also occasionally finds a woman practicing heroic medicine. The casebooks of Anna Manning Comfort, a homeopathic physician, reveal that she sometimes bled patients with leeches. Bleeding, leeching, and other drugs were often recommended therapies in the gynecological and obstetrical theses at the Woman's Medical College of Pennsylvania. These essays refer again and again to standard therapies described in medical texts that both the female authors and their male student counterparts were reading. In 1889 Mary Putnam Jacobi herself reported a case in which she used leeches applied to the cervix to restore the flow of menstruation to a woman suffering for over three months from amenhorrea. And as we shall see below, my own comparative study of the manage-ment of obstetrical cases at a female-run and a male-run Boston hospital revealed only minor variations in the use of heroic medi-cines, but an unexpected divergence in the frequency of drug prescription.[24]

It is also important to remember that patients themselves often demanded heroic treatment as proof of the physician's skill. Charles Rosenberg has observed that therapeutics played a central role in the doctor-patient interaction, and often the severity of the drug administered demonstrated to the patient and his family that something was indeed being done.[25] In fact, doctors who were skeptical of heroic dosing often complained that public expecta-tions worked against change: a physician who failed to bleed in some cases was subject to criticism. That women physicians were not immune to such pressure is illustrated by the following passage from a letter of Elizabeth Blackwell's to her sister Emily:

> Mrs. Clark is in Paris—a lady called on me today three weeks re-turned, who had boarded in the same house with her. This lady had had the red hot iron applied to the uterus by Jobert, for ulceration, (so she said) and felt so much better that she thinks there is nothing like it, and means to advise all her friends to be scorched—she came to me hoping that I would apply it to a sister-in-law! So Milly, you must be prepared to cut and burn, and practice every conceivable abomination, for it is perfectly evident to me that the more unnat-ural the applications, the more the women like it., This lady was frizzled twice, the smoke filled the room, and she is only desirous now to find some one who will practice as Jobert did.[26]

Similarly Marie Zakrzewska, writing to Elizabeth Blackwell in 1891, noted that women came to the New England Hospital beg-ging for operations "on the slightest cause." Married women "be-tween 28 and 40 years" come in asking for ovariotomies "because causing [*sic*] dismenorrhea & children were not desired." When surgeons were thus tempted, she mused, "do you wonder . . . [that they] go the whole length of disregard for Nature?" Zakrzewska felt that "material comfort, indulgence in luxurious living, dislike to work & of self abnegation are the motives which prompt women to seek operations." "Yes," she observed bitterly, "they rather die, then bring up a family of children and work & practice self denials."[27]

When discussing their conservative attitudes toward dosing, women physicians usually connected their willingness to use milder therapies to their greater emphasis on prevention over cure. Marie

Zakrzewska, remember, justified her use of placebos by her willingness to teach "people how to keep well." Similarly, Sarah Adamson Dolley expressed such sentiments in a letter to a cousin written while she was still in medical school. "Heroic treatment," she argued, was a "necessary evil" with which people could do without "if they learned to live properly." Indeed, we have seen that many women physicians took their role as teachers of hygiene extremely seriously. Scores of them gave lectures on physiology and health from the midnineteenth and into the twentieth century. Others taught hygiene in the newly established women's colleges. Still others published books and pamphlets to combat mass ignorance and the prevalence of disease.[28]

Abudant evidence also exists to suggest that the hospitals that women physicians founded in the latter half of the nineteenth century gave particular attention to the doctor's teaching role. The New York Infirmary, for example, established the office of "sanitary visitor" in 1867. This position was usually filled by a young medical graduate wishing to gain further clinical experience. The work entailed going into the homes of the poor, checking on ventilation, cleanliness, diet, and general hygiene, and giving families advice on how to keep themselves healthy.[29]

In Cleveland and Philadelphia, the Woman's Hospitals sent interns into patients' homes. Physicians, revealed the Cleveland Hospital's Annual Report of 1882, did not confine their work "entirely to curing the sick," but also offered "instruction . . . in the laws of health" and in "the care and diet of children." Similarly, the Mary Harris Thompson Hospital in Chicago had female physicians as medical visitors who did "many things for their improvement besides administering medicines for a present illness" when they went "into the homes of the poor."[30]

Let us now turn to the prevailing theories of female health in the nineteenth century, and ask how and in what ways women physicians offered an alternative to the traditional definition of woman as weak, emotional, sickly, and hysterical, governed without mercy by the vagaries of her reproductive organs, and liable to permanent physiological damage if she imprudently exposed herself to the dubious rewards of higher education.

In 1891, on the eve of the opening of Johns Hopkins Medical School, M. Carey Thomas praised the woman physician as the individual who could best guide young girls through school and college life. First, she observed, a woman doctor would be less ready than a man to preserve physical health "at the expense of intellectual development"; indeed, she would be more skeptical even that such a thing could be done. She would never "prescribe sheer idleness as a remedy . . . for the indispositions of girls" hungry to learn. But most important, believed Thomas, the woman physician would have an infinitely better "conception of the ideal or normal life of women, and will understand and know how to remove or diminish the difficulties in the way of its realization."[31]

M. Carey Thomas knew what she was about. However much women physicians differed on the details of female health, they were drawn together by the conviction that women had a right to good health, that their own role should facilitate that right, and that better health among their contemporaries and future generations of women was indeed possible. Some of them were extremely cautious about the physiological crises of puberty, childbirth, and menopause, and occasionally their prescriptions for behavior appear in retrospect strikingly similar to those of conservative men. Yet the female doctor who believed it was woman's fate to suffer indefinitely because of her physiology was a rare exception. Most would have agreed with Anita Tyng, who declared in 1880 in a paper on "Dysmenorrhea" delivered to the alumnae of the Woman's Medical College of Pennsylvania, "I do not believe that we are born to suffer, or born sick and malformed simply because we are born women."

At that meeting, Tyng called for a concerted effort by women physicians to investigate the subject of female health:

> These points and their prevention before and at the time of puberty, I desire to have women physicians study out and write upon. I also desire to have the whole subject of dysmehorrhea carefully studied, not only the mechanical, which I proposed for today, but also that arising from congestion, inflammation and nervous conditions. I hope we shall continue this subject year after year, until our united efforts will produce a series of valuable papers, to be published together as "Womans' Views of Dysmenorrhea," or some similar title.[32]

In the 1880s women physicians took up Tyng's mandate. They monitored the health of college girls and began to publish works contradicting the Clarke thesis. Most of these studies demonstrated that higher education not only did not adversely affect women's health, but made a positive contribution to good health by teaching "a proper appreciation of physiological laws."[33]

Yet it is also a mistake to claim too much innovation for the woman doctor. Especially after 1880, the majority of female physicians were committed professionals who shared a common medical education with their male counterparts, and who grew up influenced by the same social environment. Thus, it is possible to find plenty of "conservative" medical opinions among them on the subject of women's role, puberty and menopause, marriage and motherhood.

Like their male counterparts, for example, a number of women physicians, some of them strongly identified with social feminism and suffrage, revered motherhood in sentimental Victorian fashion. Though male physicians have been accused of overemphasizing woman's reproductive role in order to cement her more firmly in the home, it is hard to find much difference in the pronouncements of many women doctors on the subject. I have uncovered no woman doctor who directly challenged woman's primary role as mother, and many who devoted much attention to seeking ways to improve it. Eliza Mosher believed it "economic in the highest degree" to preserve female health because it was a great "loss to the State" when "through ill health or physical disability, women are unable to bear and properly rear children." As dean of women at the University of Michigan, Mosher enjoyed teaching home economics more than any other course because she had a chance to preach scientific motherhood. Like Mosher, Dr. Josephine Whetmore considered maternity the central event in a woman's life. She hoped women would prepare for it by "clean living from the cradle."[34]

Another defender of scientific motherhood was Dr. Mary Wood-Allen, a well-known social-purity lecturer. Though married and a mother herself, Wood-Allen thought it generally undesirable for a woman to work outside the home if a "husband's income is sufficient to maintain the home in comfort." "Motherhood is a profession most exacting in its demands," Wood-Allen wrote, "and the strength, thought, courage and patience of the wife are fully occupied in caring for the needs of the family." Dr. Josephine Griffith Davis believed that "every true wife who loves her husband is willing, nay anxious, to bear children to him"; and Dr. Helen S. Childs asserted that the best thing about a college education for women is that it made them better mothers. College women were quite as willing as non-college women to become mothers, she argued, "because the inclination toward motherhood is instinctive."[35]

All women physicians worried about the idleness and dissipation which had been brought by modern life to the lives of potential mothers. Conservative women physicians like Wood-Allen sought a solution in "professionalizing" motherhood by making it more scientific. While she discouraged work outside the home, other women doctors were bolder: Rachel Brooks Gleason urged husbands to "help their wives and daughters to some encouraging, ennobling work. Infirmities, both imaginary and real, would be lessened." Sarah Hackett Stevenson believed that "successful occupation" was "the cure for many, many sins" and that making women self-supporting would be a boon to "domestic life." She estimated that half the female population was sick from "ennui." "If Satan had a mission on earth," she wrote, "it is in finding employment for unemployed women. He starts them on a career of self-contemplation . . . they revolve from day to day around themselves . . . a sort of . . . disintegration of character takes place."[36] And yet few women doctors seemed willing to explore the logical contradiction between the idea of "scientific motherhood" and women's venturing out into the real world of work. One is never sure whether they are recommending paid work or volunteer activity, while practical solutions are generally left unexamined.

Furthermore, the importance of preserving women for healthy motherhood led many women physicians to be extremely cautious about a too casual or neglectful approach to women's biological milestones. Elizabeth L. Martin, adviser and medical examiner to women at the University of Pittsburgh, warned her colleagues that any training for woman "which in any way handicaps her for what should be her highest and happiest function—that of wifehood and motherhood" would be a wrong to society. Admitting that "brilliancy of intellect is often associated with an instability of the nervous system which makes parenthood undesirable for some of these women," Martin nevertheless believed that careful supervision by the woman physician could counteract such dangers.[37]

Margaret E. Colby, president of the Iowa Society of Medical Women in 1902, similarly viewed puberty as a dangerous time. "For a year or two . . ." she pressed, "we as physicians, should urge the necessity of fewer studies, or shorter study hours, sandwiched with manual training, in economics and out-door and indoor gymnastics, instruction in regard to the physical changes, their significance and values." Writing in the *Woman's Medical Journal,* another woman physician disapproved of competitive sports for girls, arguing that it "overworked . . . [the] heart." Mary Wood-Allen advised the avoidance of long walks, bicycling, dancing, and all physical exertion, while Anna Manning Comfort felt careful physiological instruction by mothers would ease pubescent girls onto the right track.[38]

Some women physicians subscribed to the maternal-impression theory—the idea that a pregnant mother's experience could affect a fetus—and many believed in the inheritance of acquired characteristics. Such beliefs led to the prescription of carefully chosen activity during gestation and the cultivation by women of lofty character traits. "Sometimes," wrote Mary Wenck, "a mother may force an ugly disposition on a child by her own discontented and unhappy mind during the carrying period." She urged fellow obstetricians to teach mothers the fearful effects of "mental disquietude."[39] Such an approach certainly could help to confine pregnant women to their sphere, and to encourage them to feel guilt if they felt dissatisfied with their inactivity.

Most female physicians expressed shock at the prevalence of abortion among middle-class women. "Nothing was so surprising to me during my first year of practice," remembered Eliza Mosher, "as the assurance with which women came to my office and asked for illegal operations. That's what they thought women doctors were for."[40] Yet women physicians not surprisingly displayed a particular sensitivity to women's right to control both the timing and the purpose of the sexual act. They agreed on this point, whether their attitudes toward sexuality were liberal or conservative, and whether or not they condoned family limitation. Compelling wives in sexual relations was an "outrage" to both mother and "unborn" child. "If woman has an inalienable right in this world," declared Sarah Hackett Stevenson, it is the right to become a mother "in accordance with her own desires." This conviction appeared repeatedly in the literature women doctors wrote for the lay public, although some male physicians held it as well.

Women physicians also tended to argue for a more positive interpretation of the menopause. Though they admitted that "dangers do attend the menopause," the careful supervision by a physician could avert most suffering and women "would be prepared to enjoy a healthy and useful post-climacteric period of life."[41]

One area of medical practice that seems to have drawn much critical attention from women physicians was gynecological surgery. Elizabeth Blackwell was not the only woman physician to complain about the increase in ovariotomy in the last third of the nineteenth century, others did as well. In a fit of pique in 1894, Mary A. Spink responded to a physician who had ridiculed women

doctors with the accusation that plenty of irresponsible men practiced poor medicine:

> As for removal of the ovaries the fact is, that women physicians
> object to the wholesale onslaught upon those innocent organs, which
> originated with so-called reputable physicians and has been contin-
> ued by men mountebanks to that degree that nearly every city in the
> land has several "private homes" or "sanitarioms" for the purpose of
> removing those organs, removing them for nervousness produced by
> a thousand outside causes, removing them because the husbands
> request it, removing them for everything but disease. No woman
> surgeon is capable of diagnosing a diseased ovary from a diseased
> brain.[42]

In addition, several women doctors pioneered in the growing
professional criticism of the theory of reflex irritation which
stressed uterine disease as a cause of insanity in women. In a paper
published in 1894, Anne H. McFarland welcomed the modern tendency to play down the connection between the female reproductive system and mental illness. Calista V. Luther, in a talk on the
participation of women physicians in work among the insane,
praised the pioneer activities of Margaret Cleaves in the 1880s,
though she admitted that Cleaves believed in the theory of reflex
irritation. "I differ from her in respect to uterine diseases being a
potent factor in the insanities of women," Luther explained, "yet
her opinion and the authorities are worthy of our respectful attention." Luther closed with the remark that, if Cleaves were writing
in 1900, she believed the older woman would lay much less stress
on the causal nature of uterine disease.[43]

And yet women doctors themselves occasionally performed sexual surgery, although one gets the impression they were extremely
cautious about it. Anita Tyng, Mary A. Dixon-Jones, and Elizabeth Keller all published several case studies of "Battey's Operation"—the removal of normal ovaries to cure a variety of gynecological and psychological complaints—and Anita Newcomb McGee
advocated ovariotomy for all "degraded or low-class or poor
women who will submit to it, to prevent multiplication of the race
from its dregs."[44]

Furthermore, women physicians were for the most part absolutely delighted with their achievements in the operating room.
Many believed surgery "particularly appropriate for a woman."
Their hospital reports and case studies published in the journals
proudly boasted of the number of "capital operations" performed
each year. Lilian Welsh, a graduate of the Woman's Medical Col-

lege of Pennsylvania, retrospectively summarized the attitudes of many when she recalled that "in those early days of gynecological surgery, women physicians, as a rule, were very ambitious to enter the field."[45]

It is also clear that by the 1890s a more conservative approach to ovariotomy was making headway among male physicians. In a letter to Elizabeth Blackwell written in 1896, Dr. Mary Augusta Scott, a surgical assistant to the gynecologist Howard Kelly at Johns Hopkins, reported the attempts by Kelly and several other male physicians—including the president of the AMA—to put a stop to abusive gynecological surgery. In that year Kelly published an article in the *Journal of the American Medical Association* in which he observed, "Conservatism . . . is undoubtedly the progressive spirit in gynecology: exsective and amputative gynecology has gone to its extreme limits, and the more thoughtful surgeons . . . have already sounded the keynote of the new advance." Similarly, I. N. Love accused the profession of going "mad in the direction of gynecological tinkering" after "the J. Marion Sims epoch," and praised the fact that "the surgical pendulum is swinging well in the opposite direction."[46]

It is hard not to conclude that, although women physicians had a greater awareness and sensitivity to women's issues than men, their overall medical opinions tended to reflect professional and scientific trends and their divergences among themselves often appeared to be similar to those of male doctors. Just as men lacked unanimity on many medical isues, women physicians also differed significantly with each other. As females struggling to strike a balance between science, professionalism, and their own womanhood, they were bound to develop individual solutions to the problems of female health. The historian is hard pressed, therefore, to uncover a uniform approach among these women on how to treat, diagnose, or prevent illness. Women internalized many "male" values, just as men were sometimes advocates of "female" positions.

An excellent example of such diversity may be drawn from the obstetrical literature. The persistent reader of medical journals appearing in the last third of the nineteenth century will likely discover that a debate raged among obstetricians over whether childbirth was a natural event requiring the obstetrician to "wait on nature" or a pathological crisis demanding active and vigorous intervention. Prominent male physicians can be found on both sides of the issue. The debate crystallized in the pages of the *American Journal of Obstetrics and Diseases of Women and Children* for 1888, where

William T. Byford, teacher in Rush Medical College and president of the Chicago Gynecological Society, and A. F. A. King, president of the Washington, D.C., Obstetrical and Gynecological Society, warmly contested "The Physiological Argument in Obstetric Studies and Practice." King's article had a familiar ring. Though childbirth perhaps should be natural, "in the present age, and among civilized communities," he wrote, a case of natural labor can only be "hypothetical." The bad habits of modern life had exacted their toll on parturient women. Byford, on the other hand, scorned King's distorted picture of American womanhood. The doctor's patients were not representative: "Let the author look elsewhere than in Washington and in large cities and he will find plenty of healthy women in physiological labor—he might indeed have found plenty in Washington." Byford's positive approach to female health led him to decry passionately the "meddlesome practices" of some of his colleagues.[47]

If we examine the theses on childbirth at the Woman's Medical College of Pennsylvania, we discover that they, too, reflected the thinking of the medical profession at large. In the early decades, from the 1850s to the 1870s, the theme was deference to nature, limited interference, and patience in delivery.[48] By the end of the century, however, when doctors began to worry that excessive civilization had complicated delivery for middle-class women, the women's theses reflected this change. Pregnancy, wrote Phoebe Oliver in 1869, though a physiological condition, "has the peculiarity of being in some susceptible constitutions, pathological." She recommended moderate interference, including some drugging, rather than "waiting on nature," especially when there were spasms. Other students noted the dire effects of advancing civilization on the ability of women to give birth easily.[49] Lucy R. Weaver believed that the way in which the physical system changes during pregnancy "may easily become pathological, for it borders so closely on disease." Mary Jordan Finley chided old-fashioned obstetricians reluctant to use forceps. She warned that much serious damage could be prevented by the "timely" use of both forceps and ergot to ease pain, secure the child, and conserve the strength of the mother. "A timid or incompetent practitioner," she complained, "sits by the patient waiting for nature to accomplish the delivery until the life has been crushed out of some point in the soft tissues." The result: vesico-vaginal fistula, a hole in the uterine or vaginal wall caused not by the forceps, but by the hesitation of the physician to use them.[50]

Articles on childbirth in the *Woman's Medical Journal,* established in 1893, also reflected prevailing wisdom. While old-timers such as Marie Zakrzewska reminded young practitioners that childbirth was "the most natural process in a woman's life" and decried "meddlesome interference," other women physicians shared the attitude of Agnes Eichelberger. Childbirth might be a physiological function, she conceded, but "from the moment of conception to the end of the lying-in state, our patient is in danger and it is our duty to protect her."[51]

Eliza Root recommended wide experience in the use of forceps in teaching obstetrics because of the frequency of faulty development of the reproductive system caused by modern civilization. Other women doctors were actually innovative with certain surgical procedures. Anna E. Broomall, who ran the obstetrical service at the Woman's Hospital of the Woman's Medical College of Pennsylvania, was one of the first surgeons of either sex to recommend episiotomy as a safe and justifiable procedure. When she presented her findings to the Philadelphia Obstetrical Society in 1878, she was criticized by the men for too much interference and for needlessly exposing the patient to septic poisoning.[52]

I do not believe these differences were primarily generational, although medical trends were important. It is helpful to point out that both the "natural" and the "medicalized" view of childbirth could be and in fact were used to justify both feminist and antifeminist positions. It is not surprising to learn that Dr. Byford and Dr. King's attitudes toward childbirth dovetail with other opinions they held on the subject of women. Byford was a strong supporter of women in medicine, and helped establish the Woman's Medical College in Chicago. In contrast, King opposed the admission of women to medical school, and was instrumental in seeing to it that his own institution, Columbian University, closed its doors to them in the 1890s.[53]

As for the question of childbirth, the issue was often who should be in control; male physicians who preferred interference may have done so in order to assert medical control over parturition. Women in the nineteenth century who advocated certain types of interference, however, often did so on the grounds that such interference could be liberating for patients—either from pain itself or from male incompetence. The Twilight Sleep movement in the early part of the twentieth century presents an excellent case in point. In this instance women physicians and other feminists campaigning for woman's relief from birth pain through the use of scapolomine-morphine pressured obstetricians into administering a technique of anesthesia that at the turn of the century had been rejected by male doctors as unreliable and unsafe. In contrast, antifeminist physicians often used intervention as a means of asserting professional control over the birth process and keeping women in their places.[54]

A study of the medical literature has revealed that gender played a small but not necessarily insignificant part in the approach of men and women physicians to treatment. Professional trends and shifts of opinion influenced women physicians' thinking on medical issues just as such change affected their male colleagues. Yet, unlike men, women expected to take an especial interest in female health and this interest often led them to reject the most extreme positions on woman's innate physiological infirmity. Although this meant that their differences with the majority of male practitioners would be extremely subtle, and that their opinion would usually conform to those of the more liberal wing of the profession, gender mattered, though it mattered in only obscure ways.[55]

The actual clinical records can help to strengthen these conclusions. Nineteenth-century Boston offers a unique opportunity for the study of the treatment of women. Many hospital records have been preserved and are still available. Boston also boasted one of the first hospitals for women and children staffed by women physicians. Until it began to lose its appeal in the late 1890s, the New England Hospital, founded by Marie Zakrzewska in 1862, was a showplace for quality medical care in the latter third of the nineteenth century. Ambitious women doctors longed to receive clinical training there, and its teaching program, compared to others at the time, was rigorous and demanding. Standards reflected the very highest of the day. Fortunately, medical, surgical, and obstetrical records for this institution are virtually intact, and if used along with comparable records for the Massachusetts General Hospital and the Boston Lying-In—both teaching facilities for Harvard Medical School—some interesting comparisons can be made.

My objective was to determine whether women in childbirth were likely to receive treatment from women physicians different from that given by men and to test statistically whether childbearing women received better care from female physicians. A systematic sequential sample was drawn from maternity cases at the female-run New England Hospital for the period 1873–1899 and Harvard's Boston Lying-in for the period 1887—1899.[56] Three broad areas of medical treatment and outcome were recorded: the incidence of complications among patients, the use of drugs, and the use of physical intervention techniques, particularly forceps. Any significant differences between hospitals in these areas could be attributed to the sex of the physicians involved if inherent differences in patient population and other non-gender-related institutional differences could be statistically controlled.*

For this study, this qualification was important. Nineteenth-century hospitals were institutions of the urban poor, who were by no means a homogeneous group. Nor did nineteenth-century institutions always perceive all poor people as the same. This distinction in perception was reflected in the development of two different types of hospitals. On the one hand stood the free municipal hospital, a medical almshouse which represented a refuge of last resort for the chronically ill and indigent. The private or "voluntary" hospital, in contrast, ministered to a paying clientele or to the "industrious and worthy" poor who filled its endowed beds.[57] Though Boston Lying-In and New England Hospital were both voluntary institutions, evidence reveals that there were important differences in their clienteles.

Records and annual reports indicate that the "worthiness" of patients was an appreciably more significant factor in New England Hospital's admissions policy than at Boston Lying-In's. New England Hospital patients generally paid at least a nominal fee for the medical services they received to ensure that they would not be "pauperized" by the experience. At Boston Lying-In, only 23 percent were paying patients. Like the male-run Boston Lying-In, the female-run New England Hospital normally refused obstetric service to unwed mothers bearing their second illegitimate child. Unlike Boston Lying-In, however, the ratio of single mothers to married mothers at New England Hospital declined throughout the time period studied. One of the hospital's senior physicians, Emma Call, optimistically referred to this trend when she noted that after the hospital moved to suburban Roxbury in 1871, "the class of patients was . . . a much better one, and we have never had any number of the most undesirable cases, which inevitably gravitate to an institution located in the midst of a dense population."[58] These factors, as well as comments on the physicians' charts and in the hospital's annual reports intimate that physicians at the New England Hospital showed a greater interest than the male physicians at the Lying-In in the patient amenable to moral reform and in

---

*For an essay on the methodology used in this study see Appendix.

creating a Christian atmosphere for erring women. Male physicians viewed their hospital role from a narrower perspective.

Clearly discernible here is a conflict between old and new concepts of professionalism. In the middle of the nineteenth century, doctors of both sexes believed in the medically curative powers of morality and natural living—a belief that technocratic male physicians increasingly abandoned after 1880. Male doctors apparently surrendered their concern with morality more quickly than did women, and one suspects that female physicians' traditionalism in this instance had much to do with their investment in Victorian culture's identification of women as the moral guardians of society.

The socioeconomic difference in patient populations suggests that in both hospitals patients were poor, but Boston's Lying-In's women were poorer. One infers from this that New England Hospital patients may have had an advantage, however slight, in their general medical condition. Ironically, women physicians attracted a somewhat different type of patient, with somewhat different medical and social problems, and this in turn affected the type of medicine women doctors practiced.

Another noticeable difference between the institutions was the sheer amount of information given on the hospital's patient charts. New England's records are consistently more complete. In addition to an account of actual treatment, they provided a greater amount of information regarding patients' medical background (general physical condition, number of prior miscarriages, etc.) and a more detailed indication of social status.

This meticulous record keeping reveals the self-conscious professionalism typical of women physicians, but it also indicates a "leveling" process at work in the Boston Lying-In. The women doctors at New England Hospital made an attempt to know who they were treating and distinguished, at least in their records, between various levels of poverty. The lack of similar distinctions at Boston Lying-In implies that poor women treated in an often overcrowded teaching facility may very well have represented a single category to the male physicians. Interestingly enough, case records were scrupulously complete when male Boston Lying-In physicians presided at the home deliveries of middle-class women.[59]

One's impression is that male physicians at the Boston Lying-In lumped the poor together. Additional support for such a conclusion lies in the fact that the maternal recuperative period at the hospital was a standard two weeks with very little variation. The Lying-In's annual reports express regret that overcrowding made this policy necessary. However unavoidable, it stands in marked contrast to New England Hospital practice. New England Hospital patients remained under care for from four days to three months and were, on the average, under medical supervision over one week longer than their Boston Lying-In counterparts, even during the identical time period (1887–1899). Perhaps this variation can be attributed to a greater sensitivity to individual physical considerations coupled with the availability of space. But the evidence also suggests social considerations. Single mothers normally remained under medical care longer, perhaps because they had nowhere else to go, or because the women doctors of New England Hospital felt such patients required more of the hospital's meliorative moral influence. Bits and pieces of evidence suggest that to women physicians the medical variables were measured equally with their patients' social situations when determining length of stay. This factor alone implies a very different subjective experience for each group of patients.

What about differences in actual medical treatment? The statistics revealed no significant divergence between the two hospitals regarding infant mortality or maternal outcome, particularly when the patient's general state of health was taken into account. More intriguing, however, were contrasting modes of care offered patients after delivery, particularly regarding prescriptions for relief. Here strong patterns of difference emerged.

By the 1870s heroic medicine was on the decline. Physicians conscious of changing medical trends generally avoided large doses of painful and life-threatening therapies. Nevertheless, drugs were often deemed necessary. One expected that drugs would be given in direct proportion to the severity of the complaint, and that women physicians, who had often decried heroic procedures, would be more conservative in their prescriptions. The hospital records revealed precisely the opposite pattern.

Nearly two-thirds of all Boston Lying-In patients received no medication whatever from their physicians, and the statistical correlations revealed that the use of drugs was strongly predicated on the occurrence and severity of complications. At the New England Hospital, every patient was given some form of medication by the women doctors, usually in the range of what was classified as mild to strong pharmaceuticals. Moreover, the prescription of drugs at the New England Hospital did not correlate decisively with any discernible medical factors, meaning that drug prescriptions for postdelivery women were simply standard procedure among women physicians. In short, the male Boston Lying-In physicians followed an objective model: drug prescription was dependent on the physical symptoms. Women physicians dispensed medication or supportive therapy for less codifiable and nonphysical reasons. Everyone received at least "beef tea," and more often a mild pharmaceutical.[60]

While it may be that most of the Boston Lying-In patients were protected from needless medication, it is also possible that they were virtually ignored after delivery. The scanty medical charts certainly suggest this to be the case. The New England Hospital's medication policy implies an alternative ethos concerning the needs of postdelivery women, and the greater prescription of medication by women doctors may be the objective indicator of more patient-doctor contact. If this speculation is correct, then the female physicians were again exhibiting a concept of professionalism that deemed supportive therapy as important to the patient as purely technical concerns.

Another factor under consideration was the relative use of intervention techniques, particularly forceps. This subject is easily the most controversial since it is one of the main issues on which recent historians have based their case that male physicians were arrogantly insensitive to the needs of maternity patients. The use of forceps has become symbolic of the definition of childbirth as a doctor-controlled medical crisis. Hypothetically, women physicians, because they were women, were more sympathetic to the concept of childbirth as a natural process and hence should have been less prone to resort to instrumental interference in delivery.[61]

Examined over the entire period, the data revealed no dramatic difference in the relative willingness of doctors at either hospital to resort to intervention techniques. In addition, medical criteria for forceps use were similar at both hospitals. The labors of those women involved in forceps deliveries were significantly longer than the average, probably because most were bearing their first child. Moreover, these women tended to receive stronger medication in the recuperative period. Finally, the use of forceps increased gradually at both hospitals in the last decade of the nineteenth century. This fact suggests that once sepsis could be controlled forceps deliveries became more likely.[62]

On the issue of puerperal fever, several historians have charged male physicians with negligence in correcting their role in transmitting the dreaded disease. It is true that Boston Lying-In had more difficulty controlling puerperal infection than did New England Hospital. Before the introduction of successful antiseptic techniques there in 1885, the hospital had been forced to close three times because of epidemics, in contrast to only once at New England Hospital. More lives were lost at the male-run hospital. One researcher claimed that Boston Lying-In's comparatively poorer record in preventing sepsis stemmed from the staff's stubborn reluctance to accept the nurses' and physicians' role as possible sources of infection, whereas women physicians at New England Hospital were more willing "to view themselves as fallible."[63] Careful investigation of those charges through an examination of the annual reports of the two hospitals strongly suggests that their divergent records on the fever may not have been related directly to the sex of the physicians in charge at all, but rather to complex and idiosyncratic difficulties having more to do with hospital architecture and finances, the personalities and experience of the respective resident physicians, and blind luck.[64]

As far as the mechanics of obstetric practice are concerned, the hospital studies reveal that the complication rates and frequency of forceps use within each institution indicate a rough parity between the therapeutics of male and female physicians. Drug prescription, in fact, represented the only discernible difference between the two hospitals that can be directly attributed to the sex of the physicians.

Physicians' social assumptions also influenced their medical practice, and it seems to be the case that male and female physicians' attitudes toward their role may well have been diverging. As men embraced a more "modern," technocratic approach to their patients, women physicians continued to cling to traditional holistic orientations. Thus New England Hospital sought a different type of patient from the Boston Lying-In: the "worthy poor." Its annual reports consistently emphasized the women's concern with the hospital's Christian atmosphere. That the obstetric care at the two hospitals was therapeutically similar suggests that the impact of such attitudes on patients remained indirect.

Letters, diaries, written literature, and hospital records have served to illuminate the differences between nineteenth-century male and female physicians in their approach to medical care. We see a picture certainly more penetrating than that revealed by what women physicians said and wrote about themselves. The therapeutic similarities remind us that women physicians were not only women, but physicians as well. As physicians, they operated under the dictates of their profession: they viewed themselves as full-fledged health professionals, they read the same journals as the men, and they subscribed to theories that they believed represented the collective wisdom of their group.

Nevertheless, the gender of the physician mattered in more subtle ways. Some, perhaps most, parturient women were comforted by the attendance of a professional physician of their own sex. Certainly women physicians never forgot that they were women, and it is clear that their interests within medicine as well as their affective behavior while caring for patients were influenced by that fact. Probably women physicians exhibited a different orientation toward patient care. Thus men and women doctors acted alike in most therapeutic situations, but for very different reasons and with meanings both different to themselves and to their patients. The hospital records' offer a valuable insight into this complex and as yet dimly understood relationship between attitudes and therapeutic behavior, suggesting that the polarized perspective with which historians have hitherto approached the subject of medical treatment for women must be modified.

Hopes Unfulfilled: Women Physicians and the Social Transformation of American Medicine

My experience . . . has taught me that the day has not yet come for men to yield to us equal ground with them.

Dr. Caroline Purnell, 1918

By the end of the nineteenth century women physicians could congratulate themselves for a measure of achievement which offered ample opportunity for pride and satisfaction. "The woman physician has come," wrote Dr. Mary Lobdell in the *Woman's Medical Journal* in 1905, "and she has come to stay." In numbers alone their ranks had increased by several thousand: in 1900 they comprised close to five percent of the profession, over seven thousand strong. Visionary women like Elizabeth Blackwell, Mary Putnam Jacobi, Ann Preston, Marie Zakrzewska, and Mary Harris Thompson could point proudly to the achievements of their own institutions. Even more heartening was the progress of medical coeducation. Several Midwestern and West Coast universities had begun accepting women students. By 1900, for example, the University of Michigan had already trained 394 women in its medical department. Crowning these achievements in 1893 was the opening of Johns Hopkins University Medical School as a coeducational institution.[1]

Other developments, too, provided cause for optimism. The decline of sectarian medicine meant that 75 percent or more of women doctors were regular physicians by 1900. This move toward orthodoxy gave them more credibility as a group within a profession progressing rapidly toward standardization. During the last third of the nineteenth century, most state and local medical societies quietly admitted women without objection.[2] Although the American Medical Association did not formally accept women until 1915, it indirectly recognized them when it received Dr. Sarah Hackett Stevenson as a state delegate from Illinois at the 1876 convention.

Women physicians had also made progress in securing admission to hospital clerkships, especially in New York, Philadelphia, and Chicago. Motivated sometimes by informal preference and sometimes by law, several states began to appoint them as clinicians or superintendents at state asylums for the insane in which women were confined. In addition, a handful of women surgeons had demonstrated their proficiency in a specialty that was visibly gaining status within the profession as a whole. Finally, women doctors could proudly cite a growing list of publications in respected scientific and medical journals.[3]

By the 1890s they even had a journal of their own. In 1893 a group of women physicians from Toledo, Ohio, began the *Woman's Medical Journal,* a periodical devoted to raising professional consciousness by publishing both scientific articles by and material about women physicians. The *Journal* viewed as its primary task the work of bringing the medical women of the country closer together. "Women physicians themselves, as a class," declared the editor, Dr. Margaret Rockhill,

> are not aware of the progress of other women physicians along lines but recently available to them as the work of women physicians because of the lack of numbers, has been so individual in character. The purpose of the *Journal* is to more widely spread the work of medical women, and to bring into closer relationship, the women physicians of different sections of the country. Only through the press can this result be obtained. Our columns are always open for contributions from regular women physicians.[4]

In addition to the inroads they were making among the bastions of male privilege, women physicians began to heed cries from their own ranks to formalize their professional connections. In the decades between 1890 and 1920, women's medical societies were founded in many states. Those in Boston and New York were particularly strong. In Philadelphia the alumnae association of the Woman's Medical College of Pennsylvania took great satisfaction in its activity: in 1900 it boasted of 219 members. Because it had a policy of giving honorary memberships to distinguished female graduates of other schools, this association offered much more than mere parochial contact when it gathered for its annual two-day meeting in the late spring. Members read and criticized each other's scientific papers, which were then published in the alumnae journal. They also shared case studies, debated such professional issues as fee splitting and specialization, and took positive steps to promote the interests of women in the profession.[5] Women physicians believed organization to be an important aid to integration within the profession. In 1915 the strengthening of their professional ties culminated with the founding of the American Medical Woman's Association by a group of Chicago women.[6]

Yet despite the achievements of women doctors in the last third of the nineteenth century, more than one historian has pictured the next half-century as dark years for the progress of women in medicine, years in which nineteenth-century beachheads were surrendered and lost to the champions of male backlash and institutional discrimination. The statistics confirm such a view. Though coeducation seemed to hold out enormous promise in the 1890s, the ranks of women physicians did not continue to increase. In fact, the number of women medical students actually declined from 1,280 in 1902 to 992 in 1926 out of a total of 18,840. Female physicians lost ground both in percentages and in absolute numbers. Medicine, moreover, was the only profession in which the numbers of women declined absolutely. After peaking at 6 percent of the national total in 1910, the percentages steadily shrank, and only in 1950 did women physicians again reach 1910 levels. It was not until the 1970s that dramatic increases in the numbers of women in medical schools again occurred.[7]

There were several reasons for the declining numbers of medical women in the first half of the twentieth century, but the most important was the enormous alteration that came about in the structure and content of the medical-care delivery system. While professionalization in general narrowed women's options in some fields while creating new career choices in "feminized" professions like nursing, librarianship, and social work, the overall effect of medical professionalization was to constrict women's activity as physicians, and to confine their participation to particular specialties already implicitly agreed upon in the nineteenth century.

By 1900 the changes in American medicine that were begun in the previous two decades accelerated their pace, and in the next thirty years the modern profession emerged. This was a crucial time for women physicians, for they struggled for self-definition within a field that was rapidly restructuring itself and its social role. Two developments, one taking place within medicine itself, the other external and involving significant historical shifts within the organization of society at large, converged by 1900 to shape the contours of twentieth-century medical practice. The first was the emergence of modern, "scientific" medicine and bacteriology at the end of the nineteenth century. The second was the professionalization and bureaucratization of twentieth-century society, a phenomenon that many historians have identified as a major hallmark of modernization. The growth of modern medicine was continually interwoven with the structural changes within the profession, while both took place against the backdrop of broader shifts in the society at large. All of these changes limited women physicians' options.

Although medical research flourished in France and Germany beginning in the 1830s, the American medical profession paid only nodding attention to these new developments because many of the earliest discoveries had limited application to actual practice. While pioneer researchers in France and later in Germany concentrated on differentiating diseases from each other, thus contributing to etiology and diagnosis, advances in therapeutics lagged behind, making "the inertia of traditional practice," as Charles Rosenberg has observed, "powerful indeed."[8] Even when diagnosis stimulated the use and refinement of technical aids like the improved microscope, the stethoscope, the ophthalmoscope and the laryngoscope, the progress of medicine as a more exact science was slow, and older methods of treatment passed away only gradually.

Nevertheless, laboratory scientists eventually produced findings that would not only have wide applicability to treatment, but that would revolutionize concepts of disease. While cellular pathologists such as Virchow were moving toward a theory of disease localization by the 1850s, Pasteur, Koch, and other researchers concentrated their attention on the many microorganisms that had been discovered to exist in living matter. Pasteur's work on fermentation in the 1860s and Koch's experiments with the anthrax bacillus in the 1880s eventually led them to propose that certain bacteria were the primary causes of certain categories of illness. Soon their students and followers began isolating the specific microorganisms for several diseases, including tuberculosis, diphtheria, cholera, typhoid, and tetanus. The next step, particularly important in its implications for clinical medicine, came when two of Koch's assistants, Emil von Behring and S. Kitasato, produced an antitoxin and used it successfully in 1891 to treat a child dying of diphtheria. In 1894 the era of specific immunotherapy was inaugurated when, after numerous experiments, researchers produced a diptheria antitoxin from horse serum which could inoculate successfully against the disease and be manufactured safely, cheaply, and in large quantities. The early discoveries of Pasteur also laid the foundation for surgical antisepsis and asepsis, and these techniques, combined with the discovery of anesthesia in 1846, prepared the way for the rise of gynecological and abdominal surgery in the 1880s.[9]

As Germany became the center for scientific medicine in the 1870s, some of the best-educated men and women physicians traveled abroad to study at its large clinics, excellent laboratories, and superior medical schools. It has been estimated that between 1870 and 1914, some fifteen thousand American practitioners spent time in Vienna or Berlin in some form of serious scientific study. Most men who studied abroad secured places on the medical faculties of Harvard, Yale, Johns Hopkins, and the University of Michigan when they returned to the United States.[10] Women physicians interested in bacteriology, however, were rarely hired as medical faculty except at the Women's Medical College of Pennsylvania.

With the opening of Johns Hopkins Medical School in 1892, German medical values placing emphasis on research in the basic sciences came to be implanted firmly in America. Both the medical school and the hospital so integrally connected with it were inspired by the German laboratory tradition, the "inductive" method of teaching biology, and a commitment to teaching science as a method of thinking and as an attitude of mind. The faculty at Hopkins hoped to create physicians with a generalized capacity to deal with medical problems scientifically. The great physiologist Franklin Mall, who was the most outspoken proponent of this philosophy, believed that students who had sought to assimilate information by drill must be encouraged instead to solve problems by developing their reasoning ability. A medical school, Mall believed, must carry on "perpetual warfare against drilling trades into inferior students" and ensure that the profession was filled "with learned men, and not tradesmen."[11]

This new ideology of science was greeted with skepticism by some members of the American medical community, as recent historians have made clear. The conflict was not merely one between an educated elite and the average practitioner; it reflected a disagreement in values; a debate over what it was that the physician was supposed to do. The problem was particularly apparent in the first third of the nineteenth century when the Paris School's studies in morbid anatomy contributed so little to therapeutics. One angry New York physician complained in 1836: "The French have departed too much from the method of Sydenham and Hippocrates to make themselves good practitioners. They are tearing down the temple of medicine to lay its foundations anew. . . . They lose more in Therapeutics than they gain by morbid anatomy. They are explaining how men die but not how to cure them."

In the second half of the nineteenth century the debate only intensified, as many traditional practitioners, much like Elizabeth Blackwell, sensed in the new science what they felt to be a disdain for the physician's intuition and clinical good sense. The experimental researcher's emphasis on exact numbers and empirical standards not only held out the promise that new ways of thinking would dramatically alter the physician's treatment of disease, but also threatened to remove the physician from the bedside and replace "art" with science, technology, and facts. "Out of the false pride of the laboratory, and the scorn with which the accurate man of science looks down upon medical indefiniteness," complained the prominent neurologist S. Weir Mitchell in 1877, "has arisen the worse evil of therapeutic nihilism." Like Mitchell, many physicians remained suspicious of laboratory science, and tensions between the ideals of the laboratory and the ideals of the bedside worked themselves out only haltingly.[12]

The insistence at Hopkins on basic science, however, reflected the assumption that students learned habits of thinking in the laboratory that would prove beneficial whether they remained there, moved into the clinic, or performed in the operating theater. This approach stood in opposition to the opinions of many within the profession who preferred to see only a few elite medical schools training specialists and scientists, while the rest turned out modestly knowledgeable general practitioners who could minister to the less expensive and less elaborate needs of everyday health maintenance.

Nevertheless, the new ideology of science was powerful indeed, and William Welch, one of the great prime movers at Hopkins, rejected the accusation that the Hopkins model adapted itself only to the brilliant scholar. Welch stubbornly resisted the idea of a two-track system of medical education. "The practitioner," he believed, "is all the better if he has acquired by example a precept, something of the scientific spirit and attitude of mind, and the clinician, who becomes an investigator and teacher, should become interested in patients and know how to diagnose and treat their diseases."[13] It was Welch's view of medical education that eventually prevailed.

Advances in bacteriological medicine not only affected medical education, but also catalyzed the metamorphosis of the hospital from a moralistic and caretaking institution for the urban poor to the primary locus of acute medical treatment for all classes. Urbanization and concomitant changes in family structure also had an important impact on the transformation of the hospital, while germ theory and asepsis, the professionalization of nursing, and the evolution of a whole range of diagnostic procedures, such as the x-ray, stimulated progress in surgery and other specific therapeutic regimens. As one historian has observed, germ theory narrowed the physician's perception of his patients' needs: now that diseases could be isolated and localized to some specific part of the body, the doctor no longer need be concerned with his patients' social context. The hospital offered the kind of efficiency and technological sophistication that fit well with the narrow and technocratic medical practice that emerged at the end of the nineteenth century.[14]

Yet, changes in the locus of medical care, like the coming of scientific medicine itself, threatened the practitioner at the same time that it rationalized his or her practice and radically improved efficiency. The removal of the patient from his or her home increased the emotional distance between patient and physician, while reducing the actual time both spent together. The altered setting transformed not merely the patient's experience but also the doctor's. For many physicians it meant a radical redefinition of one's professional self-image, a redefinition bound to create tension and anxiety.

Sensitive male physicians occasionally worried over the shifts in the locus and emotional ambience of medical treatment, but women physicians seem to have felt the transition more acutely. Their collective self-definition rested on their belief in their superiority over men in the "soft" and "nurturant" aspects of healing. Eliza Mosher, for example, a past president of the American Medical Women's Association, lamented the passing of the "human" in medicine, regretted the loss of "the sympathetic relation which formerly existed between doctors and their patients," and warned her colleagues to beware of "narrowing and concentrating their vision upon the purely physical to the exclusion of the psychic and human."[15]

Other spokeswomen continued to believe that women physicians in particular must exert their influence in favor of preserving holistic approaches to treatment. The president of the Alumnae Association of the Woman's Medical College of Pennsylvania spoke in defense of the general practitioner in 1901 even as she acknowledged that specialism was the wave of the future. Warning that the phrase "the healing art" should never be spoken of slightingly "as though it represented an old-fashioned idea," she worried that "a training too exclusively for the laboratory fails by leaving out the human element." "The mind that conceives of a human being as a mechanism simply and treats him as such," continued Dr. Elizabeth Peck, "is sure to fail when confronted by the needs and problems of complex human nature." Women, Peck believed, still gravitated to general practice because of their interest in family life, in children, and in "the best good of the community." Though Peck admitted that perhaps even the majority of physicians would ultimately exhibit such social concern, she felt it "to be earlier developed in the medical woman than in her brother practitioner."

Similarly, M. Esther Harding, a psychiatrist, spoke in 1930 for many women doctors when she wrote to Bertha Van Hoosen, a prominent female surgeon and the founder of the American Medical Women's Association,

> I have been struck recently more than once at the meetings of a Psychotherapeutic Society of which I am a member with a queer little difference between the attitude and approach of the men and the women . . . to the subject under discussion. . . . Usually the men lead off with scientifically arranged data, followed by statistics and rather abstract theory. Then presently a women speaks up and nearly always her voice is raised to remind the group that after all the patient is a human being and not merely the subject of certain symptoms or mechanisms. And this I think is characteristic. We women are more nearly concerned with the human problem presented to us and relatively less absorbed with the collection and classification of scientific material. Let us who write about the intricacies of the human psyche, whether in its normal functioning or in its illnesses and conflicts, remember always that in any final analysis it is the human being that matters. Knowledge of disease and its detailed investigation are not ends in themselves, they are only means to an end, namely that the human being may grow and flourish.

In agreement with Harding, both Josephine Baker and Emily Dunning Barringer expressed concern that their profession was becoming "less human," and decried the modern emphasis on "specialism."[16]

Scientific medicine, then, challenged traditional holistic therapeutics, contributed to the modernization of the hospital, and catalyzed the reform of medical education. These developments, however, were all linked to significant changes in social organization that first became apparent at the end of the nineteenth century.

Most historians generally agree with Robert Wiebe that a major organizing theme for the years between 1877 and 1920 is the decline of "community" and the rise of "society." In the late nineteenth century, the isolated, preurban "island" community, consisting of face-to-face primary group relationships, shared values, and relatively clear lines of authority, gave way to institutional centralization in nearly every aspect of life. Agriculture, industry, banking, and politics became increasingly nationalized and standardized. New bureaucratic means were devised for the modern implementation of old ethical values, and what emerged in the twentieth century was a society reordered by a reforming, professionalizing "new" middle class—an elite of technical and professional managers in business and government—a network of men and women who valued national communication through organized interest groups, and "continuity and regularity, functionality and rationalism, administration and management."[17]

In response to these developments, issues of professionalization took the center stage as professional associations, state licensing agencies, and colleges and universities gradually emerged into their modern forms. Wiebe's insights have been applied to the medical profession by a number of historians, and Wiebe himself saw the professionalization of medicine as the most important part of the emergence of the "new middle class" which he described.[18]

For example, at the turn of the century, many physicians agreed that their economic and social position, as well as the collective status of the profession itself, warned of a crisis in medicine. The interests of various competing groups—medical societies, eastern scientific elites, midwestern general practitioners, licensing agencies, and the leading bloc of medical colleges—pointed to the necessity for consolidation and reform. Common aims included the raising of professional entrance standards, the standardization of medical-school curricula, the suppression of weak proprietary institutions, the control of various sects, and the overall reduction in the number of medical graduates. The educational goal of raising standards remained intertwined with the policy of drastically reducing the number of practitioners in a field believed to be already overcrowded.

The most immediate problem facing the reformers was the large number of inferior schools. Until the 1890s the field of medical education had been characterized by competition in an open market consisting primarily of proprietary schools that vied for students by keeping down both the cost and the quality of the education they offered. Though such a situation at first threatened only a minority of elite and college-trained physicians, whose sporadic efforts at reform had been generally unsuccessful, by the 1890s, the economic pattern of unregulated competition and growth typical of the last half of the nineteenth century proved problematic for society as a whole. Saturated markets and ruinous price wars, exhausted soil, miles of unprofitable railroad track—such conditions had led forward-looking businessmen to appeal to the government for the regulation of competition and production, and to trade associations and professional societies to promote consolidation and restore order. Here the medical profession was no different: too many practitioners meant fewer patients and lower incomes for the average doctor. As an editorial in the *Journal of the American Medical Association* observed in 1901, "The multiplication of doctor factories has gone far enough in this country. It is not a dignified comparison, that of the medical graduates to output of a machine shop, but the same principles of political economy apply in a measure to both. Over production in either has its bad effects, and we have not the recourse of foreign markets enjoyed by the ordinary manufacturer." Thus rank and file physicians in the AMA favored reform much as railroad magnates looked to government for regulation: at long last it was decidedly in their self-interest to support such measures.[19]

The ideology of scientific medicine became a fitting rationale for such changes. Making medical training longer and more expensive certainly improved medical practice, but it also reduced the number of physicians in a competitive market. Fewer physicians meant predictable and more adequate incomes. As one historian suggested in his study of the rise of the discipline of biochemistry, in the unregulated market of the late nineteenth century, scientific medicine had remained the ideal of a small group of well-trained urban specialists. Indeed, its German-inspired intellectual program might well have endured as an isolated, minority style within the profession as a whole. "But in a market dominated by the new rules of regulated competition," Robert Kohler points out, " 'scientific medicine' was widely accepted as a means of improving physicians' economic and cultural status, and of promoting social progress at the same time. Thus after two decades of indifference to scientific medicine, the profession rapidly accepted it as the basis for a reorganized medical training." Indeed, no development illustrated more forcefully the ways in which science has held out to the medical profession entry into the realm of social and cultural power in the twentieth century.[20]

Working through the combined efforts of the American Medical Association's Council on Medical Education, organized in 1904, the publicity and the public pressure provided by the *Journal of the American Medical Association,* and the offices of several state licensing boards, the leaders of medical reform began the process of self-criticism. Yet, pressure from within was perhaps even less significant in the long run than pressure from without. It was in this period that large philanthropic foundations backed by Rockefeller and Carnegie wealth began to use their resources to force specific changes in medical education. From 1910 to 1930 the philanthropic foundations—which were able to provide an image of prestige and objectivity—donated over $300 million to medical education and research. Indeed, Rosemary Stevens has argued convincingly that these institutions were "the most vital outside force in effecting changes in medical education after 1910."[21]

The most important event in this new alliance between scientific medicine and corporate power was the Carnegie Foundation's publication in 1910 of Abraham Flexner's meticulous study of contemporary medical education. The Flexner report made public what medical educators had known privately and had worked to correct for a decade: American medical schools labored under appalling inadequacies. Most schools accepted inferior students, provided meager or nonexistent training in laboratory science and clinical medicine, and overproduced doctors. Only the youthful Johns Hopkins Medical School totally escaped Flexner's scathing criticism. According to Flexner's study, medical schools needed to be placed under the control of universities; preliminary education requirements needed to be enforced; curricula needed to be lengthened; and laboratory facilities needed to be improved. These changes would please both the foundations, which wanted higher standards, and the profession, which wanted less competition. Decreasing the number of doctors and consolidating medical schools reflected one important aspect of medical reform; affiliating surviving schools with hospitals and dispensaries reflected yet another. The hospital already had begun to house the complex technology that became the hallmark of modern medicine, and Flexner agreed with the leading spokesmen for scientific medicine who regarded the hospital as essential to the medical school curriculum.[22]

Flexner remained adamant on all his recommendations, and although his candid study did not launch the process of medical reform, which was already under way, it hastened the results. Between 1904 and 1915, some ninety-two schools merged with other institutions or closed their doors when confronted with higher state board requirements, poor clinical facilities, financial difficulties, or Flexner's public criticism. By 1920 only 85 out of the 155 medical schools visited by Flexner remained in existence. The better schools improved their facilities through the generous help of the foundations; other were left to fend for themselves.

By 1920, then, the basic outlines of the reform in medical education had been firmly established. Schools formerly dependent on student fees shifted to reliance on university endowments and large donations from the foundations. Medical faculties that had previously controlled appointments and finances through their corporate authority relinquished these tasks and devoted more of their time to teaching. University administrators with easy access to the philanthropic foundations assumed the task of appointments and policy. The part-time physician-teacher began to be replaced by the professor-researcher, and the Hopkins ideal of a full-time medical school faculty gradually became the reality in many, though not all, institutions. These changes in turn brought others: research work and prominence in the discipline rather than clinical performance became the new "scientific" standard for faculty promotion and high status within the profession.

In addition, the place of medical education in the entire American educational system shifted ground: In the 1890s a medical degree had been roughly the equivalent of one or two years of college, by 1920 a division of labor between secondary, college, and graduate education had been effected and a medical degree from the better schools roughly equaled the achievement of a Ph.D., a university's highest degree. Advanced courses in the biomedical sciences became a significant portion of every physician's medical education. Gradually the triumph and institutionalization of scientific medicine took hold, first in a few elite medical schools in the East and then in institutions in the Midwest and West. Thus, for the first two decades of the twentieth century a reorganized American Medical Association using scientific medicine as a reigning ideology worked closely with the large-scale philanthropic foundations to effect the modern professionalization of medicine on a national scale.[23]

These structural changes within the medical profession affected women physicians in several ways. First there was the matter of medical education. Women physicians' own commitment to separate schools was temporary. They continued to press for equal access to male institutions, and, as schools opened their doors to women, the dream of medical coeducation seemed within reach. Coupled with women's increasing preference for the coeducational setting—itself in part a function of their strong commitment to high standards for women—was the seemingly inescapable cost of modern instruction. Schools wishing to maintain standards dictated by the Council on Medical Education needed the financial backing that only universities and their large endowments, state and government funds, or sizable contributions from philanthropic foundations could provide. For all of the women's schools in existence at the turn of the century, mustering such resources proved an insurmountable barrier.

Between 1890 and 1918, women students clustered heavily in only seven states: New York, Pennsylvania, Massachusetts, Maryland, Illinois, Michigan, and California. While close to half of all regular physicians in the period between 1890 and 1918 graduated from schools located in these states, the ratio of women physicians was even higher—roughly two-thirds. In 1890, for example, 82 percent of female regulars were educated in these regions, and it was not until 1940 that their proportions from these states began more closely to approximate the figures for all students. (See TABLE 9-1.) Of further significance is the fact that prior to 1900, women were not merely clustered in these states, but were attending primarily women's medical colleges. (See TABLE 9-2.) When we remember how women's medical education in the nineteenth century took shape, this clustering is not remarkable. It was in these seven states that women made their greatest inroads prior to the 1890s. New York, Chicago, Philadelphia, and Baltimore all had flourishing women's schools. Michigan and Maryland each boasted a quality coeducational institution. Boston, of course, had an early tradition of female medical education, while California instituted its medical education on a remarkably equalitarian basis.

While the *absolute* number of women medical students increased in the 1890s, their proportional percentages compared to men hovered between 4.8 and 5 percent for the decade. While some of the absolute increase took place in the seven states cited, the growth rate in these regions was surpassed by increases in other parts of the country, particularly in the Midwest, where coeduca-

TABLE 9-1   Women Regulars in Seven Key States, 1890–1918

| | Number of Women Regulars | | | | | | |
	1890	1895	1898	1905	1910	1913	1918
Total Women Regulars	648	889	1045	835	573	526	533
Seven Key States	529	563	755	587	413	386	408
All Others	119	326	290	248	160	140	125
	Percentage of Women Regulars						
Seven Key States	81.6%	63.3%	72.2%	70.3%	72.1%	73.4%	73.4%
All Others	18.4%	36.7%	27.8%	29.7%	21.9%	26.6%	23.5%
	Percentage of All Students						
in Seven Key States	52.3%	50.1%	47.9%	46.5%	47.9%	53.1%	56.3%

Source: *Records of the Commission of Education, JAMA* "Educational Numbers" for appropriate years.

TABLE 9-2   Enrollment in Women's Medical Colleges, 1890–1899

	1890	1893	1895	1898	1899
Women in WMCs*	391	459	417	377	323
All Women	648	827	889	1045	1063
% in WMCs	60.3%	55.5%	46.9%	36.1%	30.4%

*The four WMCs are WMC of Chicago, WMC of Baltimore, New York Infirmary, and WMC of Philadelphia. There were other medical colleges for women. I have excluded them either because they were sectarian or because they were short-lived.

Sources: *Records of the Commission of Education* for appropriate years.

tion was slowly catching on. The women's colleges remained critical in this decade in educating women doctors: by 1899 they were still training nearly one-third of them. Yet the figures also reveal women's enthusiasm for coeducation: while enrollments at the four major women's medical colleges peaked around 1893, the number of students at these schools declined steadily for the rest of the decade. Though women's enrollment continued to keep pace with men's, gains were being made primarily in coeducational institutions. Dean I. N. Danforth of the Woman's Medical College of Chicago concluded that this was the case when he observed in 1898 that falling enrollments at the school resulted from the "fact that now nearly all Medical Schools not only admit women but make special provision for them." Such developments, he warned, "must be taken into account in our future calculations."[24]

Unfortunately, few women's schools could enjoy the luxury of "future calculations," because none of them were prepared to bear new financial burdens. The first to close its doors was the New

York Infirmary. In 1897 the New York Infirmary's medical college was a flourishing institution. Out of debt for the first time in its history, it boasted of a "considerable beginning of an endowment fund in our Treasury." Of all of the women's colleges, it might well have managed to connect itself in a few years with a university or a hospital while wielding considerable bargaining power. Then tragedy struck when the college building, with all its equipment, was destroyed by fire. Efforts were made to rebuild it, but the Board of Trustees quickly lost its dedication to the medical school when Cornell suddenly decided to admit women. It seemed a more suitable strategy now to build up the hospital—still an important postgraduate training center for women physicians—since opportunities for clinical positions were yet severely limited. Negotiations were completed with Cornell the following year, and in 1899 the remaining three classes at the New York Infirmary entered the university's new medical school.

In her final address to the graduating class in 1899, Dean Emily Blackwell observed wistfully that the "modern medical school, with its broad and long course of study, its army of teachers of all grades, its costly laboratories for scientific training, its systematical clinical instruction and hospital classes, is an utterly different Institution from the small, comparatively inexpensive, college of thirty years ago." Medical colleges, she continued, were beginning to "ally themselves with the universities, so as to secure the breadth of university culture, the guarantee of permanence, the prestige of a university degree." Those small colleges "that have no connection with a university, or with a great hospital," she explained, tended "to be absorbed or die out."[25]

Women physicians in New York understood from the start that Cornell's commitment to their education was equivocal. Although the school's enrollment of women students, while erratic, remained high compared to many other elite schools—roughly 16 percent—Cornell refused from the first to appoint women physicians to its faculty. For Emily Blackwell and many others this policy was a bitter pill. Fifteen years after the New York Infirmary closed its doors, the dean of the Woman's Medical College of Pennsylvania was still citing the situation at Cornell in her aggressive defense of the existence of a separate women's school. "The closing of the Woman's Medical College of the New York Infirmary . . ." Clara Marshall wrote, "was the means of cutting short the teaching career of a number of able young women; yet in Cornell University Medical School, after fifteen years (with the exception of an appointment to a minor post in 1914) not a single medical woman holds a position on the teaching staff."[26]

The fates of the other two leading women's schools were variations of the same theme. The Woman's Medical College of Baltimore, though given a respectable rating by Flexner's report, could simply not maintain the high standards set by Hopkins on its small endowment. Its shrinking enrollments led it to close shortly before Flexner published his findings. In the Midwest, the Woman's Medical College of Chicago, in a shrewd move, became part of Northwestern University in 1891. Its faculty believed that the school, which was rapidly upgrading its course of study, would especially benefit from access to the University's "extensive physiological and pathological laboratories," even as it retained its own institutional autonomy.[27]

On the part of Northwestern, the merger was one of several completed that year with a number of flourishing independent professional schools—including the Union College of Law, the University Dental College, the Illinois College of Pharmacy, and the Medical College of Chicago (a men's school). By 1890 the woman's college had erected a large new building, with two amphitheaters, each with a seating capacity of 150. It had built new laboratories and had made improvements on the old building for additional dispensary and laboratory use. "From a penniless and despised institution," wrote historian Arthur Herbert Wilde in 1905, "the Woman's Medical College had grown into a well-equipped institution with valuable property holdings, and its earnings provided for all incidental and running expenses and a fair dividend on the money expended."[28]

In 1892 Henry Wade Rogers, president of Northwestern and a staunch friend of medical education for women, optimistically told his board that taking on the women's school would be a likely financial proposition. "I am convinced that the interests of the University will be promoted by the action taken," he concluded. "The Woman's Medical College of Chicago had attained high reputation, possessed an excellent faculty, and attracted students from far and near."[29] And yet, despite the optimism of all involved, the next decade proved a fatal one for women's medical education at Northwestern. The main problem was falling enrollments. Beginning in 1897, the number of freshmen in the entering class declined precipitously, until in 1899 their ranks had dropped from thirty-two in 1895 to a mere nine. It was first believed that the change from a three- to a four-year course was the cause, but faculty members soon realized that the real culprit was the lure of coeducation. By 1899 six medical schools in Chicago admitted women, and it became clear that for a new generation of female medical aspirants, the men's schools had greater appeal, even when the woman's college could boast of high standards and a prestigious faculty.[30]

By the end of the decade, the school desperately needed to update its laboratory facilities once again. But disappointing enrollments had created an operating deficit in 1897. Although the Woman's Medical School was not the only one of Northwestern's graduate schools to run a deficit, it became clear that the university would remain committed to *women's* medical education only insofar as it was not a financial drain. Though there was some talk of sharing lab facilities and even merging with the men's division, neither solution was deemed suitable by the Northwestern trustees. Finally, in a turn of bad luck, the Woman's Medical abruptly lost a friend when President Rogers resigned in 1900. Two years later the trustees closed the women's school, while simultaneously refusing to make the men's division coeducational. Northwestern University Medical School remained closed to women students until 1926, when its faculty decided to set a female quota at four a year. Even at that time, however, the trustees were substantially influenced in their decision by a sizable donation for medical research from Mrs. Montgomery Ward, who had expressed shock and polite disapproval when she discovered that women were barred from the medical school.[31]

Because the precarious financial position created by falling enrollments caused the closing of all but one of the women's schools, it is difficult to speculate what their ultimate value would have been to women medical aspirants in the twentieth century. It is entirely possible that declining enrollments would have eventually tapered off to a respectable level. Though the Woman's Medical College of Baltimore seemed to regain some of its numbers in 1908, the very year it closed its doors, it was always the smallest and poorest of the four schools, and it could not survive in so close proximity to Johns Hopkins, even when its student body increased from sixteen in 1905 to thirty in 1908. In Philadelphia, despite the fact that the Woman's Medical College was virtually the only institution in the city to admit women until 1918, female enrollments steadily declined from 210 students in 1893 to between 90 and 120 in the 1920s. Thereafter, however, enrollments remained stable despite competition from the University of Pennsylvania, which began to accept women at the close of World War I.

The immediate impact of the closing of the women's schools was a sharp decline in female enrollments nationwide, from 5 percent in 1899 to 3.5 percent in 1905 and 2.9 percent in 1910. It took women a little more than two decades to regain their numbers in coeducational medical colleges. Furthermore, the 5 percent figure for female medical students in 1890 represents something very different from the 5 percent figure in 1928. In 1890, women were concentrated in a few states and mainly in the women's medical colleges. In 1928 they were more evenly distributed nationally and studying primarily in coeducational schools. (See TABLE 9-3)

Certainly discrimination was at work here. Yet institutional discrimination was erratic, and women fared better in some places than in others. They experienced persistent difficulties in being admitted to Southern medical schools, and Midwest enrollments also remained small. But medical education for women in California, in contrast, was remarkably integrated from 1890 and on into the twentieth century. (See TABLE 9-4.) There was neither a women's medical college nor the familiar clustering of women primarily in one or two schools. Indeed, the proportion of women students in California was roughly a consistent 10 percent—approximately twice the national average.

It is difficult to find adequate explanations for the variations. In the fall of 1917, Dr. Joseph Erlanger, a faculty member at Washington University Medical School in St. Louis, became chairman of a committee appointed to investigate the possibility of admitting women. Erlanger's first act was to poll by letter the opinions of the deans of sixty-eight Class A medical schools on the subject of coeducation. The responses he received—forty-five from schools

TABLE 9-3   Regular Schools, Male-Female Enrollments, 1890–1928

Year	Women Students	Rate of Change	Men Students	Rate of Change	Proportion Women
1890	648	(+37%)	12,873	(+38%)	4.8%
1895	889	(+20%)	17,771	(+14%)	4.8%
1899	1,063	(−21%)	20,338	(+14%)	5%
1905	835	(−31%)	23,177	(−16%)	3.5%
1910	573	(−8%)	19,410	(−21%)	2.9%
1913	526	(NC)	15,393	(−26%)	3.3%
1918	533	(+87%)	11,349	(+38%)	4.5%
1923	995	(−8%)	15,642	(+20%)	6.0%
1928	912	(+16%)	18,734	(+14%)	4.6%

Sources: Records of the Commissioner of Education 1892–1893, 1894–1895, 1904–1905, 1910–1911; *JAMA* "Educational Numbers," 1913, 1918, 1923, 1928

TABLE 9-4   Women in California Medical Schools

	1890	1895	1905	1910	1913	1918
Number of women students	28	53	67	29	47	44
Number of schools open to women	3	3	6	5	5	6
Number of schools	3	3	6	6	6	6
WMC	No	No	No	No	No	No
% of students who are women	10.9%	13.1%	12.1%	9.1%	12.2%	9.5%

Sources: Records of the Commissioner of Education 1892–1893, 1894–1895, 1904–1905, 1910–1911; *JAMA* "Educational numbers" 1913, 1918, 1923, 1928

that admitted women and eleven from schools that did not—provide a fascinating look at the uneven and complex nature of institutional discrimination against women students.

Among the schools that did not admit women, several, like Dartmouth, the University of Vermont, and Jefferson, were so conservative that the question of women students had never even been discussed. Harvard, on the other hand, conceded the fact that women were needed as practitioners, but worried over the necessity of separate anatomy instruction and felt under no obligation to admit females since "there is no great demand and ample opportunity in other schools." Others complained of the expense involved in making provision for women students, and Bowdoin and the Medical College of Virginia wondered if there was sufficient demand among them to justify the change. Still others were "considering" the question, and McGill University, the University of Louisville, and Wake Forest all expected to decide favorably in the near future.[32]

Perhaps more revealing was the variety of responses from the schools that did admit women. Indiana and Yale, having accepted a few, lodged no specific complaints, but suggested that women had trouble meeting high admission standards. The correspondent from Yale editorialized that the "courses in science in the standard women's colleges in this part of the world" had proved inferior.[33] One puzzles at such a comment, considering the fact that Vassar, Bryn Mawr, and Smith had been sending large numbers of well-prepared women to Johns Hopkins for over two decades. Colorado, Howard, and Stanford accepted their women students matter-of-factly, although only Stanford's female enrollments were significantly high. Most enthusiastic was Dr. W. S. Carter, dean of the University of Texas, who wrote that his school has always been co-educational in all of its branches. We have not had a great number of women medical students at any one time but we usually have ten or twelve in the different classes each session. Probably the number has been somewhat greater by reason of the fact that Mr. Brackenridge, a member of the Board of Regents, has been deeply interested in getting women to take up the study of medicine and to giving every encouragement to worthy young women who are ambitious in this direction, he has provided a dormitory and a loan fund for women students in the School of Medicine.

Twenty years ago when I came here I must confess that I was somewhat prejudiced against coeducation for men and women in medical schools. However, after the experience of two decades, I am free to say that I am strongly in favor of this arrangement and believe it to be the very best that can be made. It is seldom that there is any inconvenience to the teaching staff in any way in the matter of giving practical instruction. It is only in genitourinary clinics for men that there is any difficulty and women can easily be excused from parts of that. The tremendous cost of medical education at the present time makes it highly desirable that women should have the privilege of attending medical schools in good standing in different parts of the country and should not be restricted to a limited number of schools for women exclusively. I believe also that the former arrangement, i.e. the coeducation of men and woman in medical schools is the best for the maintenance of high standards of efficiency.

From my own observations the great trouble in the past has been with women, as with men, that the preliminary education required for admission to medical schools has not been sufficient to prepare them for the study of medicine. I am confident from my own observations that most of the failures in this institution were due to that fact, both among the women and men.

I cannot see any valid objection to admitting women and men to all classes in medical schools. Objections that have been raised, and that have come to my attention, have been based upon theoretical considerations and not upon actual experience. There certainly is room for women in many branches of medicine, and I believe that all educational institutions should give them the same opportunity that is extended to men. It is gratifying to see that such institutions as Columbia University and the University of Pennsylvania, which in the past have been ultra conservative in this matter, have at last come to the admission of women to their medical schools.[34]

Yet Dean Carter's unqualified approval of women proved rare. More typical was the response of Dean Thomas McKee at the University of Buffalo, who wrote that the school had always admit-

ted women. Confessing that he personally did not "regard coeducation in medicine with favor" and that his views were "shared
by a majority of the faculty," he nevertheless conceded the admission of women "to be part of the evolutionary development of the
age" and thus kept his opinions to himself. So did the dean of the
University of Pittsburgh, who felt that women should be trained at
their own schools and complained that "we were compelled to
open the doors of this school to women."[35]

Union College, Marquette, Johns Hopkins, and Cornell all tolerated coeducation, but the deans of each school warned that female
admissions should be limited, lest, in the words of M. Polk of
Cornell, the school "would be overwhelmed by women applicants."[36] The comments of J. Whitridge Williams, dean at Johns
Hopkins, are particularly noteworthy. Boasting that Hopkins could
"speak after twenty-five years experience in the matter," he nevertheless cautioned that the proportion of women to men students
should "not exceed one to four." "I am convinced," he continued,
"that the training given in such schools [where female enrollments
were limited] is quite as good as in those to which women are not
admitted." "On the other hand," he concluded, "should the proportion of women greatly increase, I feel that the effect would be
disastrous in that the school would gradually become feminized
and men would desert it in favor of others in which there were
fewer or no women."[37]

Yet even those who were more enthusiastic about women revealed hidden biases. At the University of Pennsylvania, Dean
Allen J. Smith wrote that the admission of women was proceeding
smoothly; indeed "the influence of the women in the classes has
been good." Though some faculty "grumbled" that they could
"not speak as freely to the mixed class," the majority believed "we
have done the proper thing." "The girls are good hard students
and as a class stand high," he observed. Of course they were not as
good as the best male students as a rule, "and, as you would
expect, are better 'book students' than practical workers." From
Minnesota came a similar opinion from Dean E. P. Lyon that
"women have a good effect upon men students and upon teachers." Many of the faculty favored coeducation over separate
schools for women and considered it a "manifest fact that women
physicians from the women's medical colleges were not only poorly
trained by comparison but had such false notions and such sex
limited points of view that they were much less effective in the
profession." He went on to conclude that he believed that "woman's

field in medicine is broadening" and though they would not "for a long time" be equal to men in such fields as major surgery, "there can be no doubt as to their usefulness in the profession."[38]

Finally, from Rush Medical College in Chicago came Dr. John M. Dodson's observation that women had been "no trouble" from "the day of their admission to the present time." Rush had been especially fortunate, the dean felt, "in the high type of women who had sought admission," women, who "have been in every way a credit to themselves and to us." The writer concluded his remarks with a curious paragraph which beautifully characterizes the unconscious prejudices of even women's warmest supporters:

> It will always be true, of course, that the number of women seeking to enter the medical profession will be small. A good many who do enter will be diverted into matrimony and homekeeping either before they finish or soon after graduation. That has happened to ten or twelve of our list of seventy, not counting several who were married before they entered Rush. I have noticed that no matter how superior these students may have been in their college work, nor how keen the interest of an instructor in their future development and accomplishments in medicine lies, they cannot but do otherwise than rejoice when matrimony claims them. For this reason, in my judgment, there cannot be the same interest and satisfaction in the education of women in medicine as one derives from the training of men. At the same time, as long as they are determined to enter the medical profession I feel that they ought to have the very best of opportunities. This I am sure they never could get in a school exclusively devoted to the teaching of women. Our own experience has shown that the instruction of the sexes is perfectly feasible and satisfactory.[39]

In discussing discrimination both institutional variation and regional differences must be factored into the equation. It is entirely possible that such differences may account for women physicians' own contradictory perceptions of the barriers erected against them. When the Woman's Medical College of Chicago closed, Rush Medical College and the University of Chicago showed a compensatory increase in female enrollments for several years thereafter. Consequently, female enrollments in Chicago maintained their pre-1902 levels. Such was not the case, however, in New York City, where Cornell was the only regular medical school open to women after 1899. While seventy women from the New York Infirmary entered the school in 1900, only a year later the female enrollment had dropped to twenty-one, and then to ten in 1903.

Although Cornell was ostensibly committed to coeducation, it managed to reduce the number of women students in the entering classes by requiring that women take the first two years of the medical course in Ithaca, while men were free to take them either in Ithaca or in New York City. In Dean Polk's letter to Joseph Erlanger in 1917, he admitted that the policy was deliberately intended to reduce the number of female students.[40] It took almost fifteen years for women to regain a respectable showing at Cornell. And even in the 1930s and 1940s, their numbers, though greater than at other city schools admitting women, remained erratic.

The Erlanger letters merely flesh out the statistics: medical coeducation did not fulfill its promise in the first half of the twentieth century. Well through the 1950s there remained a handful of medical schools that stubbornly refused to admit women.[41] More common were those which, in their reluctance to welcome women, grudgingly allowed them a few places each year in the freshman class—just enough, so the old joke went, to form a dissecting team. Even those schools with substantial female enrollments, such as Johns Hopkins, Cornell, Michigan, and Stanford, were not always able to provide congenial atmospheres for their women students. Discrimination in these schools, of course, remained subtle and often went by unnoticed. Yet the psychological strains of being a merely tolerated minority could often prove unbearable. Particularly difficult was the absence of female faculty role models who could provide support.

The closing of the women's medical schools caused a crucial curtailment of the numbers of women in medicine. Still unaccounted for, however, is the proportionate decline of women in medical schools *even before* the women's medical colleges shut their doors. Though the romance of women with coeducation contributed to the steady loss of *some* female students at these schools, it cannot explain why women's applications to medical school did not increase and keep pace proportionately with men's. Women's perception of the existence of institutional discrimination was certainly a significant factor. Another was that women were forced to cope with coeducation and the upgrading of standards all at once. The increasing costs of a medical education certainly hurt women more than men. Outside of the seven states we have already discussed, one finds a gradual loss of women students over time—seven women at one school, twelve at another, as enrollments for both men and women at medical schools all over the country were being drastically reduced when schools merged or closed their doors. Since the total enrollment of women in these schools were already small, every loss was critical in terms of percentages. Thus, women fell victim disproportionately to the upgrading of standards, while discrimination in coeducational schools—occasionally subtle, at times overt, proved a bitter constant.

Though the relative role of the loss of the women's medical colleges in these matters remains uncertain, one fact remains clear. When these schools closed, female medical educators lost autonomous control of institutions that, at least in the case of Chicago and New York, had been self-supporting and self-directed female communities. A loss of this kind cannot be minimized. Alice Weld Tallant, herself the product of a coeducational school, Johns Hopkins, and for many years professor of obstetrics and gynecology at the Woman's Medical College of Pennsylvania, spoke in 1917 of the contrasts in her own experience. Although she had not noticed much overt discrimination while a student at Hopkins, she claimed that in retrospect the real difficulty was the poverty of female role models. "The point that has always seemed to me the strongest for a separate school," she told her colleagues, "is that in the separate school for women, the women [*sic*] student sees women teaching and women doing the clinical work, women operating, and so on. Until I took my internship I had never seen a woman operate, and I do not think those of you who have had your training in this school can realize what it means never to have seen a woman doing that which to you seems second nature, from your student days. It must be a very great incentive to the student to see what women can do; it is almost inevitable, if you never have seen a woman doing anything, to think she cannot do it quite as well as a man, no matter how strongly you feel in favor of women." Similarly, the surgeon Dr. Clara Raven reminisced in a memorial to Dr. Bertha Van Hoosen on the importance of female role models to her own growth, especially because "my medical and premedical environment was dominated by the men."[42]

And what of the sole surviving woman's college, the Woman's Medical College of Pennsylvania? No discussion of women's medical education after 1900 can ignore its fate. While other women's medical colleges quickly surrendered to rising costs and shrinking enrollments by closing their doors, the Woman's Medical College of Pennsylvania limped along, a dissenter in the ranks. Dr. Caroline Purnell caught the emotional ambience of this effort when she reported as the alumnae's representative on the Board of Corporators to the 43rd annual meeting of the school's alumnae association in 1918. "Some years back," she began, there was quite an unsettled feeling in the minds of many of our graduates whether a small medical college should continue to exist. They were very much unsettled by the reports which were put out by the Carnegie Foundation regarding such radical changes and such high standards with such tremendous expense for every institution of medical learning. Many felt so overwhelmed by that report that they felt it not worth while to try to keep on our feet. At first I was *so* impressed. At that time I was a teacher in this institution. But finally I think I landed on my feet, and I think I landed on the right side. . . . I made up my mind, also, that there was need for the Woman's Medical College of Pennsylvania; just as much need as for Bryn Mawr, Smith or Vassar. I think women of these United States have a right to say how they shall be educated, whether in women's colleges or in coeducational institutions. . . . My experience upon committee has taught me that the day has not yet come for men to yield to us equal ground with them. . . . I think they need us, but they do not see it and therefore do not act. Therefore, I say that women should hold on to their institutions, medical colleges and hospitals. Women are capable of running these institutions. We have demonstrated that, and all we want is work.

Women had become "faint-hearted," Dr. Purnell complained, plagued too often by "words of discouragement . . . or criticism, or of doubt as to the need of our existence." She concluded with a plea to her fellow alumnae to cast aside their fears, realize that the college is now "needed more than ever" by women, and plunge themselves into new fundraising efforts.

Such appeals were standard fare at the alumnae meetings of the Woman's Medical. Despite chronic financial difficulties, and perhaps because of the peculiar slackness on the part of Philadelphia's medical schools to admit women, faculty members and graduates remained decidedly skeptical of the benefits of medical coeducation. For them the struggle was simple: to remain financially afloat *and* maintain respectable educational standards. Lilian Welsh, former president of the Alumnae Association, put it simply in 1912: "That this college stands for an idea," she observed, "will not preserve it; these must be associated with abundant financial resources."[43]

Woman's Medical faced its first financial crisis, a crisis involving its constant efforts to provide proper and abundant clinical material as part of an upgraded teaching curriculum in 1903. No element was more vital to the school's success, and no one understood the problem better than Dean Clara Marshall. Since 1861 the college had been closely connected with the Woman's Hospital, founded by Dean Ann Preston precisely to serve the purposes of clinical education. For about two decades the hospital and college had been practically one institution, but after the new college building was erected in 1875, they gradually moved apart. Aiding in their disengagement was the fact that each institution had its own separate board of trustees. Although the college administration assumed that its own professors would be appointed to the clinical staff at the Woman's Hospital, the college faculty had little direct control over hospital policy. Such a situation boded ill for the future.[44]

Besides its independent management, a second problem posed by the Woman's Hospital was that it did not admit male patients. Thus, students received excellent training in obstetrics, gynecology, and pediatrics; but their knowledge of internal medicine came only from treating women and children. In 1904 the AMA's Council on Medical Education instituted its rating system which required all accredited Class A medical colleges to be associated with a general hospital used for teaching purposes. In 1892 the college had established a small general hospital and dispensary—the Amy S. Barton Dispensary—in Philadelphia's downtown slums, which had provided additional teaching facilities to staff and students. But a decade later the Barton Dispensary was inadequate to meet new standards. Then, in 1903, the Board of Lady Managers of the Woman's Hospital suddenly decided to limit the use of its wards as a teaching facility. In an abrupt move, it refused to appoint to the hospital staff the college faculty's choice—Dr. Edith Cadwallader—as the replacement for Dr. Anna Broomall in the chair of obstetrics. To add insult to injury, not long afterward Dr. Ella B. Everitt, another faculty member, was denied the accustomed privilege of placing her postoperative patients on the hospital's wards.

Correspondence and negotiations dragged on over the next year. But the lady managers were totally unsympathetic to the clinical needs of the college and fiercely jealous of their independence as an institution. In the end, a relationship of half a century could not be salvaged, and in 1904 ties between the college and the hospital were severed.[45]

Almost immediately the college established a temporary hospital of its own by converting a small private house near the school. Next, Dean Marshall launched a campaign to raise funds for a modern structure which could provide the needed clinical material necessary to retain the school's Class A rating. In 1907 the cornerstone of the new building was laid, and six years later—through the tireless fund-raising efforts of alumnae and dedicated supporters—the hospital was completed.

During the crisis over the new hospital two members of the college faculty, Frederick P. Henry and Ella B. Everitt, were asked to explore the possibility of affiliation with another medical school in Philadelphia. Financial problems pressed so acutely that the Board of Corporators felt "the time appears opportune . . . for a comprehenseive statement of the facts bearing on this question."[46] This report was the first written statement by leaders of the college which formally investigated the benefits and liabilities of medical coeducation for all women. The results reaffirmed the importance of a woman's school.

Arguing that there was a "reactive tendency against coeducation in certain universities and colleges where formerly both sexes were admitted," the report gave as an example the closing of the Woman's Medical College of Chicago. The committee explained that the motives that had hitherto induced private men's colleges to admit women had been "largely pecuniary." It was possible, they went on, "that a medical school might be found in this city to admit women students for a sufficient monetary consideration, but that they would be admitted out of regard for the medical education of women, is highly improbable." The college did not have such funds in any event, Henry and Everitt pointed out, and, furthermore, it was doubtful whether such a course would improve women's medical education in any substantial way.

And then came the suggestion that Woman's Medical had more to offer women students than other schools. First, it afforded opportunities for personal and individual instruction—the luxury of smallness. Moreover, its course in obstetrics and diseases of women was "superior" to that of other schools, and "both are branches of prime importance to women physicians." Noting that men enjoyed the choice between separate or coeducational medical schools, the committee wondered why women should not have the same flexibility? Finally, members asked, "What teaching positions are there for women in coeducational schools?" After surveying six medical schools—Tufts, the University of Michigan, Cornell, Johns Hopkins, Rush Medical College, and the University of Texas—the committee found that among 912 teachers, only 27 were female, and these all filled "subordinate positions." "In view of the high valuation placed by men upon teaching opportunities, and the eagerness with which they are sought," the report concluded, "this showing is very significant." Raise an endowment to build a new hospital, not buy women's way into a men's school, urged the committee, and preserve the separate character of the Woman's Medical College.[47]

Though less elaborate than some others which would be produced in the future in various forms, this report stated a position that remained identified with the Woman's Medical College of Pennsylvania for the next sixty years. Each time the school faced a financial crisis, similar arguments were mustered in support of preserving a separate college for women. For a core of stubborn women and their supporters, such reasoning remained convincing.

Of course large and small crises continued to plague the school. In 1904 the college applied for state aid for the first time, petitioning the legislature for $100,000 to help defray the costs of the new hospital. After a considerable delay, the Board of Public Charities awarded only $12,500 a year for two consecutive years. Although in the future the school's state funding was increased slightly, it was never adequate.[48]

Another chronic problem was the need to upgrade the laboratories. Despite contrary trends in medical education, the college often toyed with the idea of becoming a first-rate teaching facility, while letting research lag behind. Soon after Sarah J. Morris joined the faculty in 1931 to do tuberculosis research, Dean Tracy asked her whether she thought there was a place for a "good teaching medical school, without adding the burden and expense of research." Morris replied, of course, that the future of medicine *was* research and that Woman's Medical dare not neglect it.[49] The college did its best, but again relative poverty frustrated many plans for improvement.

Despite Abraham Flexner's conclusion that the school's laboratories were "simple, but intelligently equipped and conscientiously used," and that there was "striking evidence of a genuine effort to do the best possible with limited resources," improving the laboratories became a subject of alumnae concern for several years running.[50] In 1911 Professor of Anatomy, Histology and Embryology Herbert H. Cushing put forward a four-part program to upgrade basic science teaching at the school, a program which included supporting full-time salaried instructors and graduate students engaged in full-time research. He explained that he had recently traveled to New York to see if he could induce Flexner to help him get Carnegie Foundation support for the project. Though "Mr. Flexner was courtesy itself," Cushing reported, "he was also adamant. . . . He refused to do anything. . . . He said he could not in conscience . . . because he did not believe in the separate medical education of women. He believed in coeducational medical colleges."[51]

To compound the school's difficulties, in 1912 and 1913 representatives from the Council on Medical Education made several site visits to reconfirm its class "A" rating. On 14 February 1913, Dr. N. P. Colwell, Secretary of the Council, wrote a long letter to the dean "showing the lines along which improvements could be made to the greatest advantage." Speaking to the alumnae, Dean Marshall summed up Colwell's suggestions with the observation, "The reply demonstrated what we already knew, that in order to keep in Class A, to say nothing of reaching Class A+, we need money and need it now."[52]

More specifically, entrance requirements needed to be raised from the minimum of a high school diploma to two years of college, more full-time salaried professors needed to be added to the faculty, more clinical material needed to be secured, laboratory equipment needed updating, and, finally, "medical research has not been developed as largely as obtains in the majority of Class A colleges." On this point Colwell editorialized that "one of the chief functions of the modern medical school is to add its quota to the world's knowledge of medicine and by fulfilling this function it is also in better position to carry out the other two functions, namely, that of training medical students and of giving the best treatment to such patients as may come under its care."[53]

In response, and as usual, the alumnae rallied around the dean. A campaign committee which was launched in 1911 increased its activity until it eventually collected $200,000 for the endowment fund. Most of the money came from female givers, who tended to give in much smaller amounts than their male counterparts. Indeed, the perpetual poverty of Woman's Medical eloquently demonstrates the increasing inadequacy of female philanthropy to meet twentieth century needs. Clara Hammond-McGuigan reminded her fellow alumnae of just this fact in 1913 when she observed, "I think we will all have to bear in mind that the graduates of Princeton are in very different circumstances from our graduates. A great many of them are businessmen, making not thousands of dollars, but millions. You must therefore not expect as much from our graduates."[54]

When Clara Marshall retired in 1917, Martha Tracy, a brilliant young physiological chemist who had worked with Mendel at Yale and had been since 1913 professor of physiological chemistry at the College, took her place. Tracy was a "modern" physician, well-trained in basic science and generally committed to expanding the school's role in both clinical and pure research. But she, too, was fated to steer the school through several monetary crises, including one in 1935 which threatened to remove the college from the "acceptable" list prepared by the Council on Medical Education.[55]

And yet, whatever its failings, the Woman's Medical College of Pennsylvania did give Class A medical training to several generations of women physicians. Between 1920 and 1968, when it admitted men for the first time, the school graduated between 20 and 50 women a year—between one-third and one-fifth of all women graduates. It developed distinguished programs in preventive medicine, gynecology, and obstetrics. Most important, it offered women the opportunity to study in an atmosphere that was receptive to their needs, an atmosphere in which their role models could be other women, an atmosphere in which women, and not men, were the majority. Certainly for many women physicians, the college's separatism remained suspect. But the institution's history has yet to be thoroughly explored, while the benefits of separatism as a strategy of women professionals in the early twentieth century still needs careful evaluation.[56]

The difficulties of the Woman's Medical College and the closing of the other women's schools combined to have a negative effect on female enrollments in medical school after 1900. But it is also likely that middle-class women, for a variety of reasons, found it less desirable to study medicine. The impact of these shifting career choices also must be assessed.

For example, the late nineteenth-century scientific revolution in therapeutics disarmed the arguments that earlier women physicians had used in support of female medical education. Whereas the nineteenth-century physician approached a patient with a predisposition to physiological holism, twentieth-century therapeutics transformed the doctor into a specialist whose knowledge encompassed some specific symptom or some discrete portion of the patient's body. Treatment understandably became fragmented; total patient "care" was increasingly dissociated from the specialist's concerns as he busied himself with patient "cure."[57]

Institutional developments in the early twentieth century reflected the gradual fragmentation in health care delivery. Public health nurses replaced the women interns who had defiantly entered the slums to teach the poor how to be well. In their effort to professionalize and claim nursing for women, self-conscious leaders in the field played an important part in shifting the so-called feminine and nurturing aspects of medical care from the doctor to the nurse. In 1913, while struggling to define an independent role for the tuberculosis nurse, Elizabeth Gregg, superintendent of nurses for the New York City Health Department, wrote:

> Physicians have not the time, neither is it born in many [doctors] to devote themselves to the detail that requires the patient, painstaking effort of a woman; and this detail tends to reveal the very causes or the contributing factors of tuberculosis more than in any other disease; so that the nurse, with her knowledge of home conditions and the family's principles of living, and with her instinctive woman's insight into the causes of trouble, is the physician's right hand.[58]

As long as medical practice remained more a matter of "art" than "science," women found themselves drawn to the work and armed with compelling reasons for claiming it as their own. In contrast, the organization and practice of medicine after 1900 moved from the intimacy of the home to the public arena and impersonal setting of the hospital. While it is certainly true that it became increasingly more difficult for a woman to be admitted to a first-rate school, it also seems possible to speculate that fewer woman were trying to do so.

What, then, were women doing who might otherwise have been applying to medical schools? Many chose nursing in these years. Between 1880 and 1900 the number of nurses increased from 15,601 to 120,000.[59] Another category of health workers, "physicians and surgeons attendants," showed an 86 percent increase in the census from 1910 to 1920. But because nursing generally attracted women from a different class background than that of women physicians, the declining number of women doctors after 1910 cannot be explained by the expansion of nursing alone. Statistics from these years indicate rather that social work and graduate school diverted some women's interests from medicine.

The years between 1890 and 1918 reveal sharp increases in the number of women doing graduate work. The percentage of female graduate students rose from 10.2 of all graduate students in 1890 to 41.0 in 1918. In terms of absolute numbers, this change represented a twentyfold increase, while the number of men attending graduate school increased only fivefold. After 1910, the census data suggest that many of these women were using their degrees in the new helping professions. In that year women made up about 56 percent of the welfare workers; ten years later their absolute numbers had increased almost 200 percent. In 1910 women comprised 30 percent of the "keepers of charitable institutions"; by 1920 that percentage had increased to 38 percent. Again, the increase in actual numbers is impressive, from 2,250 in 1910 to 4,900 in 1920. Unfortunately, the census information cannot indicate what percentage of the total body of educated women were choosing welfare work and its allied fields. Nevertheless, one can hypothesize that there is a distinct connection between the rising numbers of women with advanced degrees and the sharp increase in the number of women professionals in these "feminized" occupations.[60]

The census data also suggest that other cultural factors were at work. The twentieth century has witnessed unmistakable shifts in the primacy of some essential nineteenth-century values. Most notable among those changes have been the altered expectations surrounding the home, women, and family life. A prominent feature of Victorian culture was the exaltation of motherhood through the cult of domesticity. The high status afforded motherhood followed logically from the conviction that mothers were the primary agents for the transmission of culture. Yet, despite feminists' glorification of motherhood, they had expressed a particular personal disdain for the patriarchal Victorian family. In the nineteenth century, growing numbers of educated and professional women rejected marriage in favor of the pursuit of meaningful work. Opponents of higher education for women were fond of pointing out that college women married less frequently and had fewer children than did more ordinary women, and, indeed, statistics for the years between 1880 and 1920 support these claims.[61]

In the twentieth century, however, the image of woman-as-mother gradually gave way to the image of woman-as-mate. The social and economic changes in the decades before World War I created more positive attitudes toward pleasure, individual self-fulfillment, sexuality, and women's work.[62] Possibly because of this altered climate, college-educated women and professional women did not continue to reject marriage with the vehemence that they had earlier. The proportion of professional women who married, for example, doubled from 12.2 percent in 1910 to 24.7 percent in 1930.[63] Joyce Antler has convincingly argued that the early twentieth century produced a new kind of feminism, previously found only among a small minority of ninteenth-century women activists. These women chose not to shun marriage but to strive instead to "work out the large issues of feminism on an individual basis." Only if we acknowledge the existence of this brand of feminism, which Antler labels "feminism-as-life-process," can we "rescue from the lost generation of feminist endeavor after 1920 some of the women whose lives might properly be called 'feminist.' "[64]

For these women the central issue was the need to balance professional, political, or other activities with marriage and family. In their own lives, they struggled to "work out that balance of interests between the private and public [in this case, between marriage and career] that would allow them to achieve the self-determination and autonomy that they posited as their highest goal." Although more women physicians were married than other women professionals, this fact is not incompatible with the observation that it became increasingly more difficult for women who were doctors to manage both a career and family life in the high-powered world of twentieth-century medical practice. Women physicians in the twentieth century who did choose to do so were a small, exceptional, and highly motivated group, and it is quite likely that they were a different kind of woman from both their nineteenth-century counterparts and their twentieth-century sisters who chose less demanding careers. One interesting statistical confirmation of this fact is that nationally women were slightly underrepresented in Class B and C institutions, suggesting that women physicians were perhaps brighter and more motivated than many of their male colleagues. In the state of Illinois in 1913, for example, at a time when Northwestern, an A+ institution, was not even accepting women, over 51 percent of the women students were in A or A+ schools, compared with only 48 percent of the men.[65] (See table 9-5)

That these highly motivated women would continue to commit themselves to marriage was clear. The reminiscences of Bessie L. Moses about her days at Johns Hopkins and an encounter with Florence Sabin make this point particularly eloquently. Moses, who entered Hopkins in 1918, remembered Sabin as a "superb teacher and lecturer." But for a role model, the young medical student decided to look elsewhere, explaining:

TABLE 9-5   Men and Women in Illinois Medical Schools, 1913

Schools	# of men	% of total	# of women	% of total
Class "A" or "A+" (3)	1090	48.3%	63	51.6%
Class "B" (2)	991	43.9%	46	37.7%
Class "C" (1)	177	7.8%	13	10.7%

Source: JAMA "Educational Number" 1913.

My most personal association with Dr. Sabin occurred on the street car when we frequently rode over to the Medical School together. She got on the car after I did, and it was about at twenty minute ride from there to the Medical School. What she repeatedly tried to impress upon me was this idea—that no matter what happened in a woman's personal life, she should never let it interfere with her medical career. I was a young medical student at the time, and I listened attentively to her advice. She had apparently sacrificed all of her personal social relationships for her work, and for her it had apparently been a completely satisfying life. My ideas were different. I felt, and still feel, that a woman in any profession should, of course, try to do her best and achieve her ambitions, but to me the woman comes first and the profession second.

Dr. Sabin was a great feminist and had experienced the difficult struggle which was common for all women in the medical field at that time. This, of course, colored her attitude. She cared nothing for dress or personal appearance. She seemed remote in her relationships and always appeared a little impatient, as though she were wasting time unless she was working. Dr. Sabin's eminence in the field of science and medicine certainly proved that her philosophy of life for herself paid off."[66]

Bessie Moses rejected Sabin's exclusive commitment to her work, but she did not reject medicine. She married and practiced her profession with equal dedication to both. Indeed, she and many like her worked to ensure that marriage would not stand in the way of their careers. That effort alone, only partially successful, guaranteed that women physicians' numbers would remain small. For in the final analysis, they would fall victim to the social dictates of a culture still characterized by extreme sex stereotyping. The vigorous, detached, almost godlike figure of the twentieth-century physician—a product of the triumph of scientific medicine—kept all but the most determined of them from challenging cultural barriers. In the first decades of the twentieth century, women doctors would continue to develop strategies to cope with these changes and would strive to ensure for themselves a place in the professional world of modern medicine. Such strategies often bore bitter fruit.

CHAPTER 10

The Emergence of Social Medicine: Women's Work in the Profession

While the needs and interest of women physicians are inseparable from those of men, they are by no means identical; and we earnestly hope and believe that in all questions of family life, with sanitary, moral and social problems, they will raise the tone, widen the perception and alter the attitude of the profession in general, so as to make it respond more perfectly to the needs of society, and exert a high power for good in all directions. If this be realized, it will be seen that the work of women is absolutely essential and of ever increasing importance and the outlook for this in every respect most helpful.

> William H. Welch, *Women's Medical Journal*, October 1913.

The woman's movement is but a part of the evolving energy that is developing the human race. We cannot stay it if we would; we are an integral part of it.

> Margaret Colby, M.D., President of the Iowa State Society of Medical Women, July 1902.

In November 1915 a number of prominent women physicians in Chicago gathered together at a banquet organized to celebrate the fiftieth anniversary of the founding of the Mary Thompson Hospital. After the toasts and speeches praising the achievements of women physicians, Mrs. George Bass, ex-president of the Chicago women's club and a longtime trustee of the hospital, took the podium. Her words, unlike many which had been spoken that night, reflected anger and disappointment at the difficulties women physicians were having gaining proper recognition from their professional brethren. Her advice was to use separatism as a strategy: "Appreciating your inner reluctance to segregating yourselves in any way from the body of your profession," she began, "I yet ask, what have they done for you? The time is doubtless long past when they actively opposed your entrance into the profession, or openly flouted you on your way," she conceded. "But no propaganda has ever emanated from them voicing to the public your place in the profession and your especial value to the community. There has been no cordial offering of hospital and research privileges and no recognition upon boards of authority. I do not believe," she concluded, "that this is oversight."[1]

As Mrs. Bass's words suggest, women physicians continued to be plagued by conflicts between separatism and assimilation, and the professional world of twentieth-century medicine exacerbated rather than minimized tensions between the two postures. They struggled first with the problem of the continuing legitimacy of their separate organizations and institutions. Did these help or hinder the cause? Did efforts to attract women physicians to their own associations result in the inferior duplication of services they could already receive from professional organizations already in existence? Did a separate medical college for women strengthen or weaken women's position in the larger professional arena? And what of women's role in medicine itself? Did they belong in all specialties, or just those that dealt more directly with women, children and family, and community problems? The rise of modern medicine did not lay to rest the pressing issues of the nineteenth century concerning women physicians, but merely reformulated them in a different and more modern context.

Certainly the idea that women physicians needed their own organizations was not new. In the 1890s, as local women's medical societies flourished, women physicians told themselves that "the supreme force of the present age is organized effort" and that "we need our medical societies . . . for the purpose of combining our thoughts and efforts for the betterment of our own conditions and to enlarge the field of our own usefulness." "Let not the woman who enters the medical profession think for a moment," added Margaret E. Colby in her presidential address to the Iowa Society of Medical Women in 1902, "[that] she is going to have smooth sailing." Separate organizations, agreed the editor of the *Medical Woman's Journal,* offered "the power of united instead of single influence."[2]

Women physicians justified the strengthening of separate organizations in the new century on several grounds. First, they saw organized, constant pressure and disclosure of discrimination as a means to preserve their gains and to widen medical opportunities for women. In this spirit the *Woman's Medical Journal* kept them abreast of new hospital opportunities, the opening of medical schools to women, and professional achievements. Periodic reports delineating postdoctoral medical programs, possibilities for residencies, the numbers of women in medicine and their distribution in the specialties provided a good deal of information on the progress of the woman physician in the opening decades of the new century.[3]

Having their own journal also gave women a chance to publish. Bertha Van Hoosen, a prominent surgeon in Chicago who completed a number of pioneering clinical studies on the use of "twilight sleep" in childbirth, bitterly remembered her own rejections from the *Journal of the American Medical Association.* A graduate of Michigan, she admitted that sex discrimination had meant little to her until she had begun to practice medicine. Indeed, in the beginning she had even refused to subscribe to the *Woman's Medical Journal.* But when her first article was returned from *JAMA* "with a none too gracious note," she changed her mind. Despite her prominence as a surgeon, *JAMA* never published one of her papers, and she confessed in later years that she kept "a box filled with 'Jilts from the *Journal*' letters."[4]

Similarly, the Woman's Medical College of Pennsylvania justified its own existence on the grounds that it made available to many women a chance to study medicine that they otherwise would not have had. As Ellen C. Potter, a graduate of the school in 1903 and for a long time commissioner of health for the state of Pennsylvania, observed, "So many of us of that generation would never have been able to enter a medical school if it had not been for W.M.C." Even in the early years of the new century doubts lingered in the minds of many that coeducation would offer the promised rewards, and some felt, along with Eliza Root, that coeducation in medicine was "serving a term of probation." It remained to be seen, Root cautioned, whether or not women were relegating themselves to "a long and severe apprenticeship in which promotion will be painfully slow and uncertain." The separate college for women, she claimed, "still has work to do."[5]

Over and over again supporters of separate education pointed to the importance of female role models. Many women physicians, like Alice Weld Tallant, the product of a superior coeducational school, saw the significance of female role models only after they observed a woman in a position of authority for the first time. After Tallant's experience in her internship observing competent women surgeons, she understood as she never had before the role of the Woman's Medical College in providing psychological incentives to female students. In 1927 Bertha Van Hoosen reaffirmed

Tallant's observations by publishing an article in the *Medical Woman's Journal* demonstrating that all-male faculties tended to inhibit women's professional aspirations, especially in fields increasingly defined as "male preserves." Investigating the educational histories of the 51 female fellows of the American College of Surgeons, she discovered that 50 percent of them were graduated from a woman's medical college, while an additional 25 percent served internships in hospitals staffed entirely by women. Van Hoosen concluded that considerable thought should be given to the "psychological effect of being trained by women surgeons and physicians."[6]

Some were thus convinced that separate institutions at the very least lessened the corroding effects of discrimination. Others felt that separate institutions could also preserve and strengthen female "spheres of influence" within the profession as a whole, thus making an impact in a larger arena—that of medical practice. This argument merely updated Elizabeth Blackwell's contention that women had special qualities to bring to the profession, and it remained a powerful weapon in women physicians' arsenal, finding novel modes of articulation in the twentieth century.

In an address to the alumnae of the Woman's Medical College in 1912, for example, President Eleanor C. Jones suggested that co-education would never solve women's needs. "In these co-educational schools," she emphasized, "the main purpose is, of course, to fit men for the practice of medicine, and the courses have been developed to fill these masculine needs." For Jones it was decidedly a drawback that these schools subjected women to precisely the same courses of preparation as the men. The result was physicians who were "trained to carry on afterward precisely the same kind of work as men, in the same way. . . . As a consequence women in the medical profession have in a measure entered into competition with men on ground already occupied, and have, perforce adopted their methods and aims."[7] For women like Jones, nothing could be more wrongheaded than teaching women professionals to behave exactly like their male colleagues.

One important social development that gave particular credence to this point of view was the reemergence of liberal reform and the increasing visibility and influence of women reformers in the years after 1900. So conspicuous were women and women's concerns in reform activity in the decades between 1900 and roughly 1930 that many saw this period as the culmination of the long struggle by social feminists to make their impact felt in the public sphere. "As some one has said," quipped Dr. Jones, "the twentieth century has witnessed a glorious birth, and it is a girl!" New circumstances meant that women physicians too must give special thought to their own role in social change: "It is becoming recognized," she concluded, "that society needs the special feminine qualities nearly as much outside the home as in it, and it is probable that soon women can reckon on a more genuine appreciation of their special feminine gifts. When this time arrives, will they not naturally endeavor to secure a training that will emphasize their special capabilities along their own lines?" Renewed interest in the child and the family prompted Dr. Jones, like Elizabeth Blackwell before her, to conclude that it was more "practical" than ever for a woman's medical school to exist that could offer a curriculum "in the interest of women alone, that is, a curriculum which intended primarily to fit women for the practice of medicine in whatsoever way their needs in the future might demand."[8]

The difference between Blackwell and her successors was at once profound and insignificant. On the one hand, these were women who were trained in scientific medicine, and who generally accepted its implications both for the reform of medical education and for changes in practice. Consequently, they were less critical than was Blackwell, the product of another time, of the "modern" medical model, which Blackwell had equated with the victory of the male principle over the female—the triumph of "science" over "intuition." On the other hand, they still adhered to a vision of their own role that incorporated the idea of female uniqueness. Though fewer and fewer of them grounded their sense of this difference in biology, as the century progressed, many women physicians still expected that women's concerns in medicine would not be the same as men's.

One eloquent proponent of this point of view was Lilian Welsh, a graduate of the Woman's Medical College of Pennsylvania in 1889, who had spent a year abroad studying bacteriology and who had originally planned a career in research. Thwarted in these plans by the lack of opportunity, Welsh nevertheless kept eagerly abreast of scientific developments in medicine, maintaining a warm personal and professional relationship with Florence Sabin. She remained a loyal alumna of Woman's Medical, attending the yearly alumnae meetings and taking an enthusiastic interest in the fate of the school. For several years she represented the alumnae on the Board of Corporators. One can follow her initial depression regarding the fate of the school in her comments at the yearly alumnae meetings after 1900. Deeply worried about a shrinking endowment and the difficulty of keeping pace with the advancing standards of medical education, she came to doubt whether the college could be of service in any way to woman physicians. "Unless it can take its place once more with really first class schools," she warned, "its existence might even be detrimental to the position of women in medicine."[9]

In September 1911, Welsh had an experience that dramatically altered her increasingly doubtful attitude about the future of the college. She attended the International Congress for the Prevention of Infant Mortality as a representative from the United States. In Berlin she heard a great deal about European efforts to reduce infant and maternal mortality rates. There, the importance of modern instruction in pediatrics and obstetrics was repeatedly emphasized. While Sweden outshone all the other European countries in its boast of "one of the lowest rates of infant mortality in the world because it made pediatrics a distinct department of medicine over thirty five years ago," the United States with its shockingly high rates of mortality and its abysmal record on the teaching of obstetrics and pediatrics in the medical schools had been "dismissed" by all the delegates "with a word of amusement." Welsh's shame at the failings of her country's medical profession gave birth to an idea: The Woman's Medical must capitalize on the interest of progressive reformers in these subjects.

> In all the present day discussion in the feminist movement the loudest cry from the "anti" is "The function of women is to bear and rear children!" While the "pros" march proudly under the banner, "We prepare children for the world, let us prepare the world for our children!" Is it not then fitting that a well-established medical college, devoted to the medical education of women, should take a new lease on life in retaining and establishing leadership in teaching these two branches of medicine which especially concern women—obstetrics and pediatrics? I believe no pleas for increased endowment would receive greater consideration from a contributing public, than the plea that a woman's college desires to take advanced standing in teaching these two subjects, now inadequately taught in most of the schools of our country.

Trends in medicine, too, were responding to progressive ideology, and a greater emphasis on preventive medicine—an area of interest to women in the past—appeared inevitable to Welsh:

> Both research and social medicine today are opening up fields of remunerative employment, that are not only attractive to women, but that particularly need the services of women medically trained. The

field of medicine, both curative and preventive then, we may say, presents some problems that are essentially the problems of women, and for their solution special training for women students should be provided. Where can such training be better given than in a School of Medicine for Women . . . ? In my vision I see . . . a school of medicine designed especially to meet the needs of women—a school that shall primarily be a first class medical school, providing a thorough education in the fundamental medical sciences, but which shall place special emphasis on teaching obstetrics and pediatrics, and shall in addition provide adequate and special training for research, and for service in preventive medicine along those lines which women may best interpret. This school will proudly bear the inscription:[10]

The Woman's Medical College of Pennsylvania
Trains
Properly Qualified Women
for

Research in Laboratories and Institutions	Practice Especially among Women and Children	Preventive Medicine as Health Officers Teachers of Hygiene
		Social Workers

While presenting these ideas to the alumnae association in 1912, Welsh discovered that many women shared her vision. Clara T. Dercum agreed that "there certainly is a need for training women in certain lines. We do not want to be trained exactly as men. We want the same foundations in research work, etc., but when it comes to the practical application of our knowledge, we want to do it in a woman's way." Eleanor Jones, of course, concurred, speculating that perhaps the reason medicine had ceased to draw "to itself a due proportion of the finest women in the community" had something to do with the fact that scientific medicine was no longer offering them "up to the present time, just that which best satisfy their intellectual and spiritual needs. Women are so constituted," she felt, "that they can not do their work along just the same lines as men."[11]

In keeping with the suggestions of Welsh and others, the Woman's Medical College mounted a publicity campaign that emphasized its ability to meet the special educational needs of women physicians. Combined with the campaign itself was an effort to build its offerings in obstetrics, gynecology, and pediatrics. By 1915 its program, while meeting the AMA standards in terms of teaching hours in all subjects, exceeded by almost double the amount of time devoted to preparation in obstetrics and gynecology, well surpassing the programs of schools like Cornell, the University of Michigan, and the University of Illinois. As Mary Sutton Macy observed in the *Woman's Medical Journal,* "The Woman's Medical College of Pennsylvania surpasses by far all the other colleges of the selected group in the time devoted to gynecology and obstetrics."[12] In this manner the school walked a thin line between finding a convincing rationale for its continued existence without compromising the scientific standards that had become the hallmark of modern medicine. Judging from the support it received from various quarters during its periodic bouts with financial difficulties, such a strategy achieved for the college a measure of success. It remained in respectable existence as an exclusively woman's school for another half century.[13]

And yet, despite the extraordinary power of the Blackwellian tradition, women physicians in the twentieth century understandably displayed much more ambivalence toward separatism as either an ideology or a strategy. Some of this ambivalence can be detected even on the pages of the *Woman's Medical Journal,* which often took extraordinary pains to explain that its position was not segregationist. In a curious editorial in 1909, for example, Margaret Cleaves rejected "the exploitation of women physicians as a separate and distinct labor from the rest of the profession," declaring that "science knows no sex and should know none." The function of the *Woman's Medical Journal,* she wrote, "should be for the advancement of medical science without relationship to sex." And yet Cleaves felt the need to conclude her article by staking out claims for women doctors who "have shown themselves peculiarly fit" for "scientific research, treatment of the insane, social purity work and preventive medicine." A year later another editorial tackled the issue again. "We cannot state too emphatically," wrote the editors in 1910, "that we are unalterably opposed to the segregation of women physicians or of their work, since in medicine all are physicians first, women and men afterward." But once again the editors concluded with a gentle reminder to readers that "women cannot work harmoniously with men until they learn to work harmoniously with each other," and that because of discrimination in hospital appointments and academic departments "the needs of the woman in the medical profession today are somewhat different and more urgent than those of the man."[14]

The care with which the *Journal* dealt with the issue of separatism suggests that it aroused negative responses from a number of women physicians. And, indeed, younger generations of women who had come of age with the triumph of coeducation were understandably suspicious of the idea of women keeping to themselves. A poignant illustration of the shift in attitude can be found in a curious exchange which took place among the alumnae of the WMCP at their annual meeting of 1892. One of the members raised the question as to whether in the future the annual alumnae dinner should continue to be restricted to women. A debate ensued that demonstrates that for these women, the issue was not a simple one. Mary Putnam Jacobi, always suspicious of a certain kind of professional separatism, also understood women's need to gain professional self-confidence through their own organizations, and opposed the idea, suggesting with great insight that "we are not yet sufficiently familiarized with the business to invite critics from the specially dinner-giving and speech-making sex." Calista V. Luther agreed, feeling that "at present I believe we had better keep to ourselves." But many felt that inviting men would make the entire organization look more profesional. "I am very anxious," dissented Dr. Sarah Weintraub, "that we should have representative men of the city . . ." to "add to the standing of the Alumnae. . . . I think we keep to ourselves too much. If we could have some of the men who are interested and of influence," she added, "it would be a great advantage." And Dr. H. W. B. Carter confessed, "I know ladies, that we old ones do not care so much about having the gentlemen, but the younger ones do."[15]

With the achievement of coeducation after the turn of the century, militant separatism appeared to many to threaten the possibility that men would welcome women colleagues as equals. The *Woman's Medical Journal* admitted that "there has been among some the impression that united action on the part of medical women, would create a feeling of exclusion" which would result in "a change in the existing pleasant relationship" between men and women doctors.[16] It seemed to a younger generation that the battle over equal intelligence had ended, and they lacked the pioneer determination of their elders because in fact significant advances had been made. Consequently, many women rejected formal contacts with professional women's associations. Nowhere was this ambivalence played out more powerfully than in the history of the American Medical Women's Association.

The Medical Women's National Association (later changed to the American Medical Women's Association) was founded by a core of active feminists who were tired of their marginality within the profession and women physicians' weak group consciousness. A small gathering, including Drs. Marion Craig Potter, Martha Whelpton, Bertha Van Hoosen, and Mary Bates met with Mrs. George Bass, then president of both the Chicago Women's Club and the Board of Trustees of the Mary Thompson Hospital, in the offices of the Women's Club one evening in November 1915. After a select committee drew up a constitution and bylaws for the embryonic organization, the Medical Women's National Association was born, boasting a slate of officers including Dr. Bertha Van Hoosen, president; Eliza Mosher, honorary president; Marion C. Potter, first vice president; Mary Bates, second vice president; Mary McLean, third vice president; Martha Whelpton, secretary-treasurer; and Dr. Margaret Rockhill, the loyal editor of the *Woman's Medical Journal,* corresponding secretary.

Building on the custom established in 1908 of holding a banquet for women physicians at the yearly AMA meetings, the first regular meeting of the new organization took place a year later in Detroit, in conjunction with the meetings of the AMA. There, the group dedicated itself to advancing the cause of medical women, and Eliza Mosher gave a rousing address which "so thrilled the audience with her Great Personality and high ideals of love and service for other women that those present felt that indeed this National Association was consecrated to the highest service for medical women."[17] The group made the *Woman's Medical Journal* its official publication, and later published its own *Bulletin.*

In May 1916 the *Woman's Medical Journal* published one of several editorials explaining the philosophy of the new organization. Careful not to offend the assimilationists, the title read, "Amalgamation, Not Segregation." "The woman physician probably finds less restriction to her activities in the city of Chicago than in any other city in the United States," the *Journal* began.

Nevertheless, it is a fact that in that city of more than one hundred hospitals . . . there are two hospitals only whose doors are open to women internes.

The woman physician is admitted, and usually welcomed, to nearly all the State and County Societies in the United States; still, we know of no Gynecological or Obstetrical Society, national or local, which opens its membership to women.

If the women medical students desire to investigate the causes for their exclusion from these various hospitals, should the term "segregation" be applied to the young women, or to the hospitals excluding them?

If the women who are specializing in gynecology and obstetrics endeavor to overcome the conditions which prevent their admission into national or local gynecological and obstetrical societies, will the term "segregation" belong to them or to the societies excluding them?

The remedy for segregation is *organization*. Organization is the guiding star of the Twentieth Century, and leads on to Liberty, Equality, and Fraternity. Organization of women outside of the profession will be equally effective and will hasten the day when it can be truthfully said, "There is no sex in Medicine."[18]

During the next year the new president of the Medical Women's National Association created a number of important committees—on Public Health, Race Betterment, and Medical Opportunities for Women, for example—which would take liberal positions on social issues throughout the 1920s. However, the group's immediate concern quickly became war work. Interestingly enough, it was probably the ambivalent response of the United States government to women physicians' desire to aid in the war effort that virtually guaranteed the future existence of the organization.

Torn between their "professionalism" and the real attractions of their own organization, many women physicians withheld support from the National. In fact, condemnatory petitions were immediately circulated in response to its establishment, with opposition particularly strong on the West Coast. Perhaps California's uncharacteristically positive record on the admission of women to medical school accounted for the negative response of its women physicians, but, whatever the cause, disapproval of a separate organization remained strong. Then, shortly after the entrance of the United States into World War I, the surgeon general, who had been inundated with applications from thousands of patriotic women doctors, refused to commission them in the army. Almost overnight, doubts about the usefulness of a separate organization disappeared, and women from all over the country united behind Van Hoosen's efforts to challenge the surgeon general's humiliating policy. Though efforts to gain commissions for women failed, the National did create its own War Service Committee, later retitled American Women's Hospitals. One of the most successful arms of the National, this committee sent hundreds of women physicians overseas for active duty in war and postwar relief during the four major wars of the twentieth century. American Women's Hospitals still funds rural and urban clinics for the benefit of the poor and needy in Asia and Latin America.[19]

And yet, as war enthusiasm waned, so did the interest of many women physicians in the National. Prominent women, such as Florence Sabin and Alice Hamilton, maintained strong and close contacts with other women physicians, but kept aloof from separate organizations. Hamilton was always pleased to speak to the National on issues of concern to her, especially the importance of protective legislation for women and her opposition to the Equal Rights Amendment. In her private correspondence, too, she occasionally exhibited concern for "the status of women in our profession." Her primary interests always lay elsewhere, however, and not with women physicians as a group. Typically, she once declined to write a review of Kate Campbell Hurd-Mead's history of women physicians, saying, "I am a poor feminist when it comes to magnifying the achievements of women."[20]

Sabin harbored even stronger feelings on the issue of separatism, though, unless asked, she kept her opinions very much to herself. She never publicly denigrated women's institutions, and once "mildly chided" a female Hopkins student for not displaying enough respect for the Woman's Medical College of Pennsylvania. In 1922 she gave the commencement address at the women's school. Yet in 1936 she refused to allow her name to be added to a committee of supporters of the College as a fund-raising measure because she confessed that she was "sceptical as to the necessity and the wisdom of maintaining a medical school by and for women at this time." And though she maintained warm relationships with both Bertha Van Hoosen and Kate Campbell Hurd-Mead, each extremely active in the Medical Women's National Association, she declined to allow either of them to pull her in. She even shared with them her private skepticism about the necessity of the organization, writing to Mead in 1935:

> I still feel very strongly that the position which the women in the scientific branches have taken, that of joining their professional organizations and taking full part in them, is a much stronger position than could be filled by any separate organization of women. As I go to various scientific meetings and hear women read papers in the major organizations and compare that work with that of the few meetings of the Medical Women's Association that I have attended from time to time here in New York, I feel quite confident that to cast one's interest into the medical profession accomplishes much more for women than the separate and, as they seem to be, feebler organizations.[21]

Younger generations of women physicians were even more suspicious than Sabin of what they perceived as feminist militancy among the members of the National. Many shared the sentiments of Ethel Walker, a pediatric resident of Johns Hopkins Hospital, who coolly explained to Bertha Van Hoosen her reasons for declining to join the organization:

> I am strongly opposed to any organization or individual's attitude which sets women apart from men . . . instead of teaching them to lose themselves in their profession. . . . In the early days of women in medicine they no doubt had to band together, but now in most sections of the country if not all the quicker the woman physician can forget any feeling that she is in a class apart from her men colleagues the happier she will be and the better she and they will get along. In medical school and interne days I have seen it happen time and time again that the girls who were totally unconscious of any difference between themselves and their men confreres and who mingled with them on exactly the same footing achieved a professional equality and friendship which was entirely denied to the women who were always huddled together with other women and who continually made it plain to everybody that they were different and knew they were different. In my experience it has been the former group who did well in their profession . . . whereas the other group of women's women . . . seldom advanced.[22]

Coupled with the National's problems over women physicians' ideological diversity was the fact that some women were simply not joiners. In an effort not to appear in competition with the American Medical Association, the MWNA deliberately required that all members belong to the AMA's constituent county and state societies. When only 48 percent of medical women were AMA members compared to 60 percent of the men, it meant that even fewer would belong to the women's organization. Membership committees complained that women were too involved in practices to show much interest. Typical were the excuses of Rosemary Shoemaker, M.D., who wrote in 1939 that she had just opened an office in Des Moines and was still waiting for her first patient. "I think I should like to wait before requesting active membership until I see how my practice develops." Other women complained of the pull of family ties. Jane Sands Robb explained that "for the last seven years, I haven't been a member of anything." Her husband was ill, had convalesced, and then decided to study medicine. She had two children. "These responsibilities have been so great," she wrote apologetically, "that it has been necesary for me to stop all my affiliations. The only exception has been the American Physiological Society. . . . It hurts my pride to make this explanation and I trust you will regard it as a personal communication."[23]

Thus, for many different reasons, only the most militant and feminist women joined the American Medical Women's Association after 1915. Although the organization not only advanced the cause of women in medicine but also supported such various sociomedical issues as liberalized birth control laws, medical insurance, Medicaid, Medicare, and abortion reform, its membership rolls never attracted more than one-third of the women physicians in the country.[24] Lamented the *Bulletin* of the MWNA in the mid-1920s:

> But *all* our Big Women have not come in. They know that this National Society is a factor in the life and progress of Women in the profession, but for one reason or another they withhold cooperation. The same thing is true of the rank and file in the profession. Opposition has arisen from an honest opinion against sex distinguishment and also an apprehension that a Woman's Organization would seem to be a pulling away from the A.M.A. and local Societies; and apprehension that it would add to the prejudice of the men in the profession where such prejudice exists.[25]

Despite women physicians' uneven success with maintaining their separate organizations, their suspicion that coeducation would not be the answer to their dreams, and the poignant attempts of the Woman's Medical College of Pennsylvania to keep itself alive, their public pronouncements during this period indicate much optimism and high hopes for significant professional advancement. To read the minutes of the Medical Women's National Association, or the pages of the *Woman's Medical Journal,* is to discover that women physicians' major preoccupations were not with shrinking educational opportunities or the social and professional prejudice against them. On the contrary, the mood was one of buoyant optimism, marred only by the lament that good women were no longer choosing to study medicine, and this at the very moment when employment opportunities for medical women were allegedly brighter than before. In the year that Abraham Flexner published his report on medical education, the *Woman's Medical Journal* did its own survey of the status of medical women. Concluding that in many areas opportunities have "advanced by leaps and bounds" the *Journal* complained that "the number of women . . . who are entering the profession is not keeping pace with the increasing opportunities." Two years later the president of the Alumnae Association of the Woman's Medical College of Pennsylvania talked of "great opportunities," and the "crying need" for women physicians, while Marion C. Potter, president of the Women's Medical Society of New York State, deplored the fact that "numerically women physicians have their limitations," because "sociological needs of all kinds appeal to them, and make unceasing demand on time, talents, and resources." By 1919 the Committee on Medical Opportunities of the Medical Woman's National Association admitted, "We want to hunt more women to study medicine. We have not enough to fill the places. The places are waiting in every state."[26]

In reality, the situation of women physicians was far more complex and profoundly less secure than they perceived it to be. Surely we cannot take their own optimistic assessment at face value. But why did they greet the first decades of the new century with such sanguine expectations? The answer lies, I believe, in the ascendancy of a progressive ideology, and women physicians' vision of their own role in early twentieth-century liberal reform.

Characterized by the confluence of a number of different streams of reform and by a general philosophy of public good which sought to elevate the character of the American population and inculcate a higher standard of individual behavior, reform in the opening decades of the twentieth century emphasized civic responsibility and social duty. Probably Herbert Croly described its spirit best when he contrasted the old "live and let live" with the new "live and help live." The passing of the traditional community-centered social structure and the rise of large impersonal urban centers demanded thoughtful solutions to novel problems of sanitation, housing, poverty, education, recreation, and the corruption of political life. The need for innovative programs gave rise to an unprecedented burst of reform activity which spilled over into every aspect of modern life.[27]

Reformers focused their attention on a number of different symbols, but perhaps the most powerful, especially for women physicians, was the symbol of the child. Many of the campaigns for health, education, and a city environment conducive to social well-being had the improvement of life for the next generation as the goal. Insofar as there was a common commitment to means, it became manifest in absolute trust in the expert. Science, which was broadly defined to embrace both technology and medicine, provided the inspiration and authority for reform. Supposedly objective, rational, and gender-free, professional values were assumed to be informed not by narrow self-interest but by concern for social and democratic ends. It was the expert who would interpret the benefits of disinterested science for the social good. Scientific professions allegedly forswore personal gain, and for this reason professionals were particularly conspicuous in the reform movement—especially those in what we now call the "helping" professions—physicians, social workers, educators. The professional was expected to be pledged to an ideal of unselfish service and gained considerable social approbation on this account. In these years of liberal activism, the twin ideals of altruism and efficiency served to validate both private and public goals.[28]

The reorganization of medicine was part of the liberal campaign to rationalize the professions for the larger social good. Moreover, the ideology of reform meshed effortlessly with the goals of the nineteenth-century movement to train women in medicine. In the nineteenth century, women physicians had pleaded for equal opportunities in medical education on the grounds that they would bring science to bear on the daily life of the family. The woman physician had a right to exist because she benefited society, and more specifically, the large majority of women who would stay at home to raise their children. It was understood that the woman physician would always remain exceptional, but supporters claimed for her a more assiduous interest in preventive medicine, a natural ability to work with women and children, and a humanizing effect on the profession.

When progressivism made women physicians' work in the form of social medicine legitimate in the early decades of the twentieth century, they achieved a cultural validation that they had never experienced before. Their response was to throw themselves enthusiastically into every aspect of progressive reform that touched even remotely on questions that could be claimed as their own area of expertise. Far from being passive beneficiaries of the new liberalism, women physicians helped to shape the tone and content of the medical profession's own progressivism, while playing a significant role in linking medical efforts at reform with social feminism.

In 1910 President Lenna L. Meanes of the State Society of Iowa Medical Women made this connection explicit in her annual address. Agreeing with a woman writer that the reform movement ought to be dubbed "The Woman's War," and its ensign should be a "Babe in Arms," she reminded her audience that "the cause of the child has been placed foremost by philanthropy, education, science, Theodore Roosevelt and Judge Lindsay." Women physicians must be at the forefront of reform programs. "The optimism of today," Dr. Meanes concluded, "is a wide-awake, hardworking, systematic, scientific kind of optimism. It is based upon many statistics, and leaves little to chance, and it is transforming the dreams of a few years ago into very substantial fact."[29]

Women physicians' participation in public-health activity was reminiscent of an older tradition of reform broadly conceived, which was characteristic of the last two decades of the nineteenth century. When the American Public Health Association was founded in 1873, it drew its membership from a wide variety of persons with diverse lay and professional interests. Although physicians took the lead in the organization, they shared with lay members the contemporary belief in the strong relationship between good health and a clean physical and social environment. Even those individuals who were willing to incorporate into their thinking the new theories about germs did so without relinquishing their conviction that health problems demanded the generalized attention of a wide number of groups: physicians, engineers, female reformers, teachers, and educators.

As public health was professionalized in the decades after 1900, the triumph of scientific medicine transformed the movement into a more narrow group of specially interested experts whose well-defined and clearly articulated theory concentrated on the specific agents of disease. This development sharply reduced the scope of professional concern. No longer advocating broad programs of sanitation and slum clearance, these new experts reflected narrower goals more specifically influenced by bacteriological medicine. The chief concern became the control of communicable diseases through public programs of immunization and treatment. Gone was the luxury of long discussions concerning the social and environmental factors in susceptibility; the language was now the language of specific etiology.[30]

Though individual women physicians also participated in this transition, as a group women doctors were much slower to respond to the "modern" approach to public health. Their participation in social medicine was so varied and so extensive that the subject demands more attention than will be given here. Though after 1900 they remained roughly 5 percent of the profession, their visibility in various progressive programs for health reform measured far out of proportion to their actual numbers. In terms of numbers only, men would continue to dominate the field of public health, but women physicians' concerns were wide-ranging: passing wages and hours legislation, developing industrial medicine, correcting health and housing conditions in the slums, popularizing sex education and social hygiene, teaching preventive medicine and public health, preventing tuberculosis and venereal disease, improving education of midwives and obstetricians, guaranteeing clean milk and pure water, revising the system of vital statistics, promoting eugenics, amending scientifically the treatment of female delinquency, and securing school health inspection.

Women physicians claimed preventive medicine as their province well before it became fashionable in the years after 1900, and their own tradition of public-health education in the form of lecturing had its roots in the health-reform movement before the Civil War. The names of women physicians, such as Helen C. Putnam, Eliza Mosher, Mary Wood-Allen, Alice Hamilton, Mary Putnam Jacobi, Bertha Van Hoosen, Rachelle Yarros, Josephine Baker, and Annie S. Daniel are conspicuous in the early public health movement, the settlement movement, and the Association for the Study and Prevention of Infant Mortality, as well as social-purity crusades, tuberculosis-prevention campaigns, antiprostitution and antivenereal disease activity, and other lay and quasi-professional meliorist efforts which had their origins in the last two decades of the nineteenth century.

More than half of the papers delivered at the alumnae meetings of the Woman's Medical College of Pennsylvania in these years were explorations of public-health problems and women's role in particular. In 1901 the *Woman's Medical Journal* established a monthly department under the general editorship of Dr. Jennie McGowan entitled "State Medicine and Hygiene" which was devoted to keeping readers current on the problems and progress of social medicine. The pages of the *Journal* from the 1890s onward, in contrast to the *Journal of the American Medical Association,* are full with public-health concerns which formed part of the reform agenda.[31]

Women physicians also dominated public-health education out of proportion to their numbers. This was a part of medicine that they claimed as their own special province and that male physicians generally were happy to concede to them. This activity also linked women physicians to social feminism and allowed them to maintain strong connections to the women's movement. In 1905, for example, an editorial in the *Woman's Medical Journal* appealed to the profession and to the AMA to support programs in public health and preventive medicine. We are "pitiably provincial in our public efforts," the *Journal* complained, criticizing physicians for their neglect. Four years later Rosalie Slaughter Morton, a New

York surgeon and an active member of the Women's Medical Association of New York, brought the issue before the AMA. Attending the annual meeting in 1909, she was struck by an implicit consistency in the numerous papers on acute diseases given at the conference:

> In papers on tuberculosis and cancer medical men lamented the prevalent ignorance of the public regarding early symptoms which, as a result, reached the stage of futility before patients recognized them. Pneumonia, nephritis, gastritis and other acutely serious diseases developed, owing to lack of knowledge about the care of common colds, diet and other easily corrected health faults, and often progressed to almost incurable states before coming under professional care. When there was inflammation of eyes or ears, obviousness usually gained early attention, but most insidious diseases grew unnoticed or willfully neglected for years.[32]

Attending the section on Public Health, Morton observed that similar regrets were expressed by the assembly, but no one bothered to propose remedies for the situation. Impatient and frustrated, Morton rose to introduce a resolution which read,

> Whereas the American Medical Association . . . stands committed to the education of the public with respect to the nature and prevention of disease, resolved, that the women physicians, members of the American Medical Association, take the initiative individually in their respective associations in the organization of educational committees to act through women's clubs, mothers' associations, and other similar bodies for the dissemination of accurate information touching these subjects among the people, and that they be requested to submit to the House of Delegates a yearly report of such work, and elect from among their number a committee to take charge of the same."[33]

Explaining her resolution to the gathering in the midst of "masculine chuckles," she observed that she considered it "odd" that "men physicians were just waking up to preventive medicine, while women doctors had for fifty years been stressing the importance of educating mothers in the care of children's health, in pre-natal care of mothers, etc." A sympathetic male colleague added that women physicians "as members of church and lay women's organizations" were constantly being asked to lecture publicly on health issues, while "medical men almost always refused to make similar addresses," claiming that it was undignified or that they did not have time. Morton herself believed that men's orientation emphasized acute care and that they gave little thought to anything else. Dr.

William Bumby, a state health officer from Texas, rose to confirm her observations. Recounting his own disappointment with the private practitioners of his area in mustering support for a legal measure guaranteeing milk pasteurization and the testing of cows—"they all replied they were too busy to be bothered with such details"—he finally appealed to the women's clubs. "The result was electrifying," Bumby recalled. "They were delighted to help regulate a cow instead of reading Emerson to one another." With women's help, Bumby concluded, legal action swiftly ensued.[34]

Still, objections were raised to Morton's resolution. Some men worried that public lectures could be considered a form of self-advertisement, something that violated medical ethics. A few complained that if lectures on preventive medicine were successful, doctors' incomes would be reduced as people ceased to consult them as often. Still others remained suspicious of the idea of professionals cooperating so closely with lay women. Four years later at a meeting of the Woman's Medical College of Pennsylvania alumnae, Dr. Rachelle Yarros testified to a similar reaction when she recalled that when she first came to Chicago at the turn of the century, "my men colleagues in medicine rather resented my taking part in club work. They did not think it was worth my while." But a decade later, their attitude had changed, "because, whenever they are interested in any health legislation or health education, they ask their wives and friends to bring these topics before the women's clubs, feeling that this will assure their success."[35]

After a protracted debate Morton's resolution gained endorsement by the AMA in 1909, and she was appointed to organize their Public Health Education Committee. Joining her in the planning were Sarah Adamson Dolley, Evelyn Garrigue, and Alice Gregory of New York; Lillian H. South of Bowling Green, Kentucky; Sara Craig Buckley of Chicago; Rose Talbot Bullard of Los Angeles; Annie Lee Hamilton of Boston; Margaret Holliday of Austin, Texas; and Laura L. Leibhardt of Denver. Within a year a ten-member central committee consisting of six women and four men and chaired by Eleanor S. Everhard of Dayton coordinated the work of three subcommittees—on affiliated public health work, medical literature, and cooperation, respectively—and kept in contact with 42 state chairpersons, 270 county chairpersons, and 6 city secretaries, all of them women physicians. Letters were written to another six thousand women physicians, and authoritative lecture series by medical men and women were soon launched under the auspices of state and county medical societies in thirty-three states.

At the next annual meeting of the American Medical Association the committee presented a 136-page printed report in book form to every member of the House of Delegates, "giving condensed details of subjects, by whom presented, attendance at lectures, direct and indirect results, in every state in the Union and also in Alaska, Hawaii and Panama."[36]

The activities of the Public Health Education Committee continued a long-standing tradition of cooperation between women physicians, clubwomen and other feminists. From the turn of the century on, the *Women's Medical Journal* called for a closer relationship between the clubs and women physicians.[37] Women doctors were urged to join their local clubs and influence the direction of their programs toward the preservation of public health through teaching and leadership. Typically, they displayed a lively interest in euthenics—the idea of making housekeeping more scientific.[38] After the organization of the AMA Committee in 1909, they formed hygiene committees in local clubs which then cooperated with medical societies and other public welfare groups to sponsor lectures.

For example, one of the most successful and well-publicized lecture series was held between January and April 1910 at the New York Academy of Medicine. It was sponsored jointly by the Public Health Education Committee of the Medical Society of the City of New York and the Hygiene Committee of the New York Federation of Women's Clubs. Lectures by two male and two female physicians covered a wide range of topics, including fresh air treatment in the school, the nursery and the sick-room, wholesome food and diet, feeding school children, industrial diseases, hookworm, malaria and yellow fever, and dental care. A similar program sponsored by the Kings County Society took place in Brooklyn the following year. Between a third and a half of the speakers were women.[39]

The work of California women physicians with local women's groups was particularly remarkable. They lectured endlessly on the hygiene of young girls, tuberculosis, school hygiene, food and milk sanitation, and nervousness in children, preparing book lists and leading study groups. They organized pure milk campaigns, "clean up" days in local towns, and pure food and drug activity. In the San Joaquin Valley, Dr. Mary Butin formed visiting committees that inspected local dairies, and convinced her club to sponsor a district nurse. Dr. Rose Bullard, the chairperson of public health for the Los Angeles district, maintained a speakers' bureau of women physicians and hired a nurse on behalf of her club who "located every tuberculous individual" in the district to see that "certain precautions" were carried out.[40]

Rosalie Slaughter Morton summarized women physicians' various contacts with the lay women's movement in her autobiography:

> Their [the General Federation of Women's Clubs] national organization numbered nine hundred thousand intelligent, public-spirited and wealthy women who molded public opinion toward protecting the health of American citizens. We were in touch with all educational and philanthropic agencies through the United Charities Association. Our work became of service to the hundred and ninety-three thousand women in the local and national Young Women's Christian Associations through the direct cooperation of the national secretary. We likewise functioned through the Mothers' Clubs, of which there were sixty in New York City alone; with the State Assemblies of Mothers and the National Congress of Mothers; with the National and International Council of Women, the National Society of Sanitary Prophylaxis, the Ethical-Social League and with many other organizations. We learned what efforts toward preventive medicine were already being made in various states in order to be most helpful and not duplicate services. Pamphlets and lists of books were given general distribution.[41]

The Public Health Education Committee of the AMA remained in existence for four years, when it was superseded by a new body, the Council on Health and Public Instruction, which ultimately published the AMA's popular magazine *Hygeia.* Morris Fishbein, one-time president of the AMA and its historian, does not even bother to mention the Public Health Education Committee in his massive history of the organization, and he describes the primary purpose of the AMA Council on Health as one of "public relations. It conceived its principal commission to be the development of public confidence in the purposes and work of the American Medical Association and of the medical profession."[42]

Rosalie Slaughter Morton also understood that one aspect of women physicians' public-health work would be public relations for the profession. Like Fishbein and the other members of the AMA she worried that it was often the women's clubs that fell victim to "antivivisectionists and other sobbing cliques" and she understood that women physicians—both as scientific experts *and* as "members of these clubs"—were in a position to refute medical quackery. She believed, in fact, that it was primarily the accomplishments of *women* physicians in the area of public instruction that eased the relationship between the profession and the lay public. "It would have been a serious reflection upon our profession at this psychological time," she wrote, "if we had not promptly educated the public to a thorough appreciation of the doctor's role as protector of health of the community. . . . We credited the American Medical Association with all our gratuitous work in order to foster an acceptance of its altruistic concern for the health of women and their children." Similarly, Dr. Lena K. Sadler, chairperson of the AMWA Public Health Committee, highly valued work with the women's clubs for the same reason. "Why not," she asked, "intelligently guide their interest and enthusiasm along the proper channels by co-operating with them in such a way as to bring about a closer understanding between them and organized medicine?" Women doctors "as women" understood their viewpoint, while "as physicians" sympathized "with the attitude of organized medicine."[43]

Women physicians, however, valued public-health instruction not solely for what it could accomplish in positive professional public relations. They were reformers in their belief that their role in such educational activity would have even greater social significance by changing the living habits of most Americans. Thus, when the Council on Health and Public Instruction was established with no women members, women doctors perpetuated their educational activities with the women's clubs through other organizations. The Woman's Medical College of Pennsylvania, for example, offered courses of popular lectures on various health topics given by distinguished members of the faculty.[44] A number of women physicians were active leaders in the American Social Hygiene Association and worked closely with the YWCA. Throughout the 1920s the American Medical Women's Association, through its own Public Health Committee, continued to maintain strong ties with local women's groups. Argued President Grace Kimball in 1923:

> When you realize that this association is affiliated through the federation of clubs in America with eleven million organized women, you will see the duty and the opportunity of our medical women to act as authorities on health and medical information to these great bodies of lay women. . . . We must get busy.[45]

The AMWA yearly sent its representative to the meetings of the General Federation of Women's Clubs. It also attempted to coordinate its activities with the AMA Council on Health and Public Instruction; the Association of Women in Public Health, founded in 1920; the Woman's Advisory Council of the United States Public Health Service, a group first appointed in 1922 and consisting of three prominent women physicians; the Woman's Joint Congressional Committee; and the Women's Foundation for Health, founded in 1922 and consisting of lay and medical women who worked closely with the AMWA's own Public Health Committee.[46]

Directly related to their work in public health education was women physicians' active participation in a variety of other social hygiene programs. "The question of social hygiene," remarked Dr. Prince Morrow in 1910, "is a woman's question."[47] Women physicians took Morrow's statement to heart. The Woman's Medical Association of New York City, to choose one of many examples, organized a standing committee on social hygiene in 1907. Believing that the subject held special concern for women physicians because of their expertise, the group played an active role in the promotion of progressive social hygiene measures on the state level. They investigated the management of women offenders before magistrate courts, looked into the conditions under which such offenders were placed when convicted and sentenced, and concerned themselves with provisions for educational training and rehabilitation. They studied state laws governing sexuality and methods of police enforcement. They actively engaged in promoting and encouraging progressive legislation whenever possible, making personal appeals by letter to lawmakers in Albany on behalf of the Association and of women physicians in general.

Emily Dunning Barringer remembered the impact of her first visits to women offenders in the city's jails. She believed the experience "influenced my subsequent medical activities more than any others." Particularly vivid was her memory of the way male police approached these women with "disgust and disdain," in spite of the fact that "the prostitute . . . would not be in her unfortunate position if the men of the community had not put her there for their own gratification." It was then that she understood "how basically unfair the relation between the sexes was, and how much there was to be done in improving the condition of our woman criminals." Barringer later joined the National Prison Association and worked for a time among the female wards of New York City's correctional institutions.[48]

Each year the Woman's Medical Association of New York City sponsored a symposium for lay and medical professionals on the subject of social hygiene. Under their auspices, progressive reformers like Florence Kelley of the National Consumer's League, Felix Adler of the Ethical Culture Society, Katherine Bement Davis of the Bedford Reformatory, Frank Moss, assistant district attorney for New York City, and Dr. Prince A. Morrow, founder of the American Society of Sanitary and Moral Prophylaxis, were provided with a public forum consisting of lay and medical personnel for the exchange of information.[49]

Directly related to women doctors' interest in social hygiene was their promotion of the teaching of hygiene and physiology in the public schools. Helen C. Putnam, for example, devoted a good deal of her career to encouraging such teaching by professionals, preferably physicians. Putnam was a graduate of the Woman's Medical College of Pennsylvania in 1889, a cofounder, along with Dr. Abraham Jacobi, of the American Child Health Association, and former president of the American Academy of Medicine, a progressive group of doctors interested in "medical sociology." She chaired the Academy's committee on the teaching of school hygiene and represented the United States at a number of international conferences on the subject. Her articles on child hygiene, as well as those of a number of other women physicians, often appeared in the *Woman's Medical Journal*.[50]

Although Putnam was willing to see such teaching be done by trained professionals in fields other than medicine, some women physicians believed the work should be reserved exclusively for women doctors. In 1920 Lilian Welsh, also active in the cause, told the alumnae of the Woman's Medical College of her faith in the special benefits of their particular expertise. "I think teachers of hygiene should be doctors of medicine," she concluded, after completing a long discussion of the social benefits of such programs. "I have watched it taught from the physical training department. I have watched it taught from the so-called domestic science department, and the very sure background is that which comes from those who have medical knowledge. Here is the place, a specified place, for the women medically trained, who bear today the degree of doctor."[51]

In addition to their interest in school curricula, a number of women physicians, like Dr. Valeria Parker, Dr. Rachelle Yarros, Dr. Anna L. Brown, and Dr. Mabel Ulrich, had strong connections with the Bureau of Social Hygiene, spending time primarily in antivenereal disease and anti-prostitution work. The Social Morality Committee of the YWCA, founded in 1913, also maintained a staff of women physician lecturers who taught sex hygiene primarily in the normal schools.

American entry into World War I stepped up social hygiene activity concerned specifically with the problems of venereal disease and prostitution. Katherine Bement Davis of the Bedford Hills Reformatory was appointed to head the social hygiene division of the Commission on Training Camp Activities of the War Department and, though the Army refused to commission women as medical officers, the government welcomed their participation as social hygiene lecturers. Dr. Anna L. Brown of the War Work Council of the YWCA made its Lecture Bureau available to the government, and over a hundred women doctors participated in sex education and antivenereal disease programs, utilizing Davis's harshly moralistic film "The End of the Road" to illustrate to the young women of the country "the importance of physical, mental and moral hygiene."[52]

Women physicians working in social hygiene demonstrated a wide range of attitudes toward the changes in social and sexual mores that took place in the early decades of the twentieth century. Just as it is impossible to generalize in any comprehensive way about their approach to therapeutical issues, it is difficult to demonstrate that there was any single collective answer among women doctors to questions involving sexual morality. Many of them shared the beliefs of conservative social hygienists and social-purity feminists who attacked the double standard and sought to impose a single, female standard of chastity on American society. Along with other women activists, they worked to gain social and legal controls over sexuality, emphasized the importance of consensual sex for women in marriage, and fought against prostitution and its related evils. Like Dr. Inez Philbrick of Lincoln, Nebraska, many perceived an increase in venereal disease and attributed it to the "enormous exaggeration of the sex instinct" resulting from the economic dependence of women on men, and believed that women physicians had an important role to play in reversing such dangerous trends. For these women, the sexual drive and initiative were primarily male, and thus they viewed the prostitute either as a total victim of male lust or as a sexual delinquent. "Marital, as well as social continence, is a crying need of the hour," wrote Philbrick in the *Women's Medical Journal.* "And the medical profession must take the lion's share of the responsibility in pressing for these values, alongside the church and the press."[53]

A conservative approach to sexuality generally led some women physicians to support the eugenics movement. A number of them developed hereditarian ideas while serving as school inspectors or resident physicians in institutions or reformatories. The increased emphasis of many social thinkers on heredity and biology gave physicians a new authority in these institutions, and women physicians gained an even greater voice because of their presumed connection with family life, other women, and children. As the *Woman's Medical Journal* observed in 1907, "Teachers have naturally turned to medical science for help in the solution of the many problems presented, consequently the pedagogic and medical mind are beginning to look at the growing child through each other's eyes with mutual benefit to the two sciences, and we hope with benefit to the present-day child."[54]

Katherine Bement Davis, a social worker who directed the Bedford Reformatory in New York, testified to the increased use of physicians in reformatory work in a paper entitled "Delinquency and the Medical Profession" that she gave to the alumnae of the Woman's Medical College of Pennsylvania in 1917. Admitting that in the beginning of her career she believed that she needed only a staff of good teachers, she gradually had come to see that the problem of delinquency was more one of inheritance and disease. "Now the pendulum has swung so far," she declared, "that the members of the medical profession have first place on our staff."[55]

Similarly, Helen MacMurchy, Inspector of the Feeble Minded for the Department of Education in Ontario, Canada, argued in 1915 that medical expertise had become essential in the proper handling of delinquency. "Sometimes," she wrote in "The Doctor and the Children's Court,"

> one wonders whether the fault is with the doctor or with the public. Has the doctor forgotten what he or she can do for the public, or has the public no idea what the doctor can do for every person and for every institution? The home, the school, the church, and the court struggle along with problems which only the doctor can solve. They do not seem to realize that the doctor has a key that will open the doors and bars against which they hopelessly beat themselves in an endeavor to open them. One can not sit in a children's court without having this sad truth painfully beaten in upon mind and heart. The endless procession passes through faster or slower according to the skill, the insight and the ideals of the judge on the bench. About one-third or more of these boys and girls really belong to the doctor.[56]

For many women physicians, delinquency, especially among girls, usually meant some form of sexual misbehavior. Some reformers viewed eugenics as a solution that offered a chance to remedy problems that were being diagnosed increasingly as biologically induced. The American Medical Women's Association established a Committee on Race Betterment, for example, and occasionally debated the question of sterilizing criminals and the feeble-minded. A few members supported such measures, though the association never took a public stand on the issue. Numerous articles in the *Woman's Medical Journal* discussed the connection between eugenics and social reform.

Elizabeth Thompson Smart, for example, medical examiner for the mentally defective in the New York City Department of Education, published several studies declaring feeble-minded children a "*social menace.*" Most of them, she wrote,

> are, or may become, to a more or less degree sexual perverts. The sex instinct is very strong in very many of the older boys and girls. The school law protects them up to the age of sixteen years; we can do everything possible for them to better their condition up to that age, with the consent of the parents, of course, but beyond that we may not go. What is to become of this vast army of menacing humanity? Shall we, as medical women and men, sit calmly by with folded hands and permit the outrages of illegitimacy and prostitution to go on in the midst of human beings who do not know the meaning of their acts? Shall we sit by while some of these mental weaklings are granted licence to marry and reproduce their kind—or worse? This is a burning question brought home daily, I might say hourly, to the physician whose duty it is to examine and prescribe for them.[57]

In the eyes of some reformers, eugenics was a rational means of improving the social environment. But well-meaning progressivism could occasionally cross the line and become the elitist racism of the ruling class. In this, too, some women physicians differed little from other liberal reformers. In justifying their own central role in raising the question of positive eugenics Kate Campbell Hurd-Mead warned:

> We are confronted today by problems in a measure unknown a generation ago. Instead of the sturdy Irish and Swedish immigrants of the 70's, we have the underfed, undereducated and nervously irritable Italians, narrow chested neurotic Jews, and half-famished Russians whose suppressed energy may rise in anarchy as soon as it feels the unrestrained freedom of our country. From the children of such parents we must raise a nation strong in mind and body.[58]

Fears of "race suicide" and an inordinate respect for motherhood led many of these same women physicians to reject artificial birth control and to sanction only sexual continence for the sake of a woman's health. Eliza Mosher, senior editor of the *Medical*

Woman's Journal and an outspoken critic of the American Birth Control League, argued that contraception was "a menace to the population of America fifty years from now," and would "destroy in girls and young women the maternal instinct." She linked the availability of artificial contraceptives with increased sexual promiscuity among the young, suggesting that "men no longer feel" the "urge to Marriage that they formerly did . . ." because "they are able to gain all the sexual pleasure they desire with less expense and in safer companionship."[59]

Similarly, Dr. Mary L. Fitzpatrick of Milwaukee, writing in 1916, told Julia Lathrop, head of the Children's Bureau:

> Experience has taught me that what women do need to realize is this, that the bearing and rearing of as many healthy children as she can, and thereby do justice to both herself and her offspring is the most satisfactory in after life, the most worth-while, and in comparison with it all the occupations of men are dull and stale and pale into insignificance. To rear strong children and to train them so that they become useful men and woman—what more stimulating or inspiring brain work could women desire?[60]

While some women physicians rejected female sexuality, favoring legal measures to regulate the sexual behavior of the community at large, and flirted with eugenics to create a race less sexually "perverse," others joined a minority of their male colleagues in welcoming the changes in sexual mores that recognized in female sexual expression a positive personal and social good. These clinicians, often gynecologists, witnessed firsthand the vast misery in marriage caused by sexual ignorance, and entertained the notion that a more satisfying physical admustment would lead to happy, more stable marriages—an ultimate guarantee of social stability. Rather than blame the rising divorce rate on the decline in sexual standards, they preferred instead to see it as a symptom, among other things, of improper sex education.[61]

Mary E. Bates, for example, a graduate of the Woman's Medical College in Chicago in 1881 and one of the earliest women to intern at Cook County Hospital, owned a flourishing gynecological practice in Denver. In an article on phimosis in the female, published in the *Woman's Medical Journal* in 1906, she berated male physicians for not taking sufficient interest in physical handicaps that might hamper women from experiencing sexual pleasure. "Sexual undevelopment, indifference and incompetence," she believed, "is one of the most frequent causes of the 'failure of marriage.' "

Couples that were sexually "mated" were usually happy, while those that were unhappy were often "sexually mismated." Bates believed that medical silence on the sex psychology of patients was a "mockery of 'modesty.' " She urged women physicians to bring their expertise to bear on these problems. The potential for easing the difficulties of their patients was boundless. The woman physician, she suggested, must be a sex therapist.

> A woman physician . . . should carry the higher thought that the woman physician is the response to the inherent need of her sex kind for some one to comprehend her sex construction; to appreciate her sex limitations and deviations; to realize her social sex conditions, her physical, mental, and moral sex responsibilities; some one to minister to her mind, her soul as well as to her flesh; and to point the way to woman's sex freedom and sex self-respect.[62]

Another woman physician who displayed a long-standing interest in female sexuality was Clelia Mosher, a graduate of Johns Hopkins. In the 1890s, under the influence of her good friend, the sociologist Mary Roberts Smith, she began a survey of sexual behavior and attitudes first, among members of the Mother's Club of Madison, Wisconsin, and later among faculty wives and coeds at Stanford University. Although she never published the results, which revealed her subjects to be cautiously positive about their own sexuality, her questionnaire suggests that she was extremely sensitive to changing sexual mores among women, and wished to understand better the importance of sexuality to stable marriages.[63]

There was also an important group of women physicians who were active in the birth-control movement, and many of them, too, viewed artificial contraception as a means to foster positive sexual relations in order to preserve marital happiness. Some, like Rachelle Yarros, also hoped that contraceptive information would ease the burdens of working-class women and preserve the health of all women by allowing them to space their children more carefully. Others, like Lydia Allen DeVilbiss, were less sympathetic with poor immigrants and blacks, and intended contraceptive clinics primarily to control the alarmingly high fertility of "inferior" races. But for the most part, women physicians participated in the early birth-control movement—directing many of the birth-control clinics that sprung up in the 1920s—because they viewed "Constructive Birth Control" as another means of rationalizing family relationships and improving the quality of life for women, men, and children. Explained Rachelle Yarros, who ran her own clinic in Chicago:

Constructive Birth Control must concern itself frankly with marital happiness. . . . Our policy should be to dispel ignorance of men and women in sex matters, to teach them frankly and earnestly how to retain and foster love. . . . We must teach them that sex gratification in moderation plays a very important part in life, *apart from the rearing of a family,* because it is necessary to intimacy and tender affection between husband and wife. . . . A fundamental change in the mental attitude of men and women towards the sex relationship can only be brought about through the training of the individual from earliest youth in physiological science, ideals and standards of conduct. By overcoming our own inhibitions and clearly defining our own ideals we may become truly helpful in training the next generation.[64]

The establishment of the Children's Bureau in 1912 and later the passage of the Sheppard-Towner Act, intended to help reduce infant and maternal mortality, increased women physicians' opportunities to do the kind of public-health fieldwork at which they had become particularly adept. The Children's Bureau underscored reformers' concern for the child, and women physicians hailed the new agency as a "great step forward" in preventive medicine. They hoped and expected that women physicians would be integral to its work. "The medical woman," speculated the *Woman's Medical Journal,* would be of special value by virtue of her "inherent motherhood, together with the quick perceptions and keen discernment incident to her professional training." Again the argument ran that the medical woman could combine rational, scientific, and professional values with tenderness, sympathy, and "infinite tact."[65]

Even before the Bureau got under way women doctors pioneered in the work that would ultimately be identified with it. One of the earliest of these pioneers was Josephine Baker, whose accomplishments in New York City provided a model for later Children's Bureau programs. In the early 1900s she had opened a private practice with another woman physician. To supplement her income, she became an inspector for the city health department. She saw a good deal of departmental corruption, but after 1902 when Seth Low became New York City's mayor, a general house cleaning occurred and Baker began working with Dr. Walter Bensel, an energetic chief who was committed to making his department an instrument of social change. Soon Baker was appointed his assistant. In 1908 the Department created the first Division of Child Hygiene in the country, an agency designated specifically to design programs in preventive medicine, and Baker was appointed the chief.[66]

From then on, Baker published sophisticated analyses in the *Woman's Medical Journal* of the successes and failures of the Division of Child Hygiene. Such reports inspired physicians—many of them women—in other cities across the country to imitate her methods and goals. "Communities of any size," wrote Baker in one of her earliest articles, "when confronted with the problems of poverty, congested living quarters, ignorance and influx of alien races have found that in order to assure their future well being they must protect the health of the children. In public health movements proper guidance and instruction are essential. Municipalities have found that they must assume this function," she continued, "and in no other line is the need more imperative and the results of more importance in their bearing on the future national progress than in the broad, comprehensive, and consecutive care of the health of children."[67]

One of the first concerns of the new division was the legal regulation of midwives. In New York City in 1910, midwives managed over 40 percent of all births, a situation dictated largely by the cultural traditions of its large immigrant population. Unlike the majority of male physicians and even many women doctors who disapproved of midwives, Baker insisted that the employment of trained midwives was "an established necessity." "The doctors," Baker wrote in her autobiography, "were never able to understand the sort of people we had to deal with. If deprived of midwives, these [immigrant] women would rather have amateur assistance from the janitor's wife or the woman across the hall than to submit to this outlandish American custom of having in a male doctor for a confinement."[68]

Using what Baker liked to term "our mother-wit," her bureau developed ingenious methods for supervising midwives already in practice, while weeding out the incompetent. In 1911, partly as a result of Baker's support, a school for midwives was founded at Bellevue Hospital. From then on the Bureau refused to license midwives who were not graduates of either this school or a European equivalent. The six-month Bellevue course was under city control and was offered free to competent applicants. Baker believed that its graduates "knew more about delivering babies than three-quarters of the recently graduated internes entering on medical practice."[69] Though the properly trained obstetrical specialist was "of course the best possible person to bring a child into the world," Baker understood that obstetricians were often too expensive for the modest household. Moreover, specialization in obstetrics still carried with it the stigma of low status and fewer financial rewards than other branches of medicine, while few who trained as general practitioners received adequate instruction in childbirth in their four years of medical school. For Baker the experienced and well-supervised midwife remained the most practical solution.

Baker collected statistics that bore out her hypothesis. In the first year of the regulatory program, for example, eighty-four deaths from puerperal septicemia were reported. Investigation revealed that only twenty-two of these occurred under the supervision of a midwife, while sixty of the women who died were being treated entirely by physicians. In the next few years, Baker collected and published figures which proved the maternal mortality rate to be higher among mothers delivered in hospitals by doctors than among women attended in their homes by a midwife.

Her claims often caused strained relations with her professional colleagues. She remembered one "hot discussion" at the New York Academy of Medicine soon after one of her articles was published. "I had a very bad hour indeed," she recalled,

> sitting at an Academy meeting as the target of all kinds of pointed remarks—they did not exactly call me a liar, but they skirted around it much too close for comfort. Then, to prove their point, they started an investigation of their own. That was my innings. In preparing my figures I had been absurdly careful to make them as unfavorable as possible to my point of view. If a midwife had so much as walked into the room where a prospective mother was in bed, her death would be placed to the discredit of the midwife, even if it had occurred while the case was under the doctor's care. Since the Academy did not go into these details quite so carefully, their figures, when they were finally compiled, were even more favorable to the midwives than mine.[70]

As head of the Division of Child Hygiene, Baker shaped policy in her department according to the tenets of progressive health reform. Once the wrinkles in the program regulating midwives were smoothed over, she turned to other things: the education of mothers in the care of babies, a systematic inspection of all institutions involved in the care of dependent children, the comprehensive monitoring of child health in the schools through the control and elimination of contagious disease, the detection and correction of noncontagious physical defects, and controlling the worst abuses of child labor through the issuance of employment certificates to children between the ages of 14 and 16 years old.[71]

The Federal Children's Bureau elaborated and supplemented the kind of work women like Josephine Baker were doing in cities and states across the country. In the first year of the Bureau's existence it published a birth registration report, a survey of baby-saving campaigns, a pamphlet on prenatal care, one on infant care, a study of New Zealand's infant-saving techniques, a report on laws relating to mothers' pensions in the United States, Denmark, and New Zealand and an infant mortality study of Johnstown, Pennsylvania. In later years, nine more infant mortality studies were completed in a number of other communities.[72]

The Children's Bureau was distinctly a *female* agency, and like no other in the federal government. It was female voluntarism, in the form of pressure groups and lobbying, that helped create the Children's Bureau in the first place. Once organized, the Bureau imitated on a national scale the techniques of the settlement house. Much of the agency's success in the progressive period can be attributed to its ability to continue a close relationship with female voluntary organizations and muster their help in its work. In its National Baby Week Campaigns, for example, it received the cooperation and enthusiastic support of local women's clubs; groups of unpaid volunteers from these organizations worked all over the country to help the Bureau gather information for its studies. Clubwomen prepared personal reports for the Bureau about their findings. Wrote Alice Kimball, a Rhode Island woman's club member who participated in its massive birth registration campaign, "I found my investigating extremely interesting, and instructive, as well. I feel now that I know a little more about the *where* if not the *how* 'the other half lives.' "[73]

As head of the Children's Bureau, Julia Lathrop attempted to preserve for a national agency the personal touch of the settlement house. The thousands of letters written to the Bureau during this early period suggest that for many years she achieved this goal. The letters are quite remarkable for their personal tone, the confidence that a reply would be forthcoming, and what they reveal about the difficult lives of the women of the rural and urban poor. A frightened 15-year-old, for example, wrote Lathrop in 1919: "I will write to you and ask you some things a lady told me about you I am 15 years old I was married the 23rd of June it will soon be 3 months and I dont feel good I think there is something going to happen to me will you please send me information of what to do I never had a mother to tell me anything so please write me at once what to do." From Chicago, a working mother explains, "I nursed my baby mornings and night at night time after working all day then nursing my child, every drop it swallowed it would throw it up, at the same time suffering the awfull tortures with my milk, pumping it and throwing it into the sink. while my baby *starved* and my husband *refused* to provide for us."[74]

The letters were all answered personally, either by Lathrop or Mrs. Max West, an assistant who also wrote the Bureau's publication, *Infant Care*. The agency developed widespread female professional contacts—in both rural and urban areas all over the country—who often visited the troubled letter writer, or took the time to guide her to the proper agencies in her area.

A number of women physicians were part of this network. Some were paid by the Bureau to be field workers, others volunteered their time. For example, a farm wife from Andrus, Wisconsin, wrote after reading the Bureau's information on pre- and postnatal care: "Now if any of your advice covers what an ordinary farm wife can carry out I would like to have it. Most of the advice I have read says—Fruite in plenty a bath every morning—gentle exercise—coffe before dressing. music—pleasant surrounding now I have a perfectly fine husband and a loveing home but here is my day—get up at 5 a.m. hustle breakfast for 5. wash dishes help milk feed pigs clean up bakeing—scrubbing washing—(where is the gentle ex?) . . . where could I have the time for a bath every morn?" Mrs. West answered this letter by urging the writer to contact Dr. Dorothy Reed Mendenhall, a Bureau physician and author of several of their pamphlets, who traversed Wisconsin as a University extension lecturer advising pregnant women on "care of themselves and their babies."[75]

Another woman physician, Dr. Eleanor Mellen of Newton Highlands, Massachusetts, wrote to Lathrop:

> Having retired from the active practice of my profession, I have recently agreed to act as the Health Editor for a syndicate of newspapers largely among the rural districts throughout the country. Very many letters are sent to me each week and among those arriving lately was this which I copy; "My Mother never told be about myself when I am sick and so I do not know what to do when I come sick. Will you please tell me? Also I wish you would tell me how I am to tell when I am going to come sick. If you will kindly answer these few questions I will be very grateful. Please put your answer in a plain envelop so no one else will know what it contains."
>
> The child had mailed the letter in a different town from the one which she gave as her address. Of course I have given her the assistance that she desired, but I am wondering if your department in any

way meets the needs of such cases. Have you any free publications that would tell this girl and those like her what they ought to know about themselves and the life waiting for them? Or can you refer me to such? I say "free" because many of the people that I reach are pitifully poor and they could not spend even pennies without missing them somewhere else. That is why this work of mine was started. I shall be very glad for any assistance that your department may be able to give me for them.[76]

Lathrop had a keen sense of the difficult medical conditions in rural areas, and was committed to rural health reform from the beginning of her tenure. Here, too, women physicians, like Dorothy Reed Mendenhall, or Mary Bates of Denver, helped out by becoming itinerant agents for the Bureau. Probably no one, however, accomplished more in this area than Dr. Frances Sage Bradley, an early female graduate of Cornell, who settled in Atlanta, Georgia, and became one of the first specialists in rural medicine. Bradley believed that the neglect of America's rural children threatened the future of the entire nation, and in 1916 she had her chance to publicize her cause. In that year the North Carolina Board of Health requested the Children's Bureau to conduct a social-medical survey of the state, and Bradley, as the Bureau's special agent, carried it out. To this day her report remains an exemplar of its time. She spent six months investigating the conditions of tenant farmers, studying the special hazards to childbirth and the health of growing children, exploring sanitation conditions in housing and work, and observing and reporting on the particularly difficult position of rural women. In 1921, when the Sheppard-Towner Act made available federal funds for extensive programs in the prevention of infant and maternal mortality, the state of Arkansas founded a Bureau of Child Hygiene and appointed Bradley its chief.[77]

Just as the Children's Bureau can be characterized as the "women's branch" of the federal government, the Sheppard-Towner Act of 1921 might be dubbed "women's legislation." Female reformers rightly viewed the act as an important victory—one of the first results of woman's suffrage. It legitimized the activity of women physicians and lay health workers who, for almost two decades, had been working to improve the nation's health and welfare through educative preventive medicine. Under the terms of the law, the government would provide states with matching funds to establish prenatal and child-health centers. Here female professionals could teach mothers personal hygiene, infant management, proper pre- and postnatal care, and family health. Sheppard-Towner was one of the first government acts to recognize the responsibility of the State for the health of its citizenry, and it pioneered in expanding the role of the federal government in preventive medicine.

The American Medical Association opposed the passage of the bill, and lobbied against it throughout the 1920s until it failed of renewal in 1929. The official position of the AMA endorsed the goals of the legislation—to upgrade obstetrical and pediatric care—but argued against the concept of federal aid as "unAmerican," and objected to its being administered by the Children's Bureau, a lay organization.[78]

Women physicians displayed none of the ambivalence toward the Sheppard-Towner Act that characterized so many of their male colleagues. The act seemed for them to be the fulfillment of years of agitation, and in many respects the attitudes of some of their most conservative male colleagues shocked them. Josephine Baker, for example, recalled a particularly unsettling encounter with the "short-sighted psychology of a certain type of doctor, when confronted with public health work" when she was called before a Congressional committee to testify on behalf of the bill: "This New England doctor," she remembered:

> actually got up and told the committee: "We oppose this bill because, if you are going to save the lives of all these women and children at public expense, what inducement will there be for young men to study medicine?" Senator Sheppard, the chairman, stiffened and leaned forward: "Perhaps I didn't understand you correctly," he said: "You surely don't mean that you want women and children to die unnecessarily or live in constant danger of sickness so there will be something for young doctors to do?" "Why not?" said the New England doctor, who did at least have the courage to admit the issue: "That's the will of God, isn't it?"[79]

Baker understood that such thinking followed logically from the profession's overemphasis on cure rather than prevention, and she had little patience with such shortsightedness. As for other women physicians, Sheppard-Towner dramatically increased their opportunities for employment. They flocked to staff the new clinics opened under the auspices of the act. By 1924, forty states were cooperating under its provisions, and the *Medical Woman's Journal* hailed their accomplishments. In 1927 the Committee on Medical Opportunities for Women of the American Medical Women's Association revealed that a total of forty women physicians were employed full-time and three part-time in positions created by the act. In addition, four women physicians worked in the Maternity and Infancy Division of the Children's Bureau, a division directed by Martha May Eliot, professor of pediatrics at Yale Medical School. Sixteen of the forty states employed women physicians as directors, and an additional twelve employed them in a full-time capacity on the maternity and infancy staffs of the State Division of Public Health.[80]

Even in states where medical and lay opposition was so strong that state governments refused to participate, women physicians made serious efforts to devise programs that would be more acceptable. Lena K. Sadler, a member of the Public Health Committee of the AMWA, described the situation in her state to her fellow convention delegates in 1925:

> I wish to say that the Sheppard-Towner Bill, fortunately or unfortunately is not functioning in the State of Illinois. When I accepted this chairmanship, I saw the hand writing on the wall, lady physicians, that it perhaps would not function in my State because almost unanimously the medical profession is set against it.

Sadler went on to say that once she had accepted this fact she organized similar programs to which the profession would not object. "Personally," she concluded, "it is nothing to me, whether it functions or not, because I believe my record is behind me. For eighteen years I have preached preventative medicine all over the United States in the various Chatauquas. I believe in every educational feature of that Bill, but when organized medicine is against it in my state, I must do something with the clubs to take its place."[81]

Sadler's words underscore the fact that women doctors carried the tradition of what one historian has termed "social therapeutics" into the twentieth century. In a sense, they merely continued to do what they had always done, and for the first few decades of the century their work was sanctioned by a reformist ideology that considered the improved health and welfare of a modernizing nation the immediate concern of all enlightened professionals and men and women of science. Their continued optimism about their own future, at the very moment when significant barriers against women were being constructed in science and academe, and their own flexibility in the profession was being considerably narrowed by the transformation of modern medicine, can be puzzling if we do not realize how the ascendancy of liberal ideology validated their identity.[82]

It is certainly true that women physicians, because they were not as dependent on the university for employment after their training, had more autonomy than either women scientists or women in higher education. There existed a more varied market for their services. To "defeminize" medicine did not mean to rid the profession entirely of women, but merely to shunt them into "feminine preserves." Moreover, brave women could still go into private practice. Nevertheless, the numbers of women in medicine increased at a slower pace even than those for the other two fields, and in spite of women physicians' rhetoric about increasing opportunity, young women consistently chose other careers.

The numerous articles by women physicians in the first decades of the twentieth century that take it for granted that women would remain a minority within the profession also suggest that they themselves had not yet conceived of a time of real professional equality with men. Their optimism derived from the sense that they had fought and won access to the profession for a special minority. The idea that all women might somehow have jobs or careers, or that 50 percent of the profession should be female— indeed even the concept of balancing both family and career— these were visions of women's options shared only by a few, while for most, such arrangements still lay well in the future. Some women physicians, indeed, were still questioning the propriety of marriage.[83]

Moreover, the "special treatment" that women physicians received for their public-health work could often be demeaning, although such an interpretation benefits from historical hindsight and was clearly not always noticed by women at the time. For example, an enthusiastic report about the activities of women doctors in San Diego given by the chairperson of the Organization Committee at the 1924 meeting of the American Medical Women's Association boasted:

> I want to give you, as one concrete example of the organization work. . . . In San Diego County there are just nine,—I think Dr. Towle of San Diego is here, and if I am wrong she can correct me,— nine medical women. Here is what they have accomplished. They are the pet organization of the San Diego Medical Society. The men are so proud of them and so fond of them that it beams out whenever they come in contact with them. They are given every help and every cooperation, and, the men, if I were to tell the truth I think the men let them do a whole lot of the good hard work and sit back and rejoice in the spontaneity and enthusiasm with which the

Women's Medical Society does a lot of their hard work. After four years of work the San Diego County Medical Women's Association has taken over all the Chairmanships of the women's organizations in welfare work, public health work, etc. It has backed and financed the Sheppard-Towner work in San Diego County. It discusses at its meeting every two weeks for luncheon and passes upon all welfare work done in all the women's organizations. It has the cooperation of all the county and city health officers. It furnishes doctors, dentists and nurses for all the conferences of that very important society, the Parent Teachers Association, in that part of Southern California. It puts on child welfare conferences at the county fairs, in the different parts whenever they occur in the county. It has maintained centers in the schools in San Diego where conferences are held monthly. Last year they held about forty conferences and examined and reexamined over one thousand children. At each conference they have two general physicians, a specialist in eye, ear, nose and throat, a dentist and two nurses. Throughout the county in ten centers they have organized the Sheppard-Towner work. They have the full cooperation and backing of the county medical society and all organized medical groups. The standing of the women physicians has been wonderfully raised in the county, both in the profession and among the laity.[84]

And yet, as much as they valued their role as the champions of social medicine, there was in their discourse an occasional uneasiness about the unequal and confining terms of the progressive bargain. It is not always easily detected, because, as we have seen, women physicians talked a good deal *themselves* about their unique social role. They were not as sensitive to the myriad forms of discrimination as later women would be, but occasionally they chafed against it, displaying hurt and anger when it became too blatant. It is apparent, for example, in their deep disappointment over the shabby treatment they received during World War I, when their desire to serve and prove themselves as professionals was blocked by the refusal of the federal government to commission them as medical officers. Their response was to join the American Medical Women's Association, which kept up constant pressure on the government, *and* to work to fill positions left by the men who had been mobilized. In addition, they defiantly organized their own medical efforts overseas in the form of American Women's Hospitals. Explained a distraught Mary Buchanan, president of the WMCP alumnae association in 1918:

> We felt last summer, when Dr. Rosalie Morton was appointed
> Chairman of the Woman's Committee, General Medicine Board, on

the Council of National Defense, and picked a half-dozen other
women from various parts of the country to serve with her, that
before this women would be on the same footing as men in the
M.R.C.; but alas! a year has passed and despite the time, money and
energy these women have spent going to Washington, Dr. Franklin
H. Martin and his male committee are still keeping them at arm's
length with words and arguments. It is enough to make anyone but
Dr. Morton and Dr. Purnell give up in disgust.[85]

Still, Buchanan continued, all the hospitals are asking for
"women clinicians. . . . The cry is now not for positions for women
in medicine, but medical women for positions. . . . When they ask
bread, shall we give them a stone . . . ? We need successors. We
have the confidence of the community. The trail has been blazed
for the woman doctor. Shall we allow it to be lost because there
are none to "carry on?" Buchanan understood that the situation
was only temporary, and history has proved her correct. After the
war, it would be back to normal: "With the return of the men from
the C.M.C. of the A.E.F., many of our women will have to step
gracefully out and give the men the positions they had before the
war. This is not easy, but it is just—one more act of patriotism
demanded, and no one will resent it any more than the other war
sacrifices."[86]

Women physicians' discomfort with the growing inflexibility of
their role as purveyors of public medicine can also be detected in their
oversensitivity to well-meaning male physicians who occasionally
echoed back to them their own ideology. Somehow, coming from a
man, even a friend to women physicians, the ideas sounded vaguely
sinister. A curious incident illustrating their beneath-the-surface resentment occurred at the graduation ceremonies of the Woman's
Medical College of Pennsylvania in 1915. Dr. Richard Cabot of
Harvard Medical School, himself a passionately devoted pioneer of
social medicine, gave the keynote address. In his appeal to women
physicians to view themselves as peculiarly fitted for public-health
specialties, he offended every woman present. In retrospect, it is
remarkable that Cabot himself did not catch the full meaning of his
own words. Asserting that the majority of women physicians—
though equal to men in ability—were neither temperamentally nor
physically adapted for the more strenuous branches of the profession
and were often therefore "disappointed and dissatisfied," he suggested that they should instead avoid general practice and research
work in favor of social service, where they flourished and were most
needed. The women physicians present felt betrayed. Dean Marshall

responded with the angry retort that she had "been dean of the College since 1886" and she had "yet to see one woman who could be called disappointed." There ensued a public brouhaha in the form of censure and recriminations that took months to die down in the newspapers and journals.[87]

Ironically, women physicians were saying much the same thing as Richard Cabot in their public pronouncements. Nor did they cease to make similar statements after Cabot made them listen to their own words. In 1924 Lilian Welsh observed in an article entitled "The Significance of Medicine as a Profession for Women:" "The importance of preventive medicine equals or overshadows in the public mind that of curative medicine and wherever preventive medicine is studied or applied there is a call for women with medical training. . . . It is fair to predict that eventually all . . . State and municipal [health] departments will be administered by women doctors of medicine."[88]

Thousands of miles away in India, Dr. Anna M. Fullerton, an 1882 graduate of the college who served for many years on its obstetrical faculty and then became a medical missionary, viewed the Cabot affair with the honest impartiality possible perhaps only for one so removed from the fray. Her diary of 8 July 1915 speaks of having received from her brother a newspaper clipping describing the Commencement Day events in detail. After recording long summaries of Cabot's remarks and Dean Clara Marshall's heated response she mused:

> I see something of truth in the statements of both these doctors. Dr. Clara Marshall's facts are correct. Women *have* made a success of their professional work as physicians and surgeons, and have shown neither lack of intellectual ability nor strength of purpose in the way in which they have carried on their work. It is true, too, that they have carried on this work with greater sacrifice of personal happiness than men are called upon to make, and under greater strain.
>
> One source of unhappiness has, in many cases, been the fact that—being a woman—she has had to face the fact that many people still feel that *skilled* medical advice must be masculine, and she is subjected to the mortification of seeing her own advice often set aside for that of some man physician whom she knows to be her inferior professionally.
>
> Another thing that makes it difficult for her is the fact that if she would excel in her profession she must live a lonely life, and carry a double burden—her professional, and her household cares also in most cases. Whereas the man may have a help-mate to share his joys

and his sorrows and to make his home a harbor of rest after toil, the woman must do without this close companionship. Love of the personal kind, that men account none of the strongest motives for putting forth their powers in the service of mankind—must be denied her. A woman cannot undertake the duties of wife and mother, and at the same time give herself as she should to the demands of a life so strenuous both mentally and physically as that of the physician and surgeon. On the other hand, for many women who must of necessity be shut off from the occupations of home-making for their own husbands and children, the opportunities offered by medical practise for the service of their fellow-men are most satisfying, giving as they do occupation to the mind and heart which are the best compensations for what they have missed in the way of home-making.

Thirdly, because of her mother-instinct, and her faculty for looking into details, a woman doctor carries her patient on her heart as well as in her head, considering the patient more as a child in the helpless condition of disease, requiring close and constant vigilance as to nursing, food and surroundings.

Since God made mothers—and there must, necessarily—be so much of mothering in the care of the sick, one cannot but think that in the larger type of womanhood which advancing civilization has made possible, God means women both to "mother" and "doctor" the race into a healthier and happier state than that in which it now exists.[89]

As Fullerton well knew, the woman doctor combined professional values—scientific objectivity, rationalism, personal achievement—with female ideals—the nurturing of children, social concern, self-lessness, purity. The triumph of a progressive ideology and the ascendancy of social medicine in the first few decades of the twentieth century allowed women physicians to participate fully in an important segment of professional activity while maintaining their identity as women. Bringing their expertise to bear on the more private concerns of the family, women physicians, like other women professionals, became an important component of the "search for order." The participation of women professionals in the modernization process has generally been left out of the historical record, but it is no accident that the rise of what are now termed the "helping professions" coincided in time with the beginnings of women's professional activity. Women professionals helped create the liberal welfare state. The ideology of domesticity would, for a time, continue to define their work in the public sphere. Like the health reformers of the nineteenth century who wanted to "make women modern," rank-and-file female professionals in these specialties helped impose social control and middle-class values on a vastly complex and chaotic society. Whether the historian views this activity as benevolent or repressive does not detract from the fact that women physicians' participation in the process must now be made a matter of established fact.

Furthermore, the story of women physicians is connected to the story of how twentieth-century American society solved the debate over woman's nature, searching for and ultimately finding public roles for middle-class women within the professions which would not do violence to woman's primary and central connection to the family. Late nineteenth-century economic and social developments demanded a drastic expansion of welfare institutions to deal with problems of urbanization and change. The reordering of the professions was a product of the very same developments. Integrally connected to the process was the evolution of nursing, teaching, librarianship, social work, and public-health medicine. The connection is not accidental. In the future, historical accounts of professionalization must better describe the ways that women participated in the process. Women historians who have written about discrimination and defeminization after 1900 are certainly correct. There *were* concerted efforts to keep women out of some professions altogether and bar them from those intraprofessional specialties that were defined as "male." Yet other careers were simultaneously feminized, as the middle class explored new boundaries for "women's work" in a restructured, "rationalized" society.[90]

In the 1920s women physicians remained strongly identified with public health at a time when the glitter of a public health career began to fade. A changing political climate after World War I routed progressivism; the decline in public enthusiasm for social reform naturally downgraded women physicians' vision, skills, and perceptions. Finally, the defeat of the Sheppard-Towner Act in 1929 put the finishing touches on the medical profession's decade-long retreat from social activism.

At the same time, the public witnessed the rise of a new hero, the medical scientist, symbolized and celebrated in the central character of Sinclair Lewis's novel *Arrowsmith*. Martin Arrowsmith's career, as Charles Rosenberg has suggested, recapitulates in narrative form the development of modern medicine in the United States, each stage corresponding to a particular phase in its evolution. In the novel, Arrowsmith moves from his adolescent admiration for the old type of general practitioner, through encounters with various medical personalities—the dedicated clinician, the money-hungry purveyor of technology, the efficient surgeon who has traded his humanity for technical expertise. But Lewis's most biting sarcasm is reserved for Dr. Almus Pickerbaugh, the exuberant but none-too-bright public-health commissioner of the mythical midwestern town of Nautilus. Amid his own growing cynicism, Arrowsmith discovers that public-health programs were primarily matters of boosterism, politics, and propaganda, providing no role for the serious, medically trained scientist. As health commissioner, Pickerbaugh preferred writing health jingles to studying the epidemiology of disease, and under his inspiration Nautilus became "one of the first communities in the country to develop the Weeks habit. . . . " 'Better Babies Week,' was followed in succession by 'Banish the Booze Week,' 'Tougher Teeth Week,' 'Stop the Spitter Week,' 'Swat the Fly Week,' and 'Clean up Week.' " The caricature is painfully funny; even down to Dr. Pickerbaugh's silly jingles, which like the one below, written for "Clean Up Week," have a particularly insipid ring:

> Germs come by stealth
> And ruin health,
> So listen, pard,
> Just drop a card
> To some man who'll clean up your yard
> And that will hit the old germs hard.[91]

At the end of the novel Martin Arrowsmith deserts clinical medicine entirely to become the pupil of his old mentor Max Gottlieb, the pure scientist, and one of the few real seekers after truth in the book. Arrowsmith, too, becomes a heroic scientist, full of integrity but inevitably alone, doomed to withdraw even from wife and child in order to pursue his vision.[92] For Sinclair Lewis the new medical hero was a loner, a pure researcher who removed himself from the slough of human existence, and, one hardly needs to add, he was unmistakably a man. Thus, in the very same year that women physicians from Kansas could brag to the annual meeting of the Medical Women's National Association about an exemplary public-health campaign they had dubbed "Fitter Families for Future Firesides," Sinclair Lewis was holding up the Almus Pickerbaughs of the world to public ridicule.[93]

The passing of progressivism deprived women physicians of a particular kind of social validation. One might well argue that women professionals do best in periods of active social reform when women's concerns gain a more public voice. In the 1920s, a new generation of women physicians came to maturity without having had first-hand contact with a central tenet of early feminism—its commitment to an ideal of feminine purpose. Dr. Sarah Tower, a student of Florence Sabin's at Johns Hopkins and later a research scientist, remembered her own experience studying medicine in that decade:

> The days of pioneering in education for women were over. This decade, the 20's, with the first World War well behind and the depression still ahead, probably represented the least complicated period,—the period of the simplest attitudes towards education for women, especially medical education, we have yet known. We knew that when we graduated some internships would not open to us, but enough were. By and large we weren't fighting, we were simply getting educated. At the same time, the days of medical students, women or men, marrying and having babies while still in school had not yet arrived. There was a fair amount of dating between the men and the women, but by and large the main preoccupation of both was getting on with education. Some of the teachers, we knew, took a dim view of women in medicine, pointing to the "wastage" of the training when the women married, and gave up professional careers. But these attitudes troubled us little. We came in fortunate time of consolidation of a good and strong position won for us by our elders, and before the time of facing the new problems and new challenges which were to be created by the winning of that position. The spate of books on "modern women" and "American women" had not yet begun.[94]

More than ever before, women physicians in the next decades would have to learn to maneuver autonomously in a male world without either a reference group of other women or a coherent public ideology to provide them support. Battles would continue to be fought, won, and lost, but they would be viewed as private battles, irrelevant to the female community at large, with the cost measured primarily in personal terms.

CHAPTER 11

Integration in Name Only

In this effort, the most serious obstacles to be encountered are not always the most real ones. . . . People . . . ask not, Is she capable but, Is this fearfully capable person nice? Will she upset our ideal of womanhood and maidenhood, and the social relations of the sexes? Can a woman physician be lovable; can she marry; can she have children; will she take care of them? If she cannot, what is she?

Mary Putnam Jacobi,
"Shall Women Practice Medicine?" 1882.

On 16 September 1921, the *New York Times* published an editorial that enthusiastically endorsed the multiplying opportunities for women professionals in the field of public health. Observing that over 250 women held "responsible administrative positions" as chiefs or assistant directors of child hygiene, directors or assistant directors of state laboratories, school physicians, workers in venereal disease programs, inspectors of food and drugs, physicians in boarding homes for children, "and many other phases of modern life . . . which were once within the control of the housekeeper," the newspaper conceded that such work must now be "properly regulated only by educated and duly authorized agents of the government." The *Times* noted that the ten medical schools now offering degree programs in public health complained of a "want of continued interest in the subject," and urged professional women to take up the slack. The editorial concluded with an ardent reminder that public health was women's work.[1]

A month later the editor of the *Journal of the American Association of University Women* chose to make the *Times* article the subject of her own editorial. She doubted whether women physicians were losing their interest in social medicine as the *Times* had implied. If there was a falling off of their involvement in public health, the problem was not a change of attitude, "but the grim necessity of earning a living." Medical training had become "extraordinarily long and expensive." "Family and social influences playing upon young women," even those brought up in families with sufficient economic resources, were not conducive to encouraging a daughter to choose a medical career. Furthermore, women physicians still encountered discrimination, even in the field of public health. "It may be doubted," the editor concluded, "whether the experience of the few women who have trained themselves for positions of the very highest type . . . has been such as to encourage their sisters to follow in their footsteps." The AAUW *Journal* confessed "to a less roseate view of the situation so far as the opportunity open to women is concerned," and wondered about "the exact character of the 'responsible administrative positions' " held by the 250 women mentioned by the *Times*.[2]

The editor of the AAUW *Journal* did not have statistics at her fingertips, but she was more prescient than she could possibly have known at the time. By the end of the 1920s the position of women in public-health medicine had begun to reflect the precariousness of their position in medicine in general. Though the situation did not become readily apparent until the 1930s and 1940s, two events presaged women physicians' future marginality, even in their "own" fields of public health and preventive medicine. The first concerns the recruitment of Dr. Josephine Baker to teach at New York University Medical School in 1915, the second, the appointment in 1920 of Dr. Alice Hamilton to the faculty of Harvard.

In 1915 Dr. William Park, both dean of the New York University Medical School and laboratory director for the New York Department of Health, invited Baker to lecture on child hygiene for a recently developed course leading to the new degree of Doctor of Public Health. Realizing that she did not have an actual degree in the field of public health and would soon be hiring male Doctors of Public Health in her own Department of Child Hygiene, Baker offered to teach in return for the right to earn the diploma herself. Park demurred, arguing that the medical school did not admit women. Baker responded by refusing the appointment, later commenting, "I can hardly be accused of acting unreasonably because I declined to act as teacher in an institution that considered me unfit for instruction." For a year Park searched for an instructor he felt could equal Baker. In the end, the school conceded defeat, admitting Baker to its public health course and opening it to other women as well, all in order to gain her services on the faculty. Although Baker taught at NYU for fifteen years thereafter, every lecture she gave was greeted by hostile clapping from the male students because she was a woman.[3]

Five years later, Harvard Medical School, wishing to legitimize the field of public health by offering courses in industrial medicine, ended a vigorous search for an appropriate faculty appointee by settling reluctantly on Alice Hamilton, a pioneer in industrial toxocology. Harvard had never appointed a woman to its faculty, and would not appoint another for decades to come, but even the most ardent opponents of women in medicine had to admit that Hamilton was the best in her field. When Dean David Edsall approached her, however, he offered Hamilton only an assistant professorship, making clear that she could not march in the commencement along with other professors, would be barred from the Harvard Club, and must never expect to claim her quota of football tickets.[4]

Thus, though women doctors and other contemporary analysts viewed the period between 1910 and 1930 as one of increased opportunity and expansion, history suggests that the suspicions of the editor of the *Journal of the American Association of University Women* were closer to the mark. In spite of a spate of magazine articles that appeared to legitimate, even glorify, the ambitious career woman who began to work outside the home, and in spite of the falling away of most formal barriers against women in medicine (by 1930 all but six medical schools were coeducational) women doctors made even fewer gains than women in other professions. At a time when the number of female law students doubled from 1920 and 1930, and the number of women who received Ph.D.'s tripled, enrollments for women at medical schools rose at a snail's pace. While male students increased their numbers by 59 percent, the female growth rate was 16.7 percent. Moreover, the 1920s set the pattern for the next forty years. Except for sharp but temporary upsurges in female medical school enrollments at the end of World War II, the numbers of women in medical schools fluctuated between 4 and 5 percent until the beginning of the 1960s.[5]

By the middle of the 1930s, women doctors themselves were beginning to concede that the promise of the early decades of the twentieth century had been elusive. In June 1936 the AMWA Committee on Medical Opportunities for Women reported that female physicians had lost ground even among Departments of Child Hygiene, where they had originally been so numerous. When Sheppard-Towner was first inaugurated in 1921, forty-five states created positions of chief of Child Hygiene, and only three of those appointments were given to men. Little more than a decade later, all forty-eight states were operating such departments under the provisions of the Social Security Act, but only seventeen women, compared to thirty-one men, were state chiefs. Even more disappointing, the position of chief of the Division of Maternity and Infancy of the Children's Bureau, traditionally a woman's job, was also now held by a man. Just as the original AMA Woman's Committee on Public Health had gradually given way to the Council on Health and Public Instruction in 1913 with no women members, so the field of social therapeutics, where women physicians had been so visible, was absorbed into the institutional mainstream of American medicine with a resulting limitation on women's participation.[6] Women would continue to find low-paying, low-status and part-time public-health work, but public-health administration would pass into the hands of male physicians, trained in the new public-health schools connected to prestigious medical schools.

In 1939 a saddened Josephine Baker surveyed the results. "Not long ago," she wrote,

> I went to Washington to attend a dinner for state-directors of Federal child-welfare work. Fifteen years ago, when those jobs were first established by the administration of the Sheppard-Towner Act, only three out of forty-eight of these state-directors were men. Today three-quarters of them are. . . . I am not impugning the capacity of any of those men as individuals when I say that that looks very strange in a line of activity which was invented and developed by women.[7]

What, exactly, was going wrong? For one thing, women doctors misperceived the extent to which social attitudes had changed in their favor. And who could really blame them? No one would deny that the formal barriers to their entrance into the profession had been unequivocably diminished. Only a handful of medical schools still refused to open their doors to women by the 1920s. Older women who could still recall a dramatically different climate marveled at the contrasts. "When I was starting the study of medicine," wrote Rosalie Slaughter Morton, a graduate of the Woman's Medical College of Pennsylvania in 1897, "I was going into what had been considered by the ruling forces . . . a man's profession. . . . And then came what seems a miracle. The world speeded up its revolutions, bringing changes overnight. . . . We women who are now fifty are the first generation which has felt the click of progress in the making." Similarly, Josephine Baker recognized that women physicians were no longer viewed by the public as oddities. "When I think back to those years so long ago," she wrote in 1939, "it is difficult to keep proper sequence in mind. The idea of women in the medical profession is so familiar and commonplace to me now, and it was so strange and unconventional then."[8]

Younger women who had attended coeducational medical schools were even more likely to believe that much had changed. "The age is past when one expects to find in coeducation schools the difficulties the pioneers . . . had to contend with," Alice Weld Tallant, professor of obstetrics at the Woman's Medical College of Pennsylvania and a graduate of Johns Hopkins, told her colleagues in 1917. "From my experience it is perfectly fair to say the opportunity is absolutely equal for men and women throughout."[9] "The woman who works hard and is seriously interested in becoming a very good doctor is as much recognized as any one," agreed Connie Guion, a graduate of Cornell, and the newly appointed chief of Cornell Clinic in 1929. Even Florence Sherbon, active in the American Medical Women's Association and deeply concerned in 1925 about her "definite impression that the ratio of women to men in medicine is not increasing," was shocked to hear from a group of female college students that they dreaded male prejudice. Though not their only concern, this fear still contributed substantially to their decisions to steer clear of a career in medicine. "I had the good fortune," she told them, "to attend a medical school where women always had been received on an equal footing with men. . . . There were no traditions of anything else. . . . I hate to give up my conviction that essential sex prejudice is rapidly becoming a thing of the past."[10]

Indeed, successful women physicians clung so doggedly to the belief that in general the profession now welcomed women that sometimes they tended to blame the victim by voicing their disappointment in younger women's career choices and lecturing college students about their frivolity. Florence Sabin, for example, commented testily in 1924 to an eager first-year Hopkins student that "the females in the Johns Hopkins Medical School used to be serious-minded women, but now they are just nice girls." Similarly, Anna Voorhis, president of the Women's Medical Society of New York State, worried that men took "their profession more seriously than do women," and Rachelle Yarros urged women physicians to stop complaining "any more that we are not getting opportunities, but let us recognize the fact that we are not making opportunities." Florence Sherbon, concerned to discover the reasons for a lack of interest in medicine among female college students, suggested that they were perhaps mistaking for sex prejudice the replacement of "chivalry and sex privilege" with "equality and justice." "We do have to learn to be 'good sports but perfect ladies' in the necessarily vigorous give and take of professional association and competition," she urged tactfully. "We have to divest ourselves of the age-old idea that the perfect gentleman should give a woman a handicap start because she is a woman."[11]

It was not that women physicians were necessarily naive about the continued existence of institutional discrimination. Bertha Van Hoosen, who headed the AMWA Committee on Medical Opportunities for Women throughout the 1920s, periodically published even-handed and detailed reports concerning the status of women in medical schools, internships, and residency programs. She was never reluctant to expose bias when and where she found it: in the refusal of many AMA-approved hospitals to open up their internships and residencies to women, in the excruciatingly low number of female medical faculty throughout the country, in the fact that "many schools limit the number of women regardless of the number of applicants," in the surgical tracking systems which insured that the majority of women surgeons would be those trained at a woman's school, and even in the leadership of the profession, where through the year 1927, only one woman physician had held national office in the AMA.[12]

Other women physicians besides Van Hoosen were equally outspoken in their conviction that the profession was dominated by men who refused to grant women equal status. "Men do not want women in their institutions and organizations except as subordinates and auxiliaries," wrote Inez Philbrick in the *Medical Woman's Journal* in 1929. "As assistants, technicians, nurses, and stenographers, they are greatly appreciated and most indispensible. As competitors for equal recognition men simply tolerate us under compulsions."[13] Thus, medical women knew quite well that there were still significant vestiges of public and professional opposition. But the important battles had been won. The remaining task was straightforward: to investigate and expose the persisting forms of institutional discrimination. Apparently far more difficult for them to tackle was a much more insidious problem: the fact that a public debate over the "working woman" which took place in the 1920s was being resolved in a manner that would continue to make it hard for a woman to commit herself equally to career and family.

Though the achievement of female suffrage may have brought an end to a particular brand of public feminism, and the appearance of the flamboyant, devil-may-care flapper may have misled many analysts into the observation that feminism in the 1920s had lost its constituency, historians now know that what really occurred in this decade was that feminism changed its focus and direction. Barnard Professor of Economics Emilie Hutchinson correctly characterized the shift when she observed that the center of concern had moved from education and suffrage to the more basic problem of economic opportunity. And, indeed, Americans in the years after World War I began to wrestle with the question of the future position of the homemaker in American society. The most fundamental issue was whether or not to grant public acceptance and approval to the gainfully employed married woman.[14]

From 1890 to 1920 the proportion of married women workers rose from 3.3 to 7.3 percent, an increase of from 12 to a little over 21 percent of all women workers. In the 1920s working wives continued to participate in the labor force, and by 1930 they comprised 28 percent of all female workers. By the middle of the decade feminist concerns began to reflect these significant changes when a group of self-styled "New" feminists—primarily educated women professionals, some of whom had little emotional attachment to the nineteenth-century suffrage campaign—focused their public concerns on the conflicts middle-class women were experiencing when trying to balance marriage, family, and work. These new feminists rejected the notion of nineteenth-century social feminists that women could rightfully function in the public sphere only if their work made a significant contribution to the good of the community and claimed for themselves the personal and individual self-fulfillment that allegedly accrued to people who enjoyed satisfying work lives. In addition, they insisted that women need no longer be forced to choose between marriage and a career. The modern woman, wrote the journalist Dorothy Dunbar Bromley in an outspoken article in 1927 which became a kind of manifesto, was tired of "old school . . . fighting feminists who wore flat heels and had very little feminine charm." Such women were "zealous" and their methods "inartistic." The present generation of feminist—"new style"—believed "that a full life calls for marriage and children as well as a career." Like many older feminists, she valued her "economic independence . . . above all else," but was also "hard put to it to understand the sex antagonism which actuates certain advanced women." Excited at the prospect of combining work with a career, the new feminist, according to Bromley, hadn't the time to concern herself with silly details like whether or not she should keep her maiden name. Her purpose was to "emerge from a creature of instinct into a full-fledged individual who is capable of molding her own life." Thus, she would freely admit that "home and children may be necessary to her complete happiness," but she would no longer let men and children totally "circumscribe her world."[15]

Feminists like Bromley believed that they had the new psychology and Freudianism on their side when they cited a genre of 1920s literature that linked the modern woman's social isolation in the home with neurotic housewives and poorly socialized children. Picking up the argument of earlier theorists Charlotte Perkins Gilman and Olive Shreiner, new style feminists, too, stressed the connection between economic independence and individual self-esteem in more "modern" terms. Educator Ethel Puffer Howes worried that training women and then underutilizing their real abilities augured physical and emotional disequilibrium. "Probably no man who has not experienced it," wrote the advice columnist of *Woman's Home Companion,* "can conceive the ravages of financial dependence on character, the having nothing in the world he could call his own, except as a gift from someone else." Both the psychologist Lorine Pruette and the radical feminist Suzanne La Follette, anticipated the concerns of feminists in the 1960s when they argued that uninterrupted domesticity was leading to mental deterioration. In *Concerning Women* La Follette accused consumerism, technology, and advertising of hypnotizing American women so that the majority of them lived "without the exercise of the reflective intellect, without ideas, without ideals, and in a proper use of the word without emotions." Pruette worried that the monotony of domestic labor sapped energy and self-esteem, and prescribed part-time work as an antidote.[16]

"Modern" feminists militantly rejected the single life in favor of companionate marriage. Though increasingly from 1900 on small numbers of middle-class women had attempted to combine children, careers, and a marital relationship of shared intimacy and mutual support, new feminists correctly accused their forbears of viewing family life and public life as mutually exclusive. By the 1920s experiments in fusing work and family life were talked about publicly. Career feminists viewed themselves as a new kind of pioneer, insisting that their choices were a break from the past. They rejected what they termed the "self-assertive and antagonistic feminism of the past," where women "worked against heavy odds and usually had to buy success at the price of marriage and children, sometimes charm and personal appearance, of being considered queer—as some of them undoubtedly were," with nary a glance behind them.[17]

Arrogant, perhaps, in their unwillingness to acknowledge the struggles of older women who shared their goals and desires, career women in the 1920s had in fact experienced some important cultural changes. Unlike their mothers, who had lived in an age more tolerant of female bonding and the intimate friendships between women that often spanned an entire lifetime, the women of the new generation grew up in a cultural climate that vehemently stressed heterosexuality and downplayed female relationships. These attitudes reflected a radical redefinition of female sexual nature. The new feminist could be a man's pal as well as his willing and eager sexual partner. She felt little compulsion to defend or extol female capabilities in the abstract, admitting that American women had "so far achieved but little in the arts, sciences and professions as compared with men." Gone was the assumption of female superiority and natural guardianship, the sense of sisterhood. The new feminist, indeed, preferred to work with men because their methods were allegedly "more direct," "their view larger," and she could deal with them on the basis of real companionship. "Woman usually prefers to work with man, of a truth," admitted Dr. Luella Astell, president of the Wisconsin Medical Women's Society, "but that is no one's fault. If it were not so, the marriage institution would become obsolete. To admit such a preference is simply to declare oneself a normal woman with healthy sex instincts. It's nothing to be ashamed of."[18]

Indeed, only paid employment for women could presumably alter the power relationships within marriage and make it truly a union of equals. Satisfying work, with intellectual stimulation and healthy contact with the outside world, would give women the same opportunities for self-development that their husbands enjoyed. The result would be female competence and creativity in both spheres, with a particularly beneficial influence on the home. "May it not be possible," mused the economist Chase Going Woodhouse, with a nod in the direction of Elizabeth Blackwell,

> That with the right help and a bit of direction the present-day college woman with her wide interest, her ambition to continue her professional work, her refusal to be tied to a house, will be the one to reform the home and make it a more desirable and efficient place in which to develop future generations?[19]

For a time the advocates of career and marriage looked on expectantly as magazines and journals of all sorts took up the cause of the new breed of woman. Articles on "fifty-fifty" marriages and "the home-plus-job-woman" dotted the pages of the *Woman Citizen,* the *Atlantic Monthly, Woman's Home Companion,* the *New Republic,* and even the *Ladies Home Journal,* which only a few years earlier had opposed women's suffrage. Statistics suggest that growing numbers of young women were not quitting their jobs after marriage, but were extending their period of employment at least until the birth of their first child. For example, the number of married professional women rose from 12 percent in 1910 to 27 percent in 1930. Yet perhaps as a response to the literature on working wives, the 1920s were also a decade that renewed its interest in the mother-child relationship. John B. Watson's manual *Psychological Care of Infant and Child,* published in 1928, held for this generation the same fascination that Benjamin Spock's *Baby and Child Care* would for the next. Watson's emphasis on rigid schedules and the rational control of affection between mother and child still assumed that the mother's role was "second to none." "The having of children," he wrote, "is almost an unsuperable barrier to a career."[20]

Spotlighting women's central role in child rearing exposed the Achilles heel of the new feminism. Not only did the work of psychologists like Watson reinforce the ideas of those who were threatened by the desire of new feminists to restructure family life, but it also split the ranks of those eager to facilitate matters for working wives. A number who advocated combining marriage with gainful employment were careful to distinguish between working wives and working mothers. Many new-style feminists believed that working wives should become full-time mothers once their children were born. "At the present time," admitted Henrietta Rodman, a leader of the radical Greenwich Village Feminist Alliance, "the care of the baby is the weak point in feminism. The care of children, particularly those under four or five years of age, is the point at which feminism is most open to attack."[21]

Despite the best efforts of feminists in the 1920s, the problem of balancing motherhood and careers remained unsolved. Mary Ross reasoned that women had but one choice, to subordinate their careers to those of their husbands or to pursue work only at intervals guided by childbearing. The journalist Eva Hansl of *Harper's Monthly Magazine,* wrote that " 'Being there' is the greatest contribution we mothers can make in the lives of our children." Some feminists found private solutions by marrying but not having children. Of the seventeen women who were invited by Freda Kirchwey in 1927 to explore the personal sources of their feminism on the pages of the *Nation*—"to discover the origin of their modern point of view toward men, marriage, children, and jobs"—only five were mothers. Most of the childless women in the group worked only part time, carefully choosing jobs which gave them the flexibility needed to run a household. Others hired full-time nurses and housekeepers. Similarly, a study of professional women by Virginia MacMakin Collier in 1926, revealed that the overwhelming majority left their children in the care of servants.[22] Women physicians, of course, for whom professional success did not afford the luxury of moving in and out of active participation at will, were practically forced into such a solution.

Also painful and confusing to the growing number of women seeking to combine marriage and work was the feeling that their efforts attracted neither the admiration nor the interest of most of the young women who came of age in the 1920s and who chose marriage over work. From 1900 on, in fact, fewer and fewer women were deciding to remain single. College-educated women, unlike their predecessors, who had rejected marriage so emphatically at the end of the nineteenth century, were increasingly recording their preferences for marriage over a career. Whereas estimates have found that roughly 25 percent of the women in 1900 who had received bachelor's degrees remained unmarried, and 75 percent of the women who earned Ph.D.'s between 1877 and 1924 were spinsters, polls taken in the 1920s reflected the heightening popularity of marriage for all women. Educated young women's reported preference for marriage over jobs seemed particularly troubling to feminist observers. In 1927 Lorine Pruette admitted that most of these young women were "frankly amazed at all the feminist bother and likely to be bored when the subject comes up." Her own research on middle-class teenage girls revealed that of the third who would have considered giving up marriage for a career only a small proportion of them understood the implications of such a choice. The others talked about careers in Hollywood or fantasized unrealistically about glamorous jobs. Polls taken at various colleges revealed similar trends. A canvass of Vassar women in 1923 found that 90 percent wanted marriage, "the biggest of all careers." Seven years later 70 percent of the graduates of New Jersey's College for Women rated husbands and families as their top priority.[23]

The good-natured willingness of college women to steer clear of career commitments that appeared to threaten future home and family life confounded women physicians, just as it did other female professionals. But they hardly knew how to solve the dilemma. For the most part, they contented themselves with identifying and publicizing the problem. Florence Sherbon's article in 1925 enjoined the readers of the *Medical Women's Journal* "to begin vigorously to think our way through this question." Believing that the present age was witnessing "a reaction from female celibacy" as a "refreshing number of young college women declare with conviction that they want to have children," Sherbon urged her female medical colleagues to look to themselves for role models. "How many medical women marry? How many have children, and how many children? How do those that do marry and have children manage to make a home and do their duty by husband and children?"[24]

Some female medical educators only hesitantly endorsed marriage and medicine. Dean Martha Tracy of the Woman's Medical College of Pennsylvania announced in 1932 that marriage, medicine, and motherhood could be combined, but she emphasized that self-control, poise, and maturity were needed in order to achieve success. She confessed a strong aversion to young women who had already married in medical school and felt family life should be postponed until a woman completed her medical studies and her internships. "The matter of young married internes is a serious one," she cautioned. "I've known many who expect to thoroughly disorganize hospital regime and secure for themselves unusual privileges in order to be with the newly acquired husband." As a member of the Board of Internes for the College Hospital, she confessed a hesitation to appoint young married couples. "You see sentiment and sentimentality may overcome science, if only temporarily," she explained, "but during that period it is a dangerous element for disorganization."[25]

Tracy's ambivalent attitudes reflected how women physicians struggled with the issue. Individual women continued to worry about the "matrimonial mania that possesses both young men and young women" and believed that it had a great deal to do with the difficulty of recruiting good women students. Others were more accepting. Adelaide M. Brown, herself the daughter of a pioneer woman physician and for a long time connected with the San Francisco Children's Hospital which her mother helped found, was more optimistic. "Marriage comes into open competition in many women's lives," she admitted. "The woman physician seldom realizes the double tug on her brain and her emotions which this double demand will make." But Brown, much less cautionary than

Martha Tracy, encouraged medical marriages nevertheless. She did admit, however, that the married women doctors who had the most successful careers were those who chose medical fields with "less responsibility," namely, clinical and laboratory positions, work in pathology or part-time social service, psychiatry, and salaried hospital jobs.[26]

Even the Woman's Medical College of Pennsylvania offered no easy solutions to this central dilemma of women's lives. Marion Fay, later dean of the college but in the 1930s and early 1940s the head of the Department of Physiological Chemistry, remembers that she was considered "a disgrace by some of the women faculty members" because of her approval of women's combining marriage and medicine. "Some of the older M.D.'s on the faculty," she recalled, "thought I was simply outrageous, that I was promoting matrimony. I can remember one dear soul who just announced to all and sundry that no woman could possibly be a doctor and be married. . . . I was accused of being a marriage counselor." When a married student came to Fay in tears with the news that she was pregnant, expecting to be chastised and thrown out, Fay's response, "Oh, isn't that wonderful!" nearly knocked the poor girl from her chair. But in the end, the college did not dismiss the young woman, as a coeducational school might have, and after some difficulty arranging things she graduated with the rest of her class.[27]

Thus, solutions were private and piecemeal. Of the twelve women physicians who attended medical school in the 1920s and 1930s interviewed for the Medical College of Pennsylvania's Women in Medicine Oral History Project, the single women all had full-time careers. Of those who married, only two, Irene Koeneke and Katherine Sturgis, continued steady medical work after receiving their degrees. Koeneke married a man twenty-seven years her senior who was a major figure in the medical profession in Kansas, and she remained childless. Sturgis attended medical school after her children were of school age, but even then was forced by circumstances to have them live for many years with her ex-husband and his new wife. What is more, Sturgis had originally wanted to attend medical school after college, but was diverted from her goal when she fell in love with a young engineer and eloped with him at the end of her freshman year. She resumed premedical studies only after her divorce. Although none of the other women gave up medicine entirely, all of them worked at medical "odd jobs" while their children were young. Natalie Shainess, whose career in psychiatry gathered momentum after her children were grown, maintained a limited private practice. Caroline Bedell Thomas began to make her most important contributions to epidemiological research only when she was in her late fifties and sixties, and worked at a series of fellowships and part-time clinical appointments when raising her three children. Finally, Louise de Schweinitz practiced no medicine at all for the first three years after her children were born. Returning to medical work part-time, she held a variety of positions, including clinician at a pioneering birth control clinic; nursing instructor; physician to a school district, a summer camp, and a university student health service; health lecturer; and attendant in a number of well-baby clinics. Significantly, all of the women married fellow physicians. The contrasts in the professional lives of the married and unmarried women suggest that Florence Sherbon's warning, "We have got to settle all this before a large number of serious and brainy young women are going to matriculate in medical schools," hung over medical women like a pall.[28]

Lack of adequate solutions meant that large numbers of women, even those whose aspirations had been for a full and intense professional life, would falter in the attempt to balance career and family. When such women "failed," they tended to blame themselves. Louise de Schweinitz, for example, felt that her inactivity in medicine after the birth of her five children occurred because "there was something lacking in me." Though she never discussed the problems of staying professionally active with her husband, she believed years later that he "was sorry I hadn't done more in medicine at the end of my career."[29]

By the end of the 1920s, confessions of failure from many working women began to appear in a number of magazines. Articles by "ex-feminists" told sad, funny, and often self-deprecating stories of the slow death of their idealistic goals in the face of familial demands. One such "confessional" entitled "Men are Queer That Way; Extracts From the Diary of An Apostate Woman Physician" was published in *Scribner's Magazine* in 1933 by a graduate of Johns Hopkins, Dr. Mabel Ulrich. The diary began with an excited and hopeful entry in the last year of medical school:

S. and I have decided to get married next year when we get through medicine. Of course we shall be fearfully poor at first, but as long as we are both going to work we shall make twice as much as we could alone, and anyway we don't care. I told him I didn't know a thing about housekeeping, and he said why should I? That he could see no more reason for a woman's liking cooking and dishwashing than for a man's liking them. That since our education has been precisely similar, we are starting out exactly even, therefore there would be no justice at all in my having to do all the 'dirty work'. . . . So we have decided that one week I shall take over all the duties connected with the running of our house and the next week he will. Of course we are going to have an office together and be partners in every sense of the word. I was so happy I couldn't speak. Then after a long time we talked about our children. We are going to divide up the care of the children exactly as we divide the housework.[30]

Only months after the marriage, however, the experiment faltered. "It is no go," Ulrich wrote. "We have given up the 50-50 housekeeping plan. We tried for a month, but by the end of one week I knew S. is a fearful mess as a housekeeper. . . . Could never remember the laundry. . . . But then of course he is busy and I am not."

For the next seven years Mabel Ulrich struggled to balance private practice, family, and children. But even with servants the job proved a difficult one:

Twenty-five today—a quarter of a century old. A doctor, a wife, and a mother—yet I don't seem to have learned anything. Am just as mixed up as ever. Tried staying awake last night to see if I could size things up a bit. But it was no use . . . then remembered that I forgot to tell Alma that S. wants his bacon crisper, and that all S.'s buttons are off his pajamas, that I must send in the next payment on the washing-machine, that we simply must have Dr. and Mrs. S. to dinner one night this week . . .

Minor "incidents" abounded. After a visit from an unmarried female medical classmate, now a physician, Ulrich noted the contrast between her friend's "stunning" professional good looks and gay self-confidence and her own disorganization, vowing that "somehow I have *got* to get some new clothes." She gradually realized that her husband's affections for her were aroused, not when she was brilliantly diagnosing patients, but when she was "in the kitchen with an apron on, or sewing on a button." Forgiving him, she mused,

After all he can't help it. A man, it seems, may be intellectually in complete sympathy with a woman's aims. But only about ten per cent of him is his intellect—the other ninety is emotions. And S.'s emotional pattern was set by his mother when he was a baby. It can't be so easy being the husband of a "modern" woman. She is everything his mother wasn't—and nothing she was.

For a time Ulrich, discouraged in the slow development of her own practice, tried her hand at being her husband's lab technician to save money. The plan was thwarted when she discovered that he didn't trust her work and felt the need constantly to corroborate her findings. 7 August 1911, begins with the entry, "Have walked out on my job," and ends with the observation, "Verily I am no technician. But oh *what* a woman I should be if an able young man would consecrate his life to me as secretaries and technicians do to their men employers. Yet I can't rid myself of a sense of guilt and failure. My Victorian hangover at work." After turning down the offer of organizing and heading up a health service at a major university because she felt it would be too difficult for her husband to move his practice to another city, Ulrich admitted, "I don't believe a woman's work is ever so important to her as a man's is to him."

Mabel Ulrich ultimately gave up her private practice and found her niche as a lecturer in social hygiene and preventive medicine. During the years before World War I and into the 1920s she did service in antivenereal disease campaigns alongside numerous other women physicians who found health education a career choice more compatible with family life. During the Depression Ulrich became the Minnesota state director of the Federal Theater Project.[31]

Uncertain of the long-term effects on themselves, middle-class women who worked were even more doubtful concerning how their choices would touch the lives of husbands and children. Wrote one mother:

In spite of hesitations, doubts, and questionings, I hang on like grim death to my newspaper job. My reasons are simple and selfish. . . . As for the children, time alone can tell the story. . . . Whether or not they will suffer from the repeated injunction, "Now run away and play. Mother must pound the typewriter," remains to be seen.

"Nothing is settled in the woman's mind," wrote Lorine Pruette. "She is having to work out new ways of living, about which there are still many disputes. She has not the ready-made justifications of the men." What Pruette described so accurately was the tentative, trial-and-error method that women in these decades used to balance the competing demands of work and family.[32]

Thus, for all the hopeful veneer of a professional social climate which had discarded the most blatant formal barriers against women's entrance into the medical profession, the necessary changes in family life and in child-rearing practices that would have allowed the ordinarily competent but not superior woman to consider a medical career did not materialize in the 1920s, or, for that matter, for half a century thereafter. Women who wished to solve the dilemma were generally left to themselves to devise individual solutions. No wonder they remained unsure of themselves when they made the attempt.

By the end of the 1920s, the factionalization of the woman's movement after 1925, the subsequent disappointment of many that women's suffrage did not bring the hoped for "gender gap" on political issues, and the increasing ineffectiveness of the reform coalition in the face of conservative political reaction meant that there would be no coherent, centralized feminist coalition to help interpret the problems encountered by women "trying to be modern." Most troubling of all, the continued absence of effective solutions to the private and personal dilemmas of those young women who wished to combine marriage with gainful employment outside the home obscured the fact that the problems they encountered in fulfilling those intentions resulted not from some personal inadequacy, but from a fundamentally inegalitarian social structure which persevered despite the enormously compelling but ultimately cosmetic changes which the 1920s had wrought.

Medical practice, then, exhibited none of the characteristics that began to be associated with women's work by the end of the 1920s. It demanded an investment in time and educational training that far exceeded the typical white collar, clerical, service, and sales occupations growing more popular with middle-class women. Even positions as managers and proprietors and jobs in the feminized professions of nursing and social work required shorter training and provided more flexible work schedules.[33] Finally, continuous structural and professional changes within the organization of medicine itself also helped keep down the numbers of women in medicine.

Efforts to reform medical education and raise the entry requirements to medical school continued throughout the 1920s. By 1930 only seventy-six medical schools remained in existence, all of them with A ratings, compared to 166 in 1904. In another development, schools began to increase the number of college credits required for admission. In 1930 some 70 percent of medical students had baccalaureate degrees, while twenty years earlier only 15.3 percent had completed college. Then, in 1921, Johns Hopkins Medical School decided to limit the size of its freshman class rather than to admit all qualified applicants. By 1924 fifty-four schools had followed suit. Such a policy made acceptance much more competitive and gave school officials more control over admission policy. Equally significant was the growth of specialization and the consequent lengthening of medical education first to an internship year and then to several years additional training in approved residency programs.

In the early decades of medical reform, the longer term of study and the higher standards caused a noticeable drop in both male and female enrollments. But as was demonstrated in Chapter 9, female enrollments dropped more precipitously than did men's. By the 1920s, overall applicant numbers seem to have adjusted to the more stringent requirements and began to increase steadily, but female growth rates were excruciatingly slow. Though up from 3.4 percent to 5.9 percent in 1920, numbers fell back to 5.4 in 1924 and fluctuated thereafter from between 4.5 and 6.5 percent until the 1960s.[34]

These structural changes in medical education combined with the cultural prejudices against women professionals which we have discussed to work against female medical aspirants in several crucial ways. First, there was the matter of cost, a problem touched on by the editor of the AAUW *Journal* in her 1921 article. Medicine was the most expensive of the professions to enter. Yet even well-to-do families were only rarely willing to finance a daughter's medical training. Medicine's demanding schedule also made it the hardest professional training to combine with part-time work. Finally the unequal job structure meant that women would generally have fewer opportunities for self-support, and, when they could work, their wages would be lower. No wonder the college women Florence Sherbon interviewed in 1925 complained of the high cost of medical education and the difficulties of self-support as a deterrent to a medical career.[35]

Katherine Sturgis, interviewed in connection with the Women in Medicine Oral History Project, had come from a wealthy family reluctant to support her medical career. She remembered teaching Sunday school, running the school bookshop, and taking on other odd jobs to earn money. Living with her two children during the first years of medical school in Philadelphia, she recalled that sometimes "we were so broke . . . we once had the electricity turned off and sometimes we ran out of coal." Another interviewee, Pauline Stitt, a student at the University of Michigan, babysat, ironed shirts "in interesting faculty homes," cooked and cleaned, and gave blood in order to save up for medical school.[36]

Statistics confirm that women found it more difficult than men to put themselves through school. A 1929 government study revealed that in 1927–1928, 45 percent of the male undergraduates to only 25 percent of female coeds earned part of their college expenses, suggesting that most women either received full support from their families or didn't attend school at all.[37]

Medical women were aware of these financial constraints. In 1918 Martha Tracy, dean of the Woman's Medical College of Pennsylvania complained that,

> It has become the registrar's painful duty to hand me, all too frequently from the same mail, letters calling in distress for women physicians to fill vacant places in hospitals or private practice, and letters from young women, college graduates, from Bryn Mawr, Cornell, Goucher, Syracuse, Swarthmore and elsewhere, ready and anxious to study medicine, but without funds to do so.[38]

Women also obtained scholarships with greater difficulty than did men. Of the 24,328 educational scholarships available both to women and men in 1927–1928, funds were awarded to only 8,834 women. Seven hundred forty-seven of the scholarships available were exclusively for medical education, and women received only 7 percent of them. Even these were inadequate because they covered tuition only, without any allowance for living expenses. Attempting to remedy the problem, women doctors and other women professionals called for women's organizations to "make possible the provision of adequate financial assistance to women of outstanding promise in the medical field. This aid is needed at both the undergraduate and post-graduate levels." Both the Alumnae Association of the WMCP and the AMWA had scholarship funds, but the money was never adequate.[39]

Competition for places in medical schools heightened as schools took steps to hold down attrition rates and admit only those outstanding students whom they could be certain would finish the medical course. By the end of the 1920s applicants presented credentials that often exceeded most of the schools' official requirements. While still only two institutions insisted on a baccalaureate, in 1929 45 percent of the applicants had bachelor's degrees, while 49 percent had at least four years of college credit. After 1925 Johns Hopkins instituted a policy of looking only at the best students from the best schools, and requiring a deposit of $25 and a personal interview with the application. Anticipating that this move would curtail their enrollments for several years, Hopkins officials were amazed to learn that over a hundred outstanding students applied in 1927 for their 75 places. Hopkins's new policy helped to reduce its attrition rate substantially, and in time other schools adopted its methods. Analyzing these changes in the applications statistics, Dean Burton Meyers of the Indiana University Medical School observed,

> The schools of medicine of America occupy a position that is unique—unprecedented. No other school of any university is forced by applications greatly exceeding school capacity to select so discriminatingly the membership of its classes.[40]

At first glance the application statistics do not reveal overt discrimination against women. Indeed, Dean Meyers of Indiana University declared that they even hinted at a slight female bias. In 1929, for example, 65.5 percent of the women applicants were accepted to medical school, while only 51.0 percent of the men were admitted. Overall, roughly half of the applicants of each gender were admitted each year for the next four decades. In the 1970s the number of women admitted exceeded half temporarily for a few years. Not all the medical schools pursued a coordinated policy of institutional discrimination. Quotas, when they existed, were scattered and inconsistent, with some schools having very few or no women students and others, including some of the better institutions like Stanford, Columbia, University of Chicago, and Johns Hopkins, admitting up to 10 percent. However Meyers's conclusion that women received slightly preferential treatment ignored the fact that female applicants were even more qualified than their male counterparts—something he himself admitted in his report. "We are probably justified in assuming," he wrote, "that a higher percentage of women who present themselves for matriculation in medical schools are well prepared for the study of medicine."[41]

Of course such an observation was no surprise to women doctors. Grace Goldsmith, who edged out the future heart surgeon Michael E. Debakey for the top position in her 1932 graduating class at the Tulane University School of Medicine, and who later did important nutrition research and ultimately retired as dean of her alma mater, believed, as did many of her successful female colleagues that "on the whole, women have to work harder and do more, and seldom are equally paid." Goldsmith was one of six women students in a class of 108. Similarly, Martha Tracy, in her study of female medical graduates published in 1927, reported that most of them agreed "that a woman must be about 50 per cent superior in the quality of her work to receive the same consideration as a medical man."[42]

Evidence suggests that once women were accepted to medical school, they performed as well if not better than their male counterparts. Bertha Van Hoosen polled over forty medical colleges and found that women equalled the men as students. But her inquiry also revealed a widespread assumption among administrators that women dropped out of medicine to marry. One of her official respondents judged the attrition rate among women to be as high as 50 percent, concluding that "the education of women medical students [was] about twice as expensive as men." Indeed, the general disappointment in women's commitment to medicine was often so pervasive that women physicians themselves voiced doubts. In a letter to Florence Sabin, Adelaide Brown, who in 1923 was considering endowing a fellowship for women in gynecology and obstetrics at one of the California medical schools, worried that women students she had observed were not performing as they should. Disappointed with the career choices of female medical graduates in the last ten years, she had noticed that most wound up in "Anaesthetics & Pediatrics . . . Infant Feeding . . . or Matrimony." "I had a talk with Dr. Edsall about Harvard Medical School & the possibility of its being opened to women students," she informed Sabin. "He told me . . . the general opinion . . . that women were *far* less likely to contribute to the world by active work in medicine and . . . they felt it was more valuable to train more men as the number was necessarily limited." In a commencement address to the graduating class at the Woman's Medical College of Pennsylvania that same year, Sabin herself urged the audience not to give up medicine when they married because it contributed to prejudice against women doctors. "Indeed," she concluded, "one of the next steps in the feminist movement is for educated married women to claim and to carry on a share of professional work."[43]

In 1938 Martha Tracy reported the overall dropout rate for medical students at 25 percent. There is no conclusive evidence to suggest that the attrition rate of women medical students was considerably higher than men's, but it might have been. It is true that the proportion of female students decreased in the 1920s, but one historian has argued that enrollment figures in these early years do not account for women who transferred schools or took leaves of absences. Also absent from the statistics is any adjustment for the variance in program length. However, a study of medical student attendance between 1949 and 1958 does find women dropping out of medical school twice as often as men (15 percent to men's 9 percent). By this decade the overall dropout rate for all students had declined to a little over 8 percent. Moreover, female medical students' attrition rate was considerably lower than the dropout rate for women in other professional occupations like law, academia, or engineering.[44]

Discriminatory assumptions about women's commitment to the profession continued to make it difficult for them to receive equal treatment. By the end of the 1920s female medical educators had begun to complain that "the increased competition hurt women." The 1928 AMWA report of the Organization Committee included Mary McKibben Harper's warning that "covert opposition, of a dangerous variety" was visible in "the increasing difficulty with which women enter medical colleges." "Study carefully the actual and relative numbers of women students admitted to the university medical schools," agreed Martha Tracy a year later. "Awake anew to the fact that these schools are not increasing their opportunities to women students and do not intend to do so, for competition for places by men is too great."[45]

Although women physicians might disagree on the relative equity of their chances for admission to medical school, few of them would dispute the fact that good internship and residency programs were extremely difficult to obtain. In 1922 Alice Hamilton, who kept herself aloof from the American Medical Women's Association and bitterly opposed the Woman's Party Equal Rights Amendment platform because of its threat to protective legislation for working women, commiserated on the question of advanced training with Dr. Mary O'Malley, an officer in both the Woman's party and AMWA.

> As for the status of women of our profession, that seems to me a very serious question, which I wish I could discuss with you some day. Do you think that any sort of legislation will help to get us the thing we need most, places on the staffs of hospitals? As it is now, a woman can obtain the same education as a man and is on an equality with him till her interneship is over. From then on she is hampered by her inability to secure the one thing that will give her aide, experience and prestige, a hospital appointment. But the hospitals are privately run and could not be forced to appoint women.[46]

The difficulty for women was especially poignant because women doctors enthusiastically accepted the rise in standards that lengthened internship and residency requirements appeared to represent, and in their struggle to be as good or better than the men, they hardly realized how higher standards and limited programs would adversely affect them. But worry about internship opportunities surfaced as early as 1901. In August of that year Helen MacMurchey published a study that revealed that there were 203 women holding hospital appointments in the United States. Although the number of women graduates from 1900 to 1922 stayed a little below 200 each year, few of the available internships were the most desirable ones. Complaints continually surfaced that the coeducational medical colleges, by their indifference to helping women obtain hospital appointments, were not following through on their commitment to educated women students.[47]

In 1926 the undefatigable Bertha Van Hoosen surveyed the internship opportunities for women once again. Though she found that a total of 1,047 internships were available for roughly 212 graduates, the figures were misleading because many of the hospitals listed would "not consider a woman intern unless it is impossible to get a desirable man." Seventeen states had no hospital at all willing to accept a woman, and most of the opportunities were concentrated in Pennsylvania, New York, California, and Illinois. Over and over again hospitals complained of the problems involved in housing women interns, although it was clear from the response of many administrators that this excuse would be set aside if a woman was really needed. Such a situation arose during World War I, when many women doctors were hired to replace men who left for the army. Margaret Castex Sturgis, for example, a graduate of the Woman's Medical College of Pennsylvania in 1915 and recently married to an army physician working at Fort McPherson who was waiting to be shipped overseas, wrote her old dean, Martha Tracy, in July 1918 that she was looking for a hospital job. After an exchange of several letters she reported excitedly that she would be replacing New York Hospital's resident physician, who was leaving for the army.[48]

After the war, however, women were not so fortunate. In 1923 Louise de Schweinitz applied to three Boston hospitals for an internship in order to be in the same city as her physician husband. All three of them turned her down because she was a woman. She wound up an intern at the New England Hospital for Women and Children without even bothering to assess the quality of its program simply because it was in Boston. For a graduate of Johns Hopkins, interning at the New England was a step down in the quality of her training. At the time it was not a teaching hospital, and de Schweinitz knew that the training was not on a par with what she had received in Baltimore. But she felt that she had no choice.[49]

Quality residency training was even more difficult to obtain than a good internship. Even at Johns Hopkins, where according to one woman faculty member, "the woman medical student is tolerated during her undergraduate days," a woman was "given early in her career to understand that she can go only so far in the department and no further." Recalling the experience of one young woman graduate when she applied for an internship there, Professor of Psychiatry Esther Richards wrote years later that the department head had responded, "Yes, I will be glad to have you, but I want you to understand you can be interne and assistant resident but you can never be resident or go any higher, no matter how good you are."[50]

In 1920 Martha May Eliot left Johns Hopkins to take a first year residency with Dr. W. McKim Marriott at the St. Louis Children's Hospital. Initially interested in staying for another year as senior resident, Eliot gave up in disgust when, after a long talk with her mentor, she realized that "it is evident that he doesn't want a woman as resident.—He constantly evaded the question but was very cordial about my coming back to do any type of research work I might desire." Eliot's only firm chief residency offer was at Detroit's Woman's Hospital, where a long and respectable line of women physicians had been before her. Instead, she decided to come East and begin a private practice in Boston. Later in the year she was offered a position as pediatric resident at Yale. Marriott, interestingly enough, eventually came through with the offer of a chief residency, but only after she had indicated her plans to return to Boston.[51]

Similarly Alma Dea Morani, the first woman to become certified as a plastic surgeon in the United States, became the first woman intern at St. James Hospital, a Roman Catholic institution in Newark, New Jersey. A graduate of the Woman's Medical College of Pennsylvania in 1931, she had hoped from the very beginning to become a surgeon. But even the WMCP did not encourage women in general surgery, although there were several gynecologists on the faculty who did surgery. The head of the Department of Surgery, Dr. John Stewart Rodman, was a man, and he had two male associates in preceptorship with him. Rodman had not yet trained a woman to become a surgeon. While still in medical school Morani told Rodman that she wanted surgery. After thinking about it for a year and monitoring Morani's performance as an intern, Rodman agreed to take her on. Morani believes that she would not have had the slightest chance of becoming a surgeon if she hadn't attended a woman's school. Even though there hadn't yet been any women assistants in Rodman's tenure, Morani felt that a woman in a woman's school at least stood the possibility of acceptance. Bertha Van Hoosen's findings that 75 percent of the women surgeons in 1926 had either graduated from a woman's medical school or had served as internes or residents at hospitals staffed entirely by women, corroborated Morani's impression.[52]

The Depression severely threatened even the slim gains that professional women had made in the 1920s. Economic dislocation, psychological disillusionment and public hostility to women working meant that women would fail to maintain their position even in the predominantly feminized fields of teaching, nursing, librarianship, and social work, where men made significant inroads for the first time. Male teachers increased from 19 percent to 24.3 percent of the total between 1930 and 1940, while the proportion of male librarians jumped from 8.7 percent to 15.1 percent during the ten-year period. Male welfare workers increased from one-fifth to one-third of all workers. Even in nursing men made such noticeable advances that the U.S. Office of Education recorded male enrollment in nursing schools for the first time.[53]

Women had made less progress in medicine than in any of the other professions in the 1920s, and it is no wonder that this stagnant position continued throughout the 1930s. The records of AMWA and the financial struggles of the Woman's Medical College of Pennsylvania reveal reduced incomes and some economic hardship, but no widespread unemployment among women physicians. In their study of Muncie, Indiana, however, Helen and Robert Lynd found that in the years between 1920 and 1935 the number of female physicians practicing there dropped from eight to two. The Lynds viewed this loss as directly related to the general precariousness in the 1930s of women's professional position relative to men's.[54]

For all these reasons, the aspiring woman physician in the twentieth century was hampered by professional and cultural handicaps which, though they appeared less visible than those suffered by the pioneer generations earlier, were no less effective in keeping the numbers of women doctors down to a tiny 5 percent of the profession. Unable to find social supports for maintaining a career and a rewarding family life, young women continued to turn away from a commitment to medicine when living in an atmosphere that encouraged "companionate marriage" as the most exciting and most creative endeavor available to the "modern" woman. Professional observers duly took note of young women's reluctance to sacrifice their personal lives to medicine, and punished them accordingly by discriminating against them in advanced training: because women were expected to drop out, administrators reasoned, there was real justification in withholding from them elite internships and residencies.

This unfavorable social and professional climate made it difficult for women physicians even to hold onto what they had so painstakingly built in the previous half-century. The loss of a coherent feminist consciousness, which had provided women professionals with a supportive and stimulating intellectual atmosphere from which to draw strength, was reflected in the disquieting history of women's medical institutions after 1930. Most illustrative of the growing ambivalence of women themselves toward separate female institutions was the manner in which the very existence of the American Medical Women's Association persistently split women physicians over the question of separatism. The membership rolls of the organization continued to reflect a lack of interest on the part of the majority of women doctors in an organization of their own. The numbers of women who belonged to AMWA fluctuated between 9 percent and 14 percent in the decades after 1920, and the annual turnover, according to one president, Dr. Kate Karpeles, was "appalling." The most important question that confronted the organization, she admitted in 1939, was "how to increase its membership."[55]

Leaders who made periodic attempts to drum up regional support for the organization wrote to each other in despair. "The work in this Region has been most unsatisfactory this year," admitted Kate Hurd-Mead, regional director for New England in 1931. "I have encountered the most dull indifference despite many letters to our members asking for help and advice. There seems to be in their minds no adequate reason for meetings of medical women at present. We have very few young women practicing here, and as they are busy with their work they do not offer papers for discussion. Many of them come from co-education schools and hence think that women alone are not interesting." Similarly, Elvenor Ernest of Kansas wrote to Louise Tayler-Jones, "This district of mine is certainly a poser. I get so discouraged sometimes that I feel like resigning my job. . . . The women in these states are so scattered, and women's medical organizations, according to their view point are so unnecessary, that it is about the hardest region to handle with my very limited resources."[56]

Laments about women physicians' lack of interest in their collective situation continued to be expressed by AMWA leaders with disquieting regularity throughout the 1940s and 1950s. In 1949, the guest editor of the *Journal of the American Medical Women's Association* fretted about the wide variety of opinions among medical women regarding "our exclusively feminine professional organizations." Some would have "us believe," she wrote, "that we are now accepted on an equal basis with men and that maintaining such groups is not only uncalled for but highly undesirable." Privately women physicians voiced similar worries about female complacency. "In my meeting with young physicians (most of them from co-education schools) and with young women thinking of studying medicine," wrote Inez Philbrick on a questionnaire from the Woman's Medical College of Pennsylvania, "I find most of them . . . knowing nothing of the struggle of women to enter the profession . . . and I do not find them resenting the limitation of numbers of admissions to coeducational schools, or discriminations shown therein." Likewise, confided one past president of AMWA to another in 1952, "I have learned that women doctors are not interested in promoting other women today. The older women who penetrated the profession by carrying a high spirit of enthusiasm for a cause have disappeared, and are succeeded by those who have a spirit of complacency and secure smugness in their personal accomplishments."[57]

And, indeed, with many women who took medical degrees after 1920, AMWA had a distinctly negative image. Although a handful of the women physicians interviewed for the Women in Medicine Oral History Project were active in AMWA, many rejected it quite consciously. To Harriet Hardy it "seemed like an old ladies' tea party," and Harriet Dustan considered it "entirely inappropriate"—a "Chowder and Marching Society." Katherine Sturgis, in spite of her connection with the Woman's Medical College of Pennsylvania, first as a student and then as a faculty member, felt AMWA was a "biased organization." Caroline Bedell Thomas saw it as "not pertinent" to her research-oriented career, and Louise de Schweinitz and Esther Bridgeman Clark both shied away from its perceived separatism. Beryl Michaelson, who took her medical degree in the mid-1940s, did join the association after graduation, and was for a time president of a local unit in Iowa, but the group soon fell apart, and "the individuals of the Iowa group that really wanted to continue it were so few that I lost interest."[58]

As one scans the pages of the *Journal of the American Medical Women's Association,* however, it is difficult to criticize the organization too severely for its failure to attract more members. AMWA continued to struggle with issues pertinent to its constituency. Though perhaps not on a par scientifically with the *New England Journal of Medicine* or even *JAMA,* the journal featured current publications by women physicians, listed job opportunities for medical graduates, and reported medical school news, news from branches, and other important information that in a different social climate might have been considered more relevant to the lives of women physicians. The group also committed itself to legislative committee work regarding health issues of interest to women; support for the Equal Rights Amendment; service to younger women physicians and students in the form of loans, scholarships, and assistance in finding jobs, fellowships, or residencies; vocational guidance to young women contemplating medical careers; and establishing ties with women physicians abroad through the American Women's Hospitals and a constituent membership in the International Medical Women's Association, founded in 1942.[59]

AMWA demonstrated continued willingness to investigate the status of women physicians and expose subtle and not so subtle forms of discrimination. In June 1946 JAMWA published a disturbing survey conducted by the New York Infirmary that revealed that 41.7 percent of available internships and 34.2 percent of available residencies were still closed to women medical graduates. Four months later an editorialist hailed a significant new study by two Barnard professors that sharply contradicted prevailing assumptions about the 50 percent drop-out rate of women physicians and demonstrated that roughly 90 percent of them and 82 percent of those who married remained in full-time medical work.[60]

The organization also continued to tackle the question of balancing marriage, medicine, and motherhood. AMWA President Rosa Lee Nemir chastised her constituency for being too silent on the issue in a 1962 article, and pointed out that since "the majority of our members are married and have children," the AMWA was "ideally suited as an organization to distribute information in this area. We must assure interested young women that marriage and a medical career combine not only successfully but profitably with enrichment to both. . . . It is time for women physicians to publicize the facts about ourselves."[61] Yet, for the most part, young women were not yet listening. Though middle-class women continued to work in increasing numbers after World War II, they were still not choosing to commit themselves to a career as demanding as medicine. Under such an unfavorable social climate, AMWA continued to speak for a tiny fraction of members within an often beleagered professional minority until feminism in the 1960s tackled the problem of the patriarchal family and exposed the hidden constraints that made it so difficult for women to balance family life and full-time careers. Only in the mid-1960s did the number of female applicants to medical school begin to rise significantly, and such change resulted directly from the revival of the feminist movement.[62]

The professional marginality of AMWA in the 1930s, 1940s, and 1950s reflected the marginality of women physicians as a group. The AMA patronized them, controlling in gentlemanly fashion their participation in its activities. A letter from Dr. Carl Henry Davis, secretary of the AMA Section on Obstetrics, written to AMWA President Frances Eastman Rose in 1926 exemplifies the attitude of polite tolerance which would continue to characterize these decades. Davis asked Rose to try and find "some distinguished woman physician whom you may wish to have for the Medical Women's National Association" to present a paper before the obstetrical section at the next national meeting. "We always like to have at least one woman physician in our Section program," Davis explained pleasantly. Neither Davis nor Rose seemed to think it odd that Davis himself knew of no such "distinguished woman" and had to appeal to the president of the AMWA to search for one.[63]

Two other issues symbolically important to women physicians who were members of AMWA became subjects of contention between the AMWA and the AMA. The first, which was finally resolved in favor of the women, was the question of their army status, something which became an especially emotional problem after the outbreak of World War II. Many women physicians were still smarting from the cavalier treatment they had received from the surgeon general during World War I, when he refused to commission them in the armed forces. In 1939 AMWA President Nellie S. Noble again announced women physicians' readiness to serve, and in 1940 a committee was formed to begin a registry of women physicians for emergency service. The committee unsuccessfully pressured the AMA to support the commissioning of women physicians on the same footing as men. The issue soon became a cause célèbre with the public, however, and women physicians eventually gained the support of the American Legion, the New York State Medical Society, and certain key congressmen, including New York's Emmanuel Celler, who volunteered to introduce a bill on women physicians' behalf into Congress. After much maneuvering and many disappointments, the Sparkman-Johnson Bill, providing for "the appointment of female physicians and surgeons in the Medical Corps of the Army and Navy," was signed into law by President Roosevelt on 16 April 1943. By the end of the war, over 130 women physicians had served.[64]

Another complaint lodged by members of the AMWA was its poor representation in the power structure of the AMA. As early as 1936 President Josephine Baker asked, "Where are the women?", and complained that women had "practically no representation, not only in the House of Delegates, but in the appointive office" of the AMA. Though one could not join AMWA unless one first belonged to the AMA, Baker felt that women were treated as an "unconsidered auxiliary." Three years later Emily Dunning Barringer took up the cause on behalf of the Association, proposing that a woman be appointed yearly to the AMA House of Delegates to represent women physicians as a group. The legislative body of the AMA, the House of Delegates, consists primarily of representatives drawn from state societies in proportion to their membership, as well as a few others from interest-group constituencies like the military. Raising the matter with her local New York branch, Barringer put through a resolution favoring the appointment of a woman delegate which was endorsed unanimously by the Women's Medical Society of New York State. Then the proposal went to the House of Delegates of the Medical Society of the State of New York, where it was passed with minor changes and was brought before the AMA House of Delegates in 1939. There it was defeated on the grounds that "our women physicians are now entitled to the representation they seek, through regular channels. They have the same opportunities for selection that other members enjoy."[65] Though AMWA attempted to reopen the question a number of times, it was only in 1983 that the AMA finally agreed to give a representative of the women's organization a seat—though only with observer status—in its House of Delegates.[66]

AMWA's difficulties in attracting younger members and its failure to dent the power structure in the AMA persisted throughout the 1960s and early 1970s. While the reappearance of feminist activism in the 1960s prompted a frontal attack on the social values that had kept so many women in the first half of the twentieth century from seeking professional goals, AMWA lay dormant. A poll taken in 1965 revealed that only 27.2 percent of its members were under forty years of age. Most had attended medical school in the 1930s and 1940s. A year earlier AMWA's president admitted that membership was still a "complex" problem.[67] Younger women physicians suspected that the organization was not responsive to their needs. One intern who attended a meeting observed wryly that "there was a lot of excitement and swapping of stories about injustices to women doctors during World War I." Several of the more youthful interviewees for the Women in Medicine Oral History Project felt similarly distant from the organization. Florence Hazeltine commented, "It hasn't been very effective for younger women; it's mainly for older women"; and Gillian Karatinos agreed, "I never really felt a part of them."[68]

Yet feminism's success in the 1970s began to be reflected in the rising application and acceptance statistics for women in medical schools across the country. By the middle of the decade women's professional organizations acquired new status and prestige. AMWA was no exception. Gradually younger women at the height of their careers did join the organization, and quickly dissatisfied with what they perceived as a lack of direction, several of them forced a major restructuring of the group at its annual meeting in 1980. In Boston that year the proposed slate of officers was hotly contested from the floor for the first time in the history of the Association, and although the challenge failed, the accompanying debate resulted in the subsequent charting of a more feminist course and the inclusion of many new faces among the group's leadership. Also significant was the hiring of a progressive executive director who had had many years experience working with the New York-based Committee of Interns and Residents. One of her first accomplishments was a communications audit of membership materials resulting in a streamlined brochure with a clearer statement of the organization's feminist and medical goals, which was sent as a direct mailing to every woman physician in the country. This major outreach effort has borne positive results. In 1983 regular membership increased by one-third. Although the percentage of AMWA members still remains only 8 percent of women physicians nationally, it is the strong hope of the present leadership that the Association's concerted efforts to regionalize and encourage grass-roots support will continue to bear fruit. Certainly the sudden willingness of the AMA House of Delegates to seat even a representative-observer from AMWA after forty years of opposition to the idea represents one proof of the group's increased visibility and political clout.[69]

Equally exciting to many younger members of the Association has been the refurbished image of its journal. In 1982 a new managing editor was appointed whose philosophy was in keeping with the more feminist direction of the organization. Since then, strong efforts have been made to investigate and expose the more hidden difficulties women physicians experience balancing home and careers, as well as to provide a balanced *female* professional approach to some of the important health issues for women which have been raised over the last decade by the women's movement. It is too soon, of course, to predict the long-term results of these changes for women themselves or for the profession as a whole, but what remains most significant is that such articles no longer fall on deaf ears. They reach a growing constituency of women physicians for whom these concerns are vitally important.[70]

Unfortunately, the revival of the women's movement in the 1960s came too late to preserve the integrity of other women's institutions which had performed such important service to women physicians in the last century. The fate of two of them are worthy of brief consideration, for their stories reflect yet another dimension of women physicians' precarious collective professional position in the twentieth century.

Because the formal and most visible barriers to women's entrance into the profession had appeared to have dissolved by 1920, those female medical leaders who still supported separate women's institutions were hard pressed to justify their continued existence. In 1909 Abraham Flexner had concluded that women's choices in medical education were "free and varied." He editorialized that "now that women are freely admitted to the medical profession, it is clear that they show a decreasing inclination to enter it." Flexner speculated that either women were not interested in medicine, or there was no strong demand for the woman doctor.[71] Moreover, he believed the women's schools had served their purpose and were no longer necessary.

Female leaders knew better, but their arguments in defense of women's institutions remained similar to those mustered by their predecessors in the nineteenth century. Many supporters continued to point to discrimination. Others concentrated on the special nature of women's institutions and the important tasks that only they performed. Both positions were timeworn and familiar, and both contentions had lost their "bite" in the more complicated atmosphere of twentieth-century medical professionalism. In the case of the New England Hospital such familiar refrains proved no match for the competing exigencies created by improvements in the standardization of the medical care delivery system. The burgeoning expenses of modern hospital operaton, the ever-rising certification requirements of professional physicians, the upgrading of residency programs and their connection with university teaching facilities, the changing demographic landscape of the modern city, and the adoption by women physicians themselves of the shared values of their professional community, all contributed to a loss of allegiance to exclusively female goals.

Like many of the women's medical institutions, the New England Hospital suffered in the twentieth century from rising costs and shrinking sources of financial aid. By 1950 it had become largely dependent on the contributions of the United Community Services—Boston's "Community Chest"—which had given the institution roughly $60,000 a year for the last decade. Though female philanthropy had helped sustain the hospital in its first half-century, it could no longer prove adequate to the task of maintaining a modernized physical plant. As a result, the hospital, much like other hospitals in Boston, drew from new, more "modern" sources of financial aid, sources which were less interested in the hospital's feminist past than in their assessment of its continued value in the general community.[72]

The New England's operating difficulties made its position precarious by the early 1950s. Economic problems worsened as its physical plant—the main building built in 1899, and enlarged in 1917 and 1931—became more and more outmoded and inefficient. Bed occupancy rates declined precipitously. While most hospitals strove for an 80 percent rate to balance the books, the New England's occupancy rate during the 1950s was only 68 percent in medicine and surgery, 49 percent in obstetrics and 10 percent in pediatrics. Equally serious was the hospital's resulting disfavor with young doctors seeking clinical experience. World War II had greatly increased internship opportunities for women in Boston. When Massachusetts General admitted women interns during the war years the number at the New England fell from ten to two. At one point the hospital actually offered an honorarium to women who chose to train there. The end of the 1940s brought no improvement in this situation. Inefficient facilities and few patients continued to make it difficult to recruit house staff. By 1952 the New England had only four residents and one intern.[73]

It is not surprising that United Community Services would choose to investigate the hospital's deteriorating conditions. In 1949 a general survey of all the Boston hospitals it supported suggested that the New England seek to improve its image by opening its active staff to men in order to attract more patients. A year later UCS reiterated its recommendation in a new report, declaring that "the old idea of a hospital for women and children, operated by women, must be abandoned and . . . the objective of the hospital should be changed to become a community hospital," and threatening to cut off funds.[74]

The ensuing decade witnessed a struggle to save the New England Hospital as a women's institution—a struggle which divided women doctors and their supporters into two camps. Initially sympathetic with some of UCS's demands, hospital Trustees sought to placate its critics in 1949 by dropping its designation "for Women and Children" and opening its doors to male patients. A year later, when the chief of surgery retired, she appointed a male physician in her place, and by the end of 1951 he had hired fourteen men to the surgical staff. But accepting male house staff had not yet been voted official policy, and in the meantime UCS continued to pressure the trustees about attending to the hospital's continued financial difficulties. In 1953 Dr. Phillip Bonnet, asked by the trustees to recommend improvements in hospital services, called for a merger with another hospital in the area to improve the New England's situation.[75]

The unofficial introduction of men onto the hospital staff, the continued insistence by the UCS that "the changed attitude of 1948 on the subject of women in medicine raises a serious question of the wisdom of continuing separate and designated hospitals in training and medical practice," and fears that financial difficulties would ultimately force the hospital to merge, led to something of a feminist revolt. Opposing the UCS and a minority of women doctors and trustees who favored hiring men, was another trustee, Mrs. Blanche Ames, a long-time feminist and suffrage activist. As leader of the rear-guard action, Ames determined to preserve the "traditions and objectives of the founders and . . . to oppose this strange resurgence of prejudice against women's aspirations which would turn the clock backwards one hundred years."[76]

For almost a decade, supporters and opponents of preserving the hospital as a woman's institution battled it out. But a minority of younger women physicians were quite willing to see the hospital open its facilities officially to male physicians. Women like Dr.

Rosemary Nelson, a staff surgeon, contended that "the addition of men to our staff for even this short period of time . . . improved" her "professional ability." She spoke for several others as well when she claimed, "Most of us have been educated in co-educational medical schools after having competed without any concessions because of our sex, for admission. We have gained our education on an equal basis of give-and-take. I have never had a reason to feel discrimination." The hospital, many concluded, need no longer discriminate in favor of women.[77]

More popular, but less effective, were the arguments of Blanche Ames and her supporters that discrimination against women doctors still existed on all levels of medical training, that a minority of women still preferred to be treated by a woman physician, and that at a woman's hospital "the scientific treatment of medicine is made so inconspicuous a patient hardly knows it is being carried out." In the end, such rhetoric could not save the New England. In a social atmosphere that cherished such professional values as impartiality, rationality, and egalitarianism, a hospital dedicated exclusively to the advancement of women physicians had become an anachronism. In 1964 the New England's bylaws were altered to accept men on its staff. Unfortunately even this change failed to save the institution, and four years later it closed its doors and became a community health center.[78]

Similar problems plagued the Woman's Medical College of Pennsylvania. Chronically short of funds, the institution's leadership nevertheless worked hard to upgrade its medical education. Marion Fay, later dean of the College but hired in 1935 as professor of physiological chemistry, remembers that "the question of finances was always present. This school has always had to get along on a very reduced budget, and you were conscious that many things that you wanted to do, you were hampered in trying to do them by the lack of money." The school's comparatively small means meant that it could not grow easily, and that well into the 1960s it would emphasize clinical education rather than research. Katherine Sturgis, for example, contemplating a medical education in the mid-1930s, sought advice from her internist, Dr. David Reisman, who was a professor of medicine at the University of Pennsylvania. When she replied "no" to his inquiry as to whether she was interested in research, he counseled, "You go up on the hill to Woman's Medical. They'll train you to be a good general practitioner."[79] The college's achievement in turning out creditable and sometimes brilliant women practitioners becomes all the more remarkable when one contemplates the implications of several studies that suggest a positive correlation between the relative wealth of a school and the ability and success of its student body.[80]

Members of the American Medical Women's Association understood the value of the Women's Medical College to all women physicians as a "bulwark for the future." "I have no quarrel with them for going to other medical schools," wrote Ellen Potter, of women who preferred coeducation, "but our continued existence is essential to them."[81] Even many male physicians respected the college's role in preserving a place in the profession for women. In 1941 the school's newly appointed dean, Margaret Craighill, wrote Florence Sabin of a conversation she had had with a mutual friend and male faculty member at Johns Hopkins, who "felt very definitely that the school should continue" because "the co-educational schools are so highly selective for women that only the supposed 'super women' have an opportunity to study medicine in them, whereas the average man can obtain this privilege. That leaves the 'average woman' no chance to become a physician except at this school. . . . Many of these . . . develop into better than average, and . . . the record of this school is proof of this statement." Given these realities, AMWA developed a close relationship with the Woman's Medical College of Pennsylvania in the years after 1920, organizing a special committee to give it financial support, and publishing reports about the school in its newsletter.[82]

But the college's path was never easy, and was too often filled with crises. One crucial juncture occurred immediately after World War II, and involved Margaret Craighill, a Johns Hopkins graduate, who was appointed dean of the College in 1940. Though Craighill was the product of a coeducational medical school, she seemed enthusiastic about her new position. Her first accomplishment was to strengthen academic standards by reorganizing the Board of Directors. Her goal was to limit the powerful lay interference of the president, Sarah Logan Wistar Starr, a loyal supporter of the school who, according to Marion Fay, "took the place as her private charity," and had repeatedly bailed the school out of its chronic financial difficulties since the 1930s. Craighill understood that upgrading and modernizing the college involved professionalizing and standardizing its power structure. Confronting Mrs. Starr was an important step in the right direction. She then devoted her energy reorganizing the hospital. In 1941 she wrote Florence Sabin, "I am under the impression that you feel there is no place for a separate Woman's Medical College. That was a very real question in my own mind when I came here last fall, but after studying it intensively for six months I have come to the conclusion that there is a needed place for such a school at present, and that with a combination of graduate study we may fill a real need for women in medicine." Craighill was convinced, she assured Sabin, "that we can hope to put this school in a position which needs no apologies." Also in that year, Craighill was able to involve yet another important and highly visible Johns Hopkins graduate in working to support the college—Louise Pearce, a fellow of the Rockefeller Institute since 1913. Pearce served as a member of the Board of Corporators until 1946, when she became president of the school, serving until 1951.[83]

But before Craighill could make substantive changes, her active tenure as dean was cut short in 1943 by the passage of the Johnson-Sparkman Bill, which commissioned women physicians in the Armed Forces. Craighill became the first woman doctor to join the military and, with the rank of major in the Army, left the college temporarily to take up new duties in the Office of the Surgeon General in Washington, D.C. In her place as acting dean she chose Dr. Marion Fay, chairperson of the Department of Physiological Chemistry. Fay took the position with many reservations, fearing that she "was going to be officiating at a funeral." Because of the war, Fay "thought very decidedly that the men's schools would be admitting many more women, and that both the quality and quantity of our applicants were bound to go down, and we would not be able to fill our class with properly qualified people." Much to Fay's surprise, the number of applicants "tripled and almost quadrupled" during these years as "women all over the country got much more interested in medicine." Fay plunged good-naturedly into her new role, kept the college running smoothly, and in 1946 handed over to the returning Dr. Craighill a "practically solvent" operation.[84]

In spite of the promising situation, Craighill's first move was to negotiate secretly a merger with Jefferson Medical College. Shortly after her return, she called the Board of Corporators together and presented the arrangement as a fait accompli, arguing that it was the only way the college could survive. Stunned, Fay and a majority of faculty members, students, and alumnae revolted. In a stormy session a few days later, they voted down the entire plan, and Craighill resigned in disgust. Once again Marion Fay replaced her as dean.[85]

Yet what Dean Craighill failed to accomplish in one bold stroke, the passage of time and the exigencies of medical education have achieved for her. Ironically, though Fay and her supporters fought hard in 1946 to preserve the identity of the college as a women's institution, they won the battle but lost the war. The subsequent history of the school demonstrated that no one could stem the tide of "progress." In the professional world of modern medicine, progress meant coeducation.

During Marion Fay's tenure as dean from 1946 to 1963, she presided over a number of important changes at the college. Like other medical schools in the country, Woman's Medical responded as best it could to the shifting demands of professionalization. Its faculty became full-time and salaried, money for a new research wing was secured, and the size of entering classes grew as facilities were improved. The trend towards specialization, which had accelerated after World War II, brought more and more men to faculty and administrative positions, because of women's still limited access to specialty training. From 1950 to 1960 the percentage of women faculty declined from roughly 50 percent to 39 percent. This development so disturbed the alumnae that in 1966 they petitioned the college administration in protest, asking that the balance be restored in favor of women.[86]

In 1963 Dr. Fay supported Dr. Glen Leymaster, long associated with the Council on Medical Education, as her successor. Not since the founding of the school more than a hundred years before had the deanship been held by a man. Fay argued that it was impossible to find a woman both qualified and available. Although some shared her view, other alumnae believed that she had become convinced that male leadership would be more forceful.[87]

Since 1969 Leymaster has been succeeded by several new deans, all of them men. Similarly, the college has had a succession of presidents. Only in 1970 and in 1976—for one year apiece—has that office been held by a woman. The only woman physician who was interviewed for the job in 1974 speculated cautiously that her interviewers doubted whether a woman could project "the kind of image" that was needed.[88]

At the time Leymaster was appointed, he had appeared to be committed to preserving the college's identity as a woman's institution. In 1965 he published an idealistic article that envisioned the Woman's Medical College of Pennsylvania as a national center for educating women in medicine. Only three years later, however, he had become discouraged. Worried about the mounting difficulties of getting proper funding for an all-woman's school, and pressured by the male faculty and members of the Board of Corporators who had little feeling for the school's history and who felt coeducation was the only way to help their students become competent physicians, Dr. Leymaster recommended that the college admit men.[89] In 1971 six men entered the freshman class, and the school dropped the word "Woman's" from its name and became the Medical College of Pennsylvania. Although there has remained an informal commitment to retaining large numbers of women students, the presence of males has become a significant one. By 1980 74 percent of the faculty was male, while the number of male students had increased from 6 to 40, roughly 40 percent of the entering class.[90]

Marion Fay believes that the change was "inevitable." Many agree with her that "the school's standards have definitely been raised." But other alumnae, emotionally attached to a school that had seemed to nurture, not dampen, their highest aspirations, lamented the passing of "Woman's Medical."[91] Some identified strongly with Barnard graduate Laura Inselman Guy, a member of one of the last all-woman classes, when she recounted her medical school experience:

> In June 1966 I entered the Woman's Medical School. . . . While in medical school and during my training, I never experienced negative feelings towards me about women in medicine. Much of this, I believe, is related to the fact that I attended a woman's medical college, where everyone is equal, where competition was kept minimal but yet standards were high, and where it was shown every day that women, femininity, medicine, careers, husbands and children can all exist happily and healthily in the same household. The college no longer exists as a woman's medical college. I consider myself quite fortunate to have been one of the women in medicine to have experienced the philosophy and teachings of the college, as these have influenced many of my ideas and attitudes about my role as a woman in medicine.[92]

The Woman's Medical College of Pennsylvania became coeducational in 1970 and as a result, the last woman's medical institution ceased to exist. In the future women doctors would struggle to develop a satisfying professional identity without the intangible psychological benefits provided for so long by institutions they could, if they so chose, call their own.

CHAPTER 12

Quo Vadis?

Regardless of whether they are culturally or biologically determined and regardless of whether society is mistaken in calling them womanly virtues, what are generally seen as psychic characteristics of women should be just what American medicine needs at present. I should count it a loss if these "feminine" qualities were not restored to medicine either because of the determination of radical women that men and women are just alike in all qualities except anatomy, or because of the determination of conservative men that because women do differ, they should not become physicians in any large number. . . . Some qualities attributed to women could well be shared by men without shame. Nurturing, for example . . . along with tenderness, caring, and empathy. So what is wrong? Women come along at a time when medicine needs these qualities.

Howard M. Spiro, M.D., 1975

What is being and can be done to neutralize the dogmatism of biomedicine and all the undesirable social and scientific consequences that flow therefrom? . . . The power of vested interests, social, political, and economic, are formidable deterrents to any effective assault. . . . The delivery of health care is a major industry, considering that more than 8 percent of our national economic product is devoted to health. . . . Professionalization has engendered a caste system among health care personnel and a peck order concerning what constitute appropriate areas for medical concern and care. . . . Under such conditions it is difficult to see how reforms can be brought about.

George L. Engel, M.D., 1977

Nineteenth- and early twentieth-century feminists struggled hard for women's right to enter what the nineteenth century liked to call the public sphere. They focused their agenda on equal opportunity to education, the reevaluation of woman's nature and intelligence, political equality, and the elimination of the most blatant aspects of institutional discrimination against working women of all classes. Ironically, they were unintentionally aided by the economic needs of a rapidly developing industrial democracy which found increasingly practical a theory of family structure favorable to educating women, and even to drawing some of them gradually into the labor force. In the nineteenth century, primarily single and then working-class married women began to work outside the home. By the end of

World War II, however, capitalism thrust so many women into the public sector as paid workers that it almost seemed as if the demands of the marketplace would accomplish what feminism alone could not.

The number of working wives, for example, had tripled in the two decades between 1940 and 1960. Before the war, most of them had come from the working class, but by the late 1950s an equal proportion was being drawn from middle- and upper middle-class homes. Indeed, white-collar wives were even more frequent jobseekers than the wives of factory workers.[1] While women worked in unprecedented numbers, after 1960 an increasing proportion of them entered male-dominated fields that had previously remained stubbornly inhospitable in spite of the best efforts of early women's-rights advocates. In some professions, women have already recouped the losses of the 1930s, 1940s, and 1950s. Medicine, for instance, has reflected such changes both in the rising numbers of women doctors and in their increasing willingness to articulate a female point of view. In 1979–1980 25.3 percent of medical students were women, and a survey of medical school deans predicted that females would eventually account for one physician out of every three.[2]

What have been the implications of these changes for women? Has capitalism really achieved what feminism could not? Certainly an important contribution to the recent influx of women into the labor corps has been the maturation of what Harry Braverman has called "the universal market"—the transformation of society into a giant exchange for labor and goods.[3] My primary concern has not been with the fascinating process by which home labor was rendered uneconomic as cheap manufactured goods produced in harsh conditions and thrust upon not-always-willing consumers drove women out of the home and into industry. Rather, I have sought to study the effect of such developments on a group of middle-class and professional women. And here perhaps one important clue has been the growing economic centrality of consumption. Capitalism, after all, teaches poeple to want more than they have. Historians of women's work have carefully noted the relationship between the growth of the female work force and the rising material expectations of the average middle-class family. As social custom, style, fashion, advertising, and the educational system created since the 1920s an increasing demand for goods and services just beyond what the ordinary middle-class man could comfortably earn, family life for many became characterized by a gnawing sense that there was never quite enough. The more a man earned, the more was needed: a second car, a new television, a vacation in Florida, a food processor, a better vacuum cleaner. Paid labor for the majority of middle-class women expanded in order to help provide families with these things.[4]

Not always aware of the economic forces propelling middle-class women into public activity, nineteenth-century and early twentieth-century feminists nevertheless laid the groundwork for women's unprecedented participation in politics, social reform, economic life, and the professions. Yet few of them successfully challenged the cultural mandate that consistently defined women's priorities as belonging primarily with the family. As we have seen, the overwhelming majority of ordinary women, who continued to marry and have children, accepted this cultural mandate as a given. While women were drawn into the marketplace as paid laborers, there was no concomitant rethinking of gender roles either at home or at work. As a result, the first half of the twentieth century has witnessed most women being "liberated" by the industrial order into more sophisticated forms of degradation: through job segregation, unequal wage differentials, and the perpetual exploitation of their unpaid household labor. Though they suffered in different and unequal ways, both working-class women and professional women were hampered by a domestic ideology that allowed them to work only as long as their labor did not overtly jeopardize family stability.

This particular solution to the problem of women's dual role took precedence over a more radical alternative offered by some feminists, particularly outspoken by the 1920s, who wished to find a better resolution to the organization of family life, one that could free women to pursue careers with the same seriousness as men. But by the opening decades of the twentieth century, the economy was already focused around the infinitely reduplicated single-family dwelling, designed for consuming goods and providing unwaged, privatized services. Traditional gender definitions were thus powerfully connected to the perpetuation of the economic status quo, and when women entered the public sphere, there were always tacit but mutually accepted limits to their participation. Our study of women physicians has suggested that for them the human cost of such a solution was visible primarily on an individual and a personal level. Women doctors struggled with their complicated lives, often only dimly aware that their difficulties arose because they were attempting to straddle two identities, the professional

and the personal. When individual women failed at this complicated task, they unwittingly reinforced the common assumption
that there were still important areas of public and professional
activity in which they simply did not belong.

Yet the social and economic conditions that I have been describing created fertile ground for the revival of feminist ideas in the
1960s, especially those ideas demanding equality of opportunity
and equal pay for equal work. As the job market became even
more rigidly sex-segregated in the decades after World War II,
while traditionally female professional occupations like teaching
and social work were invaded by men with the resulting decline of
female professional and technical positions, a mass market of over-
educated, underemployed, and underpaid women stood poised and
ready to join those bold enough to proclaim aloud their dissatisfaction. The feminism of the 1960s gave them a voice.

The civil rights and student protest movements of the 1960s also
unleashed the forces of women's discontent. The response to
"women's liberation" was electric. By 1970 hundreds of women's
groups had formed in cities across the country. *Time Magazine*
estimated that 10,000 had joined the cause. Tens of thousands
participated that summer in the Women's Strike for Equality.
When a group of New York feminists met a year later to publish a
national magazine written by and for women, they could not possibly have predicted the extent of its success: the premier issue sold
out—all 300,000 copies—within eight days. The ensuing weeks
brought over 20,000 letters to the offices of *MS. Magazine*—letters
full of praise for the new publication. Joining with groups of old-
style feminists who by the late 1960s had begun to reconstitute
themselves in organizations like the National Organization for
Women, the Women's Equity Action League, and the National
Women's Political Caucus, college-age, young-married, and professional women swelled the ranks of the movement and restored
feminism to public discourse as a powerful social force.[5]

One result of the feminist revival has been that, since the early
1970s, the attention of middle-class women has been increasingly
directed toward the pursuit of professional careers. Feminism and
the needs of the marketplace have combined to develop a new
norm that directly challenged older assumptions that a woman's
place was only in the home. Perhaps equally compelling among
young college women of today is the belief that women belong in
the money economy as well—indeed, women who voluntarily
choose to stay at home now run the risk of social disapproval in

many circles. Furthermore, the accomplishments of the civil rights movement, including the passage of Title VII of the 1964 Civil Rights Act, have ensured that the gatekeepers of the nation's professional schools would be monitored to guarantee fair admissions and hiring practices. Though enforcement of affirmative action by the Reagan Administration has been lax, for the most part the formal barriers that had lingered on since the 1920s were finally struck down. As a consequence of all these developments, middle-class women have easier access to the professional world than they have ever had before.

Ironically, women's new and unprecedented freedom to make career decisions has also made the social and structural impediments to their success more visible. For this reason those now entering the professions will have to struggle with powerfully subtle barriers to their achievement of equality with men. Though the remaining obstacles take two forms, they are interrelated. First, women must contend with the persistent social assumption that their, and not men's, primary obligation is to the family. Second, they must come to terms with the ethos of professionalism that has dominated professional life from the late nineteenth century until the present. Of all the professions, medicine has been perhaps the most eager and unrelenting proponent of this ethos. The tacit assumptions of professional ideology have been powerful indeed, and although all aspiring professionals have to make adjustments in order to conform to the demands of their occupational community, professional women experience special difficulties because those values often stand at odds with their feminine role.

Classical sociology has described the evolution of the professions into their modern guise after the Civil War. During that period of industrial and commercial expansion, medicine, law, academia, engineering, and other special occupations expanded their monopoly over esoteric knowledge, formed associations which established standards for admission, training, and the certification of members; organized systems of peer review which monitored and regulated practice; and devised codes of ethics which stressed both the importance of professionals' special knowledge, their consequently justifiable autonomy from lay interference, and their altruistic orientation not characteristic of other workers. Contemporary professionals' high status is allegedly derived from their expert training in an area of knowledge beyond the reach of ordinary lay people.[6]

In the last decade, revisionist sociologists and historians have emphasized the unique position of power enjoyed by the professions in American society. America has never had a hereditary aristocracy or rigid class system, and, as a consequence, occupational status has been one means of measuring social class. According to historians like David Rosner and Gerald Markowitz, medical professionalization in the early twentieth century involved an effort to raise the status and economic level of doctors by the conscious creation of an elite. The process involved the exclusion of blacks, women, lower-class white males, and other troublesome minority groups.[7]

In addition, the medical sociologist Eliot Friedson has noted the broad social power that accrued to physicians as they earned the right to define the scope and application of their own expertise. Until very recently, doctors' exclusive right not only to diagnose and treat illness, but to supervise the division of labor in health care and even to regulate the distribution of drugs and therapy has gone unchallenged. For Friedson and other revisionists, the claims of physicians to special altruism have been primarily a justification used to veil their extraordinary exercise of social power.[8]

Feminist thinkers have benefited from both types of analysis, but their most important contribution has been to offer their own critique of the ethos of professionalism described by sociologists. As increasing numbers of women enter the professions, feminist observers have had the opportunity to identify more carefully the subtle gender biases embedded in the ideology of professionalism itself. Indeed, they have pointed out, these biases are revealed even in the language commonly used to describe women professionals. We talk of "lady doctors," "women lawyers," and "female engineers." But more important than the language of exclusion, has been an ideology of work culture derived solely from male experience and male values. Professionals value "character": aggressiveness, scientific objectivity, careerism, individualism, commitment to work. Indeed, expertise is invested with a particular kind of moral intensity. For this reason professional work, unlike office or industrial employment, derives part of its high status from the assumption that such expertise is irreplaceable. Professionals are expected to identify with their work in ways not common to other workers. Because their activities are viewed as an important domain of self-expression and fulfillment, no one objects when professionals shut out personal considerations in the pursuit of rational and efficient devotion to a calling. But such allegiances are implicitly if not explicitly sex-typed. As an observer has noted, "A man owes to his profession what a woman owes to her family."[9]

In the past as well as in the present, such an ethos has spelled certain conflict for women physicians who wished to marry and have a family. In 1965 Alice Rossi laid the blame for the shortage of women in science squarely on the inability of most women who chose to be wives and mothers to overcome familial obstacles to a fulfilling career.[10] Medical sociologists as well connected the static numbers of women physicians and their relatively high dropout rate to the difficulties potential medical women experienced in handling two careers. Researchers have found that, though women doctors marry in the same proportion as women in the general population, they marry later and have fewer children. Twice as many choose salaried positions as compared to men. On the whole, they work fewer hours than men do. Moreover, marital status and family size was found to be inversely related to career success among women doctors. Those who had published extensively and achieved the highest academic rank of a group studied in 1970 were more likely to be single.[11]

Another comparative study of women physicians who did and who did not interrupt their careers found that those who dropped out of medicine even temporarily were likely to lead more complicated lives than the women who stayed in medicine without interruption. Struggling to juggle equally the tasks of professional, wife, and mother, temporary dropouts tended to exhibit what the researcher termed more traditionally "feminine" psychological development. They valued family life, children, and interpersonal relationships equally with or above their careers. Those women whose careers exhibited the least amount of disruption deliberately avoided the stresses of multiple roles by emphasizing their careers above all other aspects of their lives. In doing so they successfully reduced potential opportunities for conflict and were generally more satisfied as professionals. Much of their contentment stemmed from their ability to concentrate most of their energy on their careers. Nevertheless, specialty choices among both groups of women were still most often determined by a concern with whether or not work demands could be made compatible with family life.[12]

Though women physicians are presently seeking more effective ways to resolve the conflicts of the dual role, that is only part of their problem. Because most women are socialized to function primarily in the privacy of the family, where sentiment, intuition, feeling, and interrelatedness predominate, even single women who choose medicine experience unease with values purported to be rational, scientific, and gender neutral, but which are in reality masculine.

Whether they realize it or not, in this discomfort they are reconnect-
ing with the legacy of their nineteenth-century predecessors. Early
women physicians, like other social feminists, were instinctive critics
of the dehumanization inherent in industrialization. They feared the
tendency of the capitalist order to turn people into commodities,
even as they hailed the positive role of individualism in bringing
about female emancipation. Though they misunderstood the place
of class and misperceived the roots of economic exploitation, from
their vantage point as women they quickly comprehended that the
rationalization of human knowledge could be carried too far. They
brought to medicine a critique of the growing primacy of cure over
care, and though their values were ultimately lost or swallowed up
in the triumph of twentieth-century medical professionalism, this
perception, however vague and confused its articulation, formed the
basis of their criticism of the profession to which they so fervently
wished to belong. In the present decade, some feminist scholars are
again boldly challenging the ideological assumptions of the professional elite by suggesting that male and female values differ and that
the professional world would benefit from an infusion of female
concerns.

The psychologist Carol Gilligan, for example, complains that her
own discipline has consistently misunderstood female ethical development and has measured everyone against a male model. Her
work argues that women, speaking "in a different voice" from
men, prefer an ethic of care that takes into account their primary
experience of attachment and affiliation to others. Less concerned
with abstact principles of justice when they decide between right
and wrong, women are more likely to consider factors like who is
being hurt and why. Until recently psychology has labeled this
method of making ethical decisions immature. But this orientation
toward the preservation of relationships which often colors wom-
en's moral judgments can provide, according to Gilligan, an alternative conception of maturity which, if recognized as equally valid,
"could lead to a changed understanding of human development
and a more generative view of human life."[13]

Gilligan's argument has drawn criticism from other feminists for
sounding dangerously close to nineteenth-century concepts of "natural" female moral superiority which resulted in women's relegation
to a separate sphere. Yet modern feminist thinkers who admit to the
existence of differences between men and women would respond
that they are well aware of the possible conservative implications of
such an approach, and, having the benefit of an historical perspec-

tive, need not fall into such a trap. Nevertheless, an important and crucial debate now raging among feminists concerns the question of whether those virtues that have been labeled traditionally "feminine"—"maternal thinking," nurturing relationships, protective social concern, intuitive respect for nature, the high valuation of mercy over justice—are qualities inherent in female development or have emerged in Western society solely as a consequence of women's experience of subordination. For if female moral and social sensibilities are a mere result of their social status, will they not disappear if a truly gender-neutral society is achieved? No one yet has satisfactorily answered this question.[14]

Occasionally women physicians have joined in this debate, bringing to it their own perspective. In 1975, for example, Mary Howell, the first woman associate dean at Harvard Medical School, restated the belief of nineteenth-century women physicians that founding a woman's health school informed by "collaborative sharing of effort and responsibility, nurturance, care giving and personal service to others" was necessary to counter the massive resistance of the medical profession to "the beliefs and values held by women for women." At that time, Howell felt strongly that traditional medicine continued to glorify "science and technology to the detriment of face-to-face care giving." She cited

> the rigid hierarchy that teaches, both explicitly and implicitly, a status arrogance which places patients and so-called paraprofessional health workers at the very lowest level; the attraction to and fascination with machinery—both expensive and complicated to operate and maintain—that serves as a cold and impersonal interface between patients and care givers; and the elitism structured into the universe of health care, both in education and in work, that protects the privileged from the real world.[15]

Like Howell, other women physicians have criticized the masculine professional style. Seeking a more nurturing patient-physician interaction, Dr. Carola Eisenberg, dean of student affairs at Harvard Medical School, voiced the opinions of many when she praised women's tendency to show emotion and argued that it could be done without compromising professional identity. "Strength," she urged, "is not incompatible with compassion."[16] "If what is epitomized as 'a good physician' embodies a masculine set of traits and ideals," agreed Dr. Carlotta Rinke, in an article written for *JAMA*, "women will invariably suffer an identity crisis in attempting to adapt their womanhood into a male professional model."[17]

Equally forthright from spokeswomen in medicine has been the demand that the profession recognize women's family obligations and seek to alter a situation in which "women trade career advancement for time" to raise their children. Many have turned to co-parenting as a solution, demanding that husbands share family responsibilities equally and "be open [about them] with . . . colleagues at work."[18] "What can male physicians do to help their female colleagues?" asked Dr. Marilyn Heins in 1983. "They can,"

> 1) recognize the biologic imperative; 2) help to eliminate barriers put in the way of pregnant women physicians or those with young children; 3) acknowledge that slower career tracks do not indicate lower intelligence or lack of true worth or a lesser commitment to the profession, but rather may result from the choice a woman made to spend more time at home; 4) learn how to be a mentor to those with slower career tracks; and 5) learn to be comfortable doing household tasks and taking responsibility for these household tasks.[19]

There is some evidence that the profession is beginning to respond to these criticisms in various ways. Efforts to improve doctor-patient interaction in the form of courses and seminars are now standard fare in most medical schools. Equally promising has been the recent recognition that professional ideology has often stood at odds with a healthy family life, not just for women doctors, but for men as well. In 1982 the *Journal of the American Medical Women's Association* reported the results of a pioneer program at the University of Medicine of New Jersey. Directly addressing the anxiety of medical students "who sense that their career choice threatens to bankrupt their private lives," a course entitled "Parenting and Professionalism" was instituted to help them develop creative methods of solving work/career conflicts.[20]

In a particularly interesting recent incident in 1984, the chairman of the obstetrics department at Stanford University was forced to resign under intense criticism when he reprimanded a woman resident for getting pregnant. Declaring that chief resident Zena Levine's pregnancy was "presumptuous and a disservice to oneself and to one's colleagues" and warning that he would hesitate to appoint more women to the department, Dr. Lee Roy Hendricks found that he could muster little open support for his views among other faculty members. Less than fifteen years ago it would have been Dr. Levine who would have resigned.[21]

In addition to challenging traditional images of the doctor, women physicians have criticized other vestiges of medical professionalism—"old-boy" networks, rigid tracking systems, and the organization of medical training in a manner unresponsive to the female life cycle. They have demanded power in setting health-care policy, in making decisions pertaining to medical practice, and in determining how medicine is taught.[22] But difficulties persist, and it is still impossible to assess the long-range effect of the changes wrought in the last decade. What seems to be apparent is that a critical number of women have achieved professional status in medicine in the 1970s, and that the issues that were raised but not solved in the last century are being raised once again with greater vehemence and wider applicability. Clearly the rising numbers of women doctors are having an impact on the medical profession. One can hope only that at least some of the concerns that they brought to medical practice in the past—an emphasis on humane care and a concern for the profession's responsibility to the community—will occupy center stage in the practice of medicine once again. In the meantime women are taking their places beside male colleagues as full-fledged professionals determined to demonstrate that leading a fulfilling private life is not incompatible with the competent practice of medicine.

Notes on Methodology

The sample of the case records of the two hospitals used in Chapter 8 was a systematic sequential sample; that is, a random sample of records from alternate years. For New England Hospital, this included a sample from the odd-numbered years, 1873–1899, with a total n of 171. For Boston Lying-In, the sample included the alternate years 1887–1899, with a total n of 305. Virtually every piece of information that was available from the case records was codified. One group of variables were related to the patient's social position and included: marital status, nationality, race, place of residence, and kind of employment (if any). The second group of variables provided the patient's medical profile and included: age, number of living children, miscarriages, stillbirths and/or abortions, general physical condition, the birth presentation of the fetus, length of labor, use of anesthetics or forceps, type of postpartum complication, drugs used after delivery, length of hospital stay, and maternal and infant mortality. Whether the woman paid for hospital services was also noted. Comments that physicians occasionally wrote on the charts were recorded, but there were too few to be of any use.

Analyzing the hospital data using multiple regression was hindered by the fact that Boston Lying-In case records were relatively less complete. The impact of a woman's prior health condition and the impact, if any, of the patient's employment status, had to be excluded from comparison since Boston Lying-In did not usually include such data on their records.

The most obvious discrepancy in the samples is the difference in the time periods studied. Data from Boston Lying-In were available beginning with the year 1887. Whether the New England Hospital data remained consistent throughout the time period or whether one could only legitimately use the data after 1887 was an important concern. Accordingly, New England Hospital data before 1887 was compared with those from 1887 and later. The data remained generally consistent, with two exceptions, and the entire sample was used. The first exception was the aggregate change in the patients' employment status. The number of employed women treated at the New England Hospital declined dramatically from the first half of the sample to the second. In 1873 only 11 percent of the maternity cases were listed as housewives; by 1899, 63 percent were so listed. Supporting the conclusion that the condition of the patients did improve at the New England Hospital toward the century's end, 44 percent were listed in poor condition in 1873; by 1899 only 12 percent were so listed.

The second change over time was the decline in the complication rate at the New England Hospital from 1887 on. This decline is most dramatically shown by comparing the first year of the sample with the last. In the 1873 sample, all patients are listed as having some type of postpartum complication; in 1899, 87 percent are complication-free. Although the decision to compare complication rates from 1887 on was dictated by the availability of Boston Lying-In case records, the time demarcation is less arbitrary than it first appears. Since successful antisepsis was instituted at both hospitals in the mid-1880s, it was possible to compare directly the complication rates during a period immediately after a significant improvement had just been made in obstetrical therapeutics.

Tables A-1, A-2, and A-3 compare the complication rates and

TABLE A-1 Proportion of Patients Suffering Complications, Boston Lying-In versus New England Hospital

	Boston Lying-In Hospital 1887–1899 n = 305	New England Hospital 1873–1899 n = 171	New England Hospital 1873–1885 (n − 72)	New England Hospital 1887–1899 (n − 99)
Proportion of Patients with No Complications	73.4%	68.4%	59.7%	74.7%
Proportion of Patients with Complications	26.6%	31.6%	40.3%	25.3%
(Proportion with Injuries)	(7.5%)	(12.3%)	(16.7%)	(9.1%)
(Proportion with Infections)	(19.0%)	(19.3%)	(23.6%)	(16.2%)

Comparison of Boston Lying-In with New England Hospital for the years 1887–1899:
chi square − .066
degrees of freedom = 1
no significant difference

TABLE A-2 Proportion of Patients Suffering Complications by Marital Status/Nationality Groups

	New England Hospital 1873–1899		Boston Lying-In 1887–1899	
	number of women in group	proportion with complications	number of women in group	proportion with complications
Single American Patients	18	27.8%	55	36.4%
Married American Patients	54	24.1%	58	25.9%
Single Foreign Patients	29	55.2%	80	26.2%
Married Foreign Patients	65	27.7%	107	21.0%
Total cases	166	—	300	—
Aggregate complication rate	—	31.3%	—	26.7%

Comparison of differences in the frequency of complications among groups within each hospital:

New England Hospital	*Boston Lying-In*
chi square = 9.39	chi square − 3.59
degrees of freedom = 3	degrees of freedom = 3
probability < .05	no significant difference

drug usage at the two hospitals. To analyze the differences in frequencies, a chi square test of independence which has the advantage of correcting for an unequal number of cases was used.

In order to analyze the relationship between complications and drugs within each hospital, the correlation between the two was computed. Complications from least to most severe were scaled in ascending order of severity. They were: (0) no complications; (1) pain in groin; (2) fever and chills; (3) lacerations of vulva; (4) other—constipation, ulcerations; (5) ruptured perineum; (6) hemorrhaging; (7) vaginal fistula; (8) puerperal fever. In similar fashion, drugs were scaled from mildest to strongest prescription: (0) no drugs; (1) general supportive (teas, rubs); (2) mild pharmaceutical; (3) strong; (4) heroic; (5) combination of the preceding. The scaling is open to debate, especially the classification of teas and rubs as drugs. However, the scaled variables did in fact correlate significantly at both hospitals though there was an enormous difference in the relative predictive values of the correlations. When a multiple regression was done on drug usage at New England Hospital, only 4.5 percent of the variance in drug prescription on the basis of complications (multiple R = .21375) could be explained. In comparison, the same regression performed on the Boston Lying-In data revealed that 38 percent of the variance could be explained solely on the severity of the complication (multiple R = .61691). In neither regression did any other variable add much to the explanation of the variance in a direct—that is, logically causal—way. In this regard, though one would have liked to pursue the question of whether complications were related to the patient's prior medical history and/or her socioeconomic status, the gaps in the Boston Lying-In data precluded this line of analysis.

Tables A-4 and A-5 analyze the differences in complication rates between the group at each hospital that received neither forceps nor anesthetics and the group that received one or both intervention treatments. Once again, a chi square test of independence was used to test for significant differences in frequency of complications.

Finally, by using the scaled complications and a t-test for differences in means, it was also possible to calculate whether any intervention group suffered more severe complications than those patients that received neither anesthetic nor forceps.

At New England Hospital there was no significant difference in mean complication severity among the intervention groups. At Boston Lying-In the mean complication for the groups that received forceps or both forceps and anesthetic was significantly higher. For the group labeled "no intervention," the mean on the severity scale was .9. For "anesthetic only," "forceps only," and

TABLE A-3   Post-delivery Drug Prescription, New England Hospital versus Boston Lying-In

	New England Hospital 1873–1899		Boston Lying-In 1887–1899	
	number of patients	proportion of patients	number of patients	proportion of patients
No Medication Prescribed	0	0%	194	63.6%
General Supportive Treatments	1	.6%	5	1.6%
Mild Pharmaceuticals	89	52.0%	60	19.7%
Strong Medication	74	43.3%	42	13.8%
Heroic Medication	6	3.5%	4	1.3%
Combination of Above	1	.6%	0	0%
Total Cases	171	100.0%	305	100.0%

Comparison of the frequency of drug prescription at the New England Hospital and Boston Lying-In:

chi square − 189.86
degrees of freedom = 5
probability < .05

TABLE A-4   Frequency of Complications among Patients with Different
Intervention Treatments, New England Hospital, 1873–1899

	number of patients	number suffering complications	proportion with complications
Patients with No Intervention Treatment	139	45	32.4%
Patients with Intervention Treatment	31	8	25.8%
(Anesthetic Only)	(15)	(4)	(26.7%)
(Forceps Only)	(5)	(1)	(20.0%)
(Both)	(11)	(3)	(27.3%)

Comparison of the frequency of complications between the group of patients with no
intervention treatment and the group with one or both types of intervention:

chi square = .51
degrees of freedom = 1
no significant difference

TABLE A-5   Frequency of Complications among Patients with Different
Intervention Treatments, New England Hospital, 1887–1899

	number of patients	number suffering complications	proportion with complications
Patients with No Intervention Treatment	244	58	23.8%
Patients with Intervention Treatment	61	23	37.7%
(Anesthetic Only)	(20)	(7)	(35.0%)
(Forceps Only)	(20)	(8)	(40.0%)
(Both)	(21)	(8)	(38.1%)

Comparison of the frequency of complications between the group of patients with no
intervention treatment and the group with one or both types of intervention:

chi square = 4.86
degrees of freedom = 1
probability < .05

"both," the means were 1.2, 1.7, and 1.8 respectively. The latter
two means are significantly higher at the .05 level. Thus I concluded that at Boston Lying-In, patients who were delivered by
forceps were more likely to experience complications and, moreover, were likely to have more severe complications than other
patients.

Bibliography

MANUSCRIPT SOURCES

Ann Arbor. William L. Clements Library, University of Michigan
Harriet Hunt-Angelina Grimké Correspondence, Weld-Grimké Papers

Ann Arbor. Michigan Historical Collections, Bentley Historical Library, University of Michigan
Mary T. Green Papers; Eliza Mosher Papers; Bertha Van Hoosen Papers

Bethesda. National Library of Medicine
Catalogues and Announcements of the Woman's Medical College of Baltimore; Catalogues and Announcements of the Woman's Medical College of Chicago; Catalogues and Announcements of the Woman's Medical College of the New York Infirmary

Boston. Boston University Library
New England Female Medical College Papers

Boston. Countway Library, Harvard Medical School
Boston Lying-In Hospital Patient Records; Boston Obstetrical Society Papers; Henry I. Bowditch Papers; James C. Chadwick Papers; Edward H. Clarke Papers; Samuel Gregory Scrapbook; Massachusetts General Hospital Patient Records; Massachusetts Homeopathic Medical Society Papers; New England Hospital for Women and Children Patient Records

Boston. Massachusetts Historical Society
Caroline Dall Papers

Cambridge. Schlesinger Library, Radcliffe College
Alger Papers; Blanche Ames Papers; Elizabeth Blackwell Papers; Martha May Eliot Papers; Alice Hamilton Papers; Sarah Ernestine Howard Papers; Edith Banfield Jackson Papers; Mary Putnam Jacobi Papers; Sara Murray Jordan Papers; Margaret Noyes Kleinert Papers; May-Goddard

Papers; Helen Morton Papers; National Women's Party Papers; New England Hospital for Women and Children Papers; Eliza Taylor Ransom Papers; Anna Wessel Williams Papers

Chicago. Northwestern University Medical School Library

Evanston. Northwestern University Library Special Collections
Frank B. Crandon Papers; Northwestern University Archives; Woman's Medical College Archives

Ithaca. Cornell University Special Collections
American Medical Women's Association Papers

Minneapolis. Abbott Northwestern Hospital Archives

Minneapolis. Social Welfare Archives, University of Minnesota
American Social Hygiene Association Papers

New Orleans. Rudolph Matas Memorial Library, Tulane University
Women in Medicine Collection

New York City. Rare Book and Manuscript Library, Columbia University
Elizabeth Blackwell Papers; Emily Blackwell Diary

New York City. New York Academy of Medicine Special Collections

New York City. New York Infirmary Archives

Northampton. Sophia Smith Collection
Connie Guion Papers; Margaret Long Papers; Dorothy Reed Mendenhall Papers; New England Hospital for Women and Children Papers; Florence Rena Sabin Papers; Alice Weld Tallant Papers; Emma Walker Papers; Women Physicians File

Philadelphia. American Philosophical Society
Maria Mitchell Papers (microfilm); Florence Rena Sabin Papers

Philadelphia. Archives and Special Collections on Women in Medicine, Medical College of Pennsylvania
Alumnae Files; American Medical Women's Association Papers; Hannah Longshore Papers; Ada Pierce McCormick Papers; Ellen Potter Papers; Martha Tracy Papers; Bertha Van Hoosen Papers; Woman's Medical College of Northwestern University Archives; Woman's Medical College of Pennsylvania Archives; Women in Medicine Oral History Project

St. Louis. Washington University Medical School Library
Joseph Erlanger Papers

San Francisco. San Francisco Historical Society
Charlotte Blake Brown Papers

San Marino. Huntington Library
Dorothea Rhodes Lummis Moore Papers

Stanford. Stanford University Medical School Archives

Stanford. Stanford University Archives
    Clelia D. Mosher Papers
Syracuse. Syracuse University Library
    Anna Manning Comfort Papers
Washington, D.C. Library of Congress
    Blackwell Family Papers; Anita Newcomb McGee Papers
Washington, D.C. National Archives
    Children's Bureau Central Files

AN ESSAY ON SELECTED SECONDARY SOURCES

Students of the history of women physicians would profit by first
consulting the important general works on the history of the medical profession in America. For the nineteenth century see Richard
Harrison Shryock, *Medicine and Society in America, 1660–1860*
(Ithaca: Cornell University Press, 1960); William Rothstein, *American Physicians in the 19th Century: From Sects to Science* (Baltimore: Johns Hopkins University Press, 1972); Joseph Kett, *The
Formation of the American Medical Profession: The Role of Institutions* (New Haven: Yale University Press, 1968); William Frederick Norwood, *Medical Education in the United States* (Philadelphia:
University of Pennsylvania Press, 1944); Martin Kaufman, *American Medical Education: The Formative Years, 1765–1910* (Westport, Conn.: Greenwood Press, 1976); Barbara Rosenkrantz, *Public Health and the State* (Cambridge: Harvard University Press,
1972); and Donald Fleming, *William Welch and the Rise of Modern
Medicine* (Boston: Little, Brown, 1954). Important general surveys
that include a discussion of the modern period are Rosemary Ste-
vens, *American Medicine and the Public Interest* (New Haven:Yale
University Press, 1971); John Duffy, *The Healers: The Rise of the
Medical Establishment* (New York: McGraw-Hill, 1976); Morris
Vogel and Charles Rosenberg, eds., *The Therapeutic Revolution*
(Philadelphia: University of Pennsylvania Press, 1980); Judith
Walzer Leavitt and Ronald Numbers, eds., *Sickness and Health in
America: Readings in the History of Medicine and Public Health*
(Madison: University of Wisconsin Press, 1976); Susan Reverby
and David Rosner, eds., *Health Care in America: Essays in Social
History* (Philadelphia: Temple University Press, 1979); George
Rosen, *The Structure of American Medical Practice, 1875–1941*
(Philadelphia: University of Pennsylvania Press, 1983); and the
most recent and most comprehensive, Paul Starr, *The Social
Transformation of American Medicine* (New York: Basic Books,

1982). On the subject of professionalization, Burton Bledstein, *The Culture of Professionalism* (New York: W.W. Norton, 1976); Eliot Friedson, *Profession of Medicine* (New York: Dodd, Mead and Company, 1975); Megali Larson, *The Rise of Professionalism* (Berkeley: University of California Press, 1977); and E. Richard Brown, *Rockefeller Medicine Men, Medicine and Capitalism in America* (Berkeley: University of California Press, 1979), provided guidance.

Works in women's history that contain essential background material are Laurel Ulrich, *Good Wives: Image and Reality in the Lives of Women in Northern New England, 1650–1750* (New York: Oxford University Press, 1982); Mary Beth Norton, *Liberty's Daughters, The Revolutionary Experience of American Women, 1750–1800* (Boston: Little, Brown, 1980); Linda Kerber, *Women of the Republic: Intellect and Ideology in Revolutionary America* (Chapel Hill: University of North Carolina Press, 1980); Nancy Cott, *The Bonds of Womanhood: "Woman's Sphere" in New England, 1780–1835* (New Haven: Yale University Press, 1977); Kathryn Kish Sklar, *Catharine Beecher, A Study in American Domesticity* (New Haven: Yale University Press, 1973); Mary Hartman and Lois Banner, eds., *Clio's Consciousness Raised: New Perspectives on the History of Women* (New York: Harper and Row, 1974); and Carl Degler, *At Odds: Women and the Family in America from the Revolution to the Present* (New York: Oxford University Press, 1980). Important especially for the twentieth century are William Chafe, *The American Woman: Her Changing Social, Economic and Political Role, 1920–1970* (New York: Oxford University Press, 1972); Sheila M. Rothman, *Woman's Proper Place: A History of Changing Ideals and Practices, 1870 to the Present* (New York: Basic Books, 1978); Lois Scharf, *To Work and to Wed: Female Employment, Feminism and the Great Depression* (Westport, Conn.: Greenwood Press, 1980); and Winifred D. Wandersee, *Women's Work and Family Values, 1920–1940* (Cambridge: Harvard University Press, 1981).

For work on women professionals see Jessie Bernard, *Academic Women* (University Park: Pennsylvania State University Press, 1964); Cynthia Fuchs Epstein, *Woman's Place: Options and Limits in Professional Careers* (Berkeley: University of California Press, 1970); Helen Astin, *The Woman Doctorate in America: Origins, Career and Family* (New York: Russell Sage Foundation, 1969); Patricia Hummer, *The Decade of Elusive Promise, Professional Women in the United States, 1920–1930* (Ann Arbor: Research

Press, 1976); Frank Stricker, "Cookbooks and Lawbooks: The Hidden History of Career Women in the Twentieth-Century America," *Journal of Social History* 10(Fall 1976):1–19; Barbara Harris, *Beyond Her Sphere: Women and the Professions in American History* (Westport, Conn.: Greenwood Press, 1978); and Jonathan Cole, *Fair Science: Women in the Scientific Community* (New York: Free Press, 1979).

Recent studies of particular professions have been especially cogent. See for example, the comprehensive overview by Joan Jacobs Brumberg and Nancy Tomes, "Women in the Professions: A Research Agenda for American Historians," *Reviews in American History* 30(June 1982): 275–96. Also significant are Joyce Antler, "Feminism as Life Process: The Life and Career of Lucy Sprague Mitchell," *Feminist Studies* 7 (Spring 1981):134–57; Cynthia Fuchs Epstein, *Women in Law* (New York: Basic Books, 1981); Rosalind Rosenberg, *Beyond Separate Spheres: Intellectual Roots of Modern Feminism* (New Haven: Yale University Press, 1982); and Margaret Rossiter, *Women Scientists in America* (Baltimore: Johns Hopkins University Press, 1982).

Women physicians themselves wrote the first historical accounts of women's struggle to enter the medical profession, and these works consequently display both the advantages and disadvantages of "insider's history." They are full of much pertinent information for the researcher, but often lack analytical sophistication. The one exception is Mary Putnam Jacobi's penetrating essay, "Woman in Medicine," in Annie Nathan Meyer, ed., *Woman's Work in America* (New York: Henry Holt, 1891). Also useful, however, is Rachel Bodley, *The College Story: Valedictory Address to the Twenty-Ninth Graduating Class of the Woman's Medical College of Pennsylvania, March 17, 1881* (Philadelphia: Grant, Faires & Rogers, Printers, 1881); Emily F. Pope, C. Augusta Pope, and Emma L. Call, *The Practice of Medicine by Women in the United States* (Boston: Wright & Potter, 1881); and Clara Marshall, *The Woman's Medical College of Pennsylvania: An Historical Outline* (Philadelphia: P. Blakiston & Son, 1897).

Two amateurish but helpful general histories, both by ex-presidents of the American Medical Women's Association, Kate Campbell Hurd-Mead, *Medical Women of America* (New York: Froben Press, 1933), and Esther Pohl Lovejoy, *Women Doctors of the World* (New York: Macmillan, 1957), provide selected facts and figures for the twentieth century as well as the nineteenth. Similarly informative is *The History of the Woman's Medical College of*

Pennsylvania (Philadelphia: J.B. Lippincott, 1950), written by an alumna, Gulielma Fell Alsop. Frederick C. Waite, Ph.D., for many years the emeritus professor of histology at Western Reserve Medical School, contributed much toward retrieving the little-known past of nineteenth-century women physicians through his devoted detective work. Waite authored the *History of the New England Female Medical College, 1848–1874* (Boston: Boston University School of Medicine, 1950) and several articles on women doctors, including "Dr. Martha A. (Hayden) Sawin, The First Woman Graduate in Medicine to Practice in Boston," *New England Journal of Medicine* 205(November 1931):1053–55; Waite, "Dr. Nancy E. (Talbot) Clark, The Second Woman Graduate in Medicine to Practice in Boston," *ibid.* (December 1931): 1195–98; Waite, "The Three Myers Sisters—Pioneer Women Physicians," *Medical Review of Reviews* 39(March 1933):114–20; Waite, "Medical Education of Women at Penn Medical University," *ibid.* (June 1933):255–60; Waite, "Dr. Lucinda Susannah (Capen) Hall, The First Woman Doctor to Receive a Medical Degree from a New England Institution," *New England Journal of Medicine* 210 (March 1934): 644–47; Waite, "Dr. Lydia (Folger) Fowler, The Second Woman to Receive the Degree of Doctor of Medicine in the United States," *Annals of Medical History* 4 (May 1942): 290–97; Waite, "Two Early Letters by Elizabeth Blackwell," *Bulletin of the History of Medicine* 21(January–February 1947): 110–12; and Waite, "Early Medical Service of Women," *Journal of the American Medical Women's Association* 5(May 1948):199–203.

Biography, autobiography, and published letters can furnish much helpful information for both the nineteenth and the twentieth centuries. See especially but not exclusively Elizabeth Blackwell, *Pioneer Work in Opening the Medical Profession to Women* (London: Longmans, Green, 1895); Ruth Putnam, ed., *Life and Letters of Mary Putnam Jacobi* (New York: Putnam, 1925); Harriot Hunt, *Glances and Glimpses* (Boston: Jewett and Co., 1856); Agnes Vietor, ed., *A Woman's Quest: The Life of Marie E. Zakrzewska, M.D.* (New York: D. Appleton, 1924); Mary Bennett Ritter, *More Than Gold in California, 1849–1933* (Berkeley: Professional Press, 1933); *Bethenia Owens-Adair, Some of Her Life Experiences* (Portland: By the Author, 1905); Lillian Welsh, *Reminiscences of Thirty Years in Baltimore* (Baltimore: Norman, Remington, 1925); Elizabeth Putnam Gordon, *The Story of the Life and Work of Cordelia A. Greene, M.D.* (Castile, N.Y.: The Castilian, 1925).

For the twentieth century see first the fine sketches of women physicians in Edward T. and Janet Wilson James, eds., *Notable American Women, 1607–1950: A Bibliographical Dictionary* (Cambridge: Belknap Press, 1971); and Barbara Sicherman and Carol Hurd Green, eds., *Notable American Women, The Modern Period* (Cambridge: Belknap Press, 1980). Also revealing are Rosalie Slaughter Morton, *A Woman Surgeon* (New York: Frederick A. Stokes, 1937); Anne Walter Fearn, *My Days of Strength: An American Woman Doctor's Forty Years in China* (New York: Harper Bros., 1939); S. Josephine Baker, *Fighting for Life* (New York: Macmillan, 1939); Alice Hamilton, *Exploring the Dangerous Trades* (Boston: Little, Brown, 1943); Bertha Van Hoosen, *Petticoat Surgeon* (Chicago: Pellegrini & Cudahy, 1974); Emily Dunning Barringer, *From Bowery to Bellevue, The Story of New York's First Woman Ambulance Surgeon* (New York: W.W. Norton, 1950); Margaret R. Stewart, *From Dugout to Hilltop* (Culver City, Calif.: Murray & Gee, 1951); Mary Martin Sloop, *Miracle in the Hills* (New York: McGraw Hill, 1953); Dorothy Clarke Wilson, *Dr. Ida: The Story of Dr. Ida Scudder of Vellore* (New York: McGraw Hill, 1959); Elinor Bleumel, *Florence Sabin: Colorado Woman of the Century* (Boulder: University of Colorado Press, 1959); Janet Travell, *Office Hours: Day and Night. The Autobiography of Janet Travell, M.D.* (New York: World Publishing Co., 1968); Elinor Rice Hays, *Those Extraordinary Blackwells: The Story of a Journey to A Better World* (New York: Harcourt Brace, 1967); Joy Daniels Singer, *My Mother, The Doctor* (New York: E.P. Dutton, 1970); Dorothy Clarke Wilson, *Lone Woman: The Story of Elizabeth Blackwell: The First Woman Doctor* (Boston: Little, Brown, 1970); and, most recently Elizabeth Morgan, *The Making of a Woman Surgeon* (New York: Berkeley Books, 1980); Michelle Harrison, *A Woman in Residence* (New York: Random House, 1982); Regina Markell Morantz, Cynthia Stodola Pomerleau, and Carol Hansen Fenichel, eds., *In Her Own Words: Oral Histories of Women Physicians* (Westport, Conn.: Greenwood Press, 1982); Barbara Sicherman, *Alice Hamilton: A Life in Letters* (Cambridge: Harvard University Press, 1984); and Judith Lorber, *Women Physicians; Careers, Status and Power* (New York: Tavistock Press, 1984).

In the decades after 1950, two prominent medical historians renewed public interest in the history of women physicians with the publication of two suggestive articles: Richard Shryock, "Women in American Medicine," *Journal of the American Medical Women's*

Association 5(September 1950):371–79, and John B. Blake, "Women and Medicine in Ante-Bellum America," *Bulletin of the History of Medicine* 39(March–April, 1965):99–123. Appearing as the tangible result of a conference on women physicians sponsored by the Josiah Macy, Jr., Foundation was Carol Lopate's *Women in Medicine* (Baltimore: Johns Hopkins University Press, 1968), an intelligent overview of the past, present, and future role of women in American medicine.

The revival of historical investigation on the subject of women doctors, however, received its greatest stimulus from the emergence of interest in the history of women. Gerda Lerner, for example, was one of the first historians to raise questions about women's declining status in the healing arts in the nineteenth century in her pioneering essay, "The Lady and the Mill Girl: Changes in the Status of Women in the Age of Jackson," *American Studies* 10(Spring 1969):5–15. Moreover, from the beginning of the new women's history one area of investigation—the treatment of women's diseases and the response of nineteenth-century women to a male-dominated medical profession—proved particularly popular. Consequently, a number of books, articles, and dissertations since inspired by the new historiography deal directly or indirectly with the subject of women physicians. Jane Donegan, *Women and Men Midwives: Medicine, Morality and Misogyny in Early America* (Westport, Conn.: Greenwood Press, 1978); Judith Barrett Litoff, *American Midwives: 1860 to the Present* (Westport, Conn.: Greenwood Press, 1978); Richard W. and Dorothy C. Wertz, *Lying In—A History of Childbirth in America* (New York: Free Press, 1977); Edna Manzer, "Woman's Doctors: The Development of Obstetrics and Gynecology" (Ph.D. diss., University of Indiana, 1979); Frances E. Kobrin, "The American Midwife Controversy: A Crisis of Professionalization," *Bulletin of the History of Medicine* 40(July–August 1966):350–63; Catherine Scholten, " 'On the Importance of the Obstetrick Art': Changing Customs of Childbirth in America, 1760–1825," *William and Mary Quarterly* 34(July 1977):426–45; and Judith Walzer Leavitt, " 'Science' Enters the Birthing Room: Obstetrics in America Since the Eighteenth Century," *Journal of American History* 20 (September 1983):281–304, all offer innovative and incisive insights into the history of obstetrics and gynecology. The role of women in health reform and the connection between the health-reform movement and feminism is pursued in John B. Blake, "Mary Gove Nichols: Prophetess of Health," *Proceedings of the American Philosophical*

Society 106(1962):219–34; Regina Markell Morantz, "Making Women Modern: Middle-Class Women and Health Reform in 19th-Century America," *Journal of Social History* 10 (Summer 1977):490–507; and "Nineteenth-Century Health Reform and Women: A Program of Self-Help," in Guenter Risse, Ronald Numbers, and Judith W. Leavitt, eds., *Medicine Without Doctors: Home Health Care in American History* (New York: Science History Publications, 1977), 73–94; Martha Verbrugge, "The Social Meaning of Personal Health: The Ladies' Physiological Institute of Boston and Vicinity in the 1850's," in Susan Reverby and David Rosner, eds., *Health Care in America: Essays in Social History* (Philadelphia: Temple University Press, 1979); Sarah Stage, *Female Complaints: Lydia Pinkham and the Business of Women's Medicine* (New York: W.W. Norton, 1979); and, most recently, William Leach, *True Love and Perfect Union: The Feminist Reform of Sex and Society* (New York: Basic Books, 1980). Ann Douglas (Wood), " 'The Fashionable Diseases': Women's Complaints and Their Treatment in Nineteenth-Century America," *Journal of Interdisciplinary History* 4 (Summer 1973):25–52; and Virginia Drachman, "Women Doctors and the Women's Medical Movement: Feminism and Medicine, 1850–1895" (Ph.D. diss., SUNY Buffalo, 1976), treat women physicians as a monolithic, self-righteously feminist group, dedicated to throwing off for all women the shackles of oppression in which a hostile male medical establishment had held them bound. Mary Roth Walsh in *"Doctors Wanted: No Women Need Apply": Sexual Barriers in the Medical Profession, 1835–1975* (New Haven: Yale University Press, 1977); and Gloria Melnick Moldow, "The Gilded Age: Promise and Disillusionment: Women Doctors and the Emergence of the Professional Middle Class, Washington, D.C., 1870–1900" (Ph.D. diss., University of Maryland, 1980), take a more balanced view of the struggle of women to enter the profession while concentrating primarily on the feminist response to the crippling effects of institutional discrimination. My own work, in "The Lady and Her Physician," in Lois Banner and Mary Hartman, eds, *Clio's Consciousness Raised: New Perspectives on the History of Women* (New York: Harper & Row, 1974), 38–53; " 'The Connecting Link' ": The Case for the Woman Doctor in 19th-Century America," in Judith Walzer Leavitt and Ronald Numbers, eds., *Sickness and Health in America: Essays in the History of Health Care* (Madison: University of Wisconsin Press, 1978), 117–28; "Professionalism, Feminism and Gender Roles: A Study of the Therapeutics of Nineteenth Century Male and Female Doctors," *Journal of American History* 67 (December 1980):568–88; "Feminism, Professionalism, and Germs: The Thought of Mary Putnam Jacobi and Elizabeth Blackwell," *American Quarterly* 34 (Winter 1982):459–78; and "From Art to Science: Women Physicians in American Medicine, 1600–1980," in Regina Markell Morantz, Cynthia Stodola Pomerleau, and Carol Hansen Fenichel, eds., *In Her Own Words: Oral Histories of Women Physicians* (Westport, Conn.: Greenwood Press, 1982), has tried to broaden the focus away from the question of male oppression and institutional discrimination to consider such factors as the role of medical professionalization and women physicians' own self-definition. I have argued that the feminism of women physicians remained highly complex and diverse, riddled with tensions between separatism and assimilation, femininity and professionalism. Virginia Drachman's most recent work, "Female Solidarity and Professional Success: The Dilemma of Women Doctors in Late-Nineteenth-Century America," *Journal of Social History* 15 (Summer 1982): 607–19, and *Hospital with a Heart: Women Doctors and the Paradox of Separatism at the New England Hospital, 1862–1969* (Ithaca: Cornell University Press, 1984), has pursued a similar line of thinking.

Other aspects of the history of women physicians have been investigated in Martin Kaufman, "The Admission of Women to 19th-Century American Medical Societies," *Bulletin of the History of Medicine* 50 (Summer 1976):251–60; Cora B. Marrett, "On the Evolution of the Women's Medical Societies," *Bulletin of the History of Medicine* 53(Fall 1979):434–49; Constance M. McGovern, "Doctors or Ladies? Women Physicians in Psychiatric Institutions, 1872–1900," *Bulletin of the History of Medicine* 55(Spring 1981): 88–107; Helena M. Wall, "Feminism and the New England Hospital," *American Quarterly* 32 (Fall 1980): 435–52; Nancy Sahli, "Elizabeth Blackwell, M.D. (1821–1910): A Biography" (Ph.D. diss., University of Pennsylvania, 1974); Mary Roth Walsh, "Images of Women Doctors in Popular Fiction," *Journal of Popular Culture* 1(Summer 1978):276–84; and Judith Walzer Leavitt, ed., *Women and Health in America* (Madison: University of Wisconsin Press, 1984). Finally, an excellent bibliographical resource for the numerous books and articles on the history of women physicians can be found in Sandra Chaff, et al., eds., *Women in Medicine: A Bibliography of the Literature on Women Physicians* (Metuchen, N.J.: Scarecrow Press, 1977).

Notes

INTRODUCTION

1. Interview with Dr. Pauline Stitt, 9 December 1977, p. 11. Women in Medicine Oral History Project, Medical College of Pennsylvania Archives.
2. Emma Walker, a graduate of Smith College and Johns Hopkins Medical School, was a member of the New York State Association Opposed to the Extension of the Suffrage to Women. See *New York Times*, 15 March 1905.
3. Bertha Selmon, "Pioneer Women in Medicine," *Medical Women's Journal* 56 (January 1949): 48.
4. Henry Hartshorne, M.D., *Valedictory Address to the Graduating Class of the Woman's Medical College of Pennsylvania*, Philadelphia, 1872, p. 6.
5. Burton J. Bledstein, *The Culture of Professionalism* (New York: W. W. Norton, 1976).

CHAPTER 1

1. Keller, Woman's Medical College of Pennsylvania Alumnae *Transactions*, 1906, 36 (hereafter cited as WMCP *Alumnae Transactions*).
2. Philadelphia *Evening Bulletin*, 8 November 1869, clipping in Eliza Jane Wood Alumnae File, Medical College of Pennsylvania (MCP) Archives.
3. See Keller, WMCP *Alumnae Transactions*, 1906, p. 36, and also Anna Manning Comfort, "Struggles and Trials of the Pioneer Medical Woman," Syracuse *Sunday Herald*, 22 February 1903, clipping in Comfort MSS, Syracuse University.
4. Clipping, n.d., Wood File, MCP Archives.
5. *Leslie's Illustrated News*, 16 April 1870.
6. Saur, "Physicians and Their Duties," Thesis, 1871; Hunt, "The True Physician" Thesis, 1851, both in MCP Archives.
7. Preston, *Valedictory Address* (Philadelphia: A. Ketterlinus, 1858), 8.
8. See Richard B. Morris, *Studies in the History of American Law* (New York: Columbia University Press, 1930), 128–29; Elizabeth A. Dexter, *Colonial Women of Affairs* (Boston & New York: Houghton Mifflin, 1924), and *Career Women of America: 1776–1840,* (Francestown, N.H.: Kelley, 1950); Julia C. Spruill, *Women's Life and Work in the Southern Colonies* (Chapel Hill: University of North Carolina Press, 1938). For more recent versions of this argument see Gerda Lerner, "The Lady and the Mill Girl," *American Studies*

10 (Spring 1969): 5–15; Roger Thompson, *Women in Stuart England and America* (London: Routledge and Kegan Paul, 1974); and Mary Ryan, *Womanhood in America* (New York: New Viewpoints), 1975.

9. O. T. Beall, Jr., and R. H. Shryock, *Cotton Mather: First Significant Figure in American Medicine* (Baltimore: Johns Hopkins University Press, 1954), 66ff.

10. Kate Campbell Hurd-Mead, *A History of Women in Medicine: From the Earliest Times to the Beginning of the 19th Century* (Haddam, Conn.: Haddam Press, 1938), 487. See also Linda Kerber, *Women of the Republic: Intellect and Ideology in Revolutionary America* (Chapel Hill: University of North Carolina Press, 1980), 58; Mary Beth Norton, *Liberty's Daughters, The Revolutionary Experience of American Women 1750–1800* (Boston: Little, Brown, 1980), 139–40.

11. Mary Putnam Jacobi, "Woman in Medicine," in Annie Nathan Meyer, ed., *Woman's Work in America* (New York: Henry Holt, 1891), 141.

12. Catherine Scholten, " 'On the Importance of the Obstetrick Art': Changing Customs of Childbirth in America, 1760–1825," *William and Mary Quarterly* 34 (July 1977): 426–45; Judith W. Leavitt, " 'Science' Enters the Birthing Room: Obstetrics in America Since the Eighteenth Century," *Journal of American History* 20 (September 1983): 281–304.

13. Quoted in Scholten, " 'On the Importance of the Obstetrick Art,' " 430. See also Richard Shryock, *Medicine and Society in America, 1660–1860* (Ithaca: Cornell University Press, 1960), 15; and Jane Bauer Donegan, *Women and Men Midwives: Medicine, Morality and Misogyny in Early America* (Westport, Conn.: Greenwood Press, 1978).

14. Norton, *Liberty's Daughters,* 139–40; Jacobi, "Woman in Medicine," 141; Donegan, *Women and Men Midwives,* 90; Shryock, *Medicine and Society,* 15.

15. Norton, *Liberty's Daughters,* and Kerber, *Women of the Republic,* both argue this point of view. See also Laurel Ulrich, *Good Wives: Image and Reality in the Lives of Women in Northern New England, 1650–1750* (New York: Oxford University Press, 1982).

16. Louis B. Wright and Marion Tinling, eds., *The Secret Diary of William Byrd of Westover, 1709–1792* (Richmond, Va.: The Dietz Press 1941), 79. Quoted in Leavitt, " 'Science' Enters the Birthing Room," 282. See also Ulrich, *Good Wives,* and Scholten, " 'On the Importance of the Obstetrick Art,' " *passim.*

17. Leavitt, " 'Science' Enters the Birthing Room," 282. See also Richard W. Wertz and Dorothy C. Wertz, *Lying-In: A History of Childbirth in America* (New York: Free Press, 1977). For female culture see Carroll Smith-Rosenberg, "The Female World of Love and Ritual: Relations between Women in Nineteenth-Century America," *Signs* 1 (Autumn 1975):1–29; and Nancy Cott, *The Bonds of Womanhood* (New Haven: Yale University Press, 1977).

18. Ulrich, *Good Wives,* 132–33.

19. Kerber, *Women of the Republic,* 58.

20. Shryock, *Medicine and Society,* 1–43; Joseph Kett, *The Formation of the American Medical Profession* (New Haven: Yale University Press, 1968), 1–31; Martin Pernick, "A Calculus of Suffering: Pain, Anesthesia and Utilitarian Professionalism in 19th-Century American Medicine" (Ph.D. diss., Columbia University, 1978), 18–21.

21. Shryock, *Medicine and Society,* 9.

22. *Ibid.*, 1–43; Whitfield J. Bell, Jr., "A Portrait of the Colonial Physician," *Bull. Hist. of Med.* 44 (Fall 1970):497–517; John Duffy, *The Healers* (Urbana: University of Illinois Press, 1979), 17–23.

23. For a more detailed discussion of English and American developments in obstetrics see Donegan, *Women and Men Midwives,* 38–88, on which much of this account relies.

24. Donegan, *Women and Men Midwives,* and Leavitt, " 'Science' Enters the Birthing Room," both skillfully describe this transition. See also Edna Manzer, "Woman's Doctors: The Development of Obstetrics and Gynecology in Boston, 1860–1930" (Ph.D. diss., University of Indiana, 1979).

25. Donegan, *Women and Men Midwives,* 132.

26. Scholten, " 'On the Importance of the Obstetrick Art' " 438–40; Leavitt, " 'Science' Enters the Birthing Room," *passim.* For an excellent article that specifically addresses the reality of women's control over parturition in the nineteenth and early twentieth centuries, see Judith Leavitt and Whitney Walton, " 'Down to Death's Door': Women's Perceptions of Childbirth in America," in Judith W. Leavitt, ed., *Women and Health in America* (Madison: University of Wisconsin Press, 1984), 155–65.

27. Kerber, *Women of the Republic, passim;* Norton, *Liberty's Daughters,* 110, 295; Mary Ryan, *Womanhood in America,* 3rd ed., (New York: Franklin Watts, 1983), 69–111.

28. Alexis de Tocqueville, *Democracy in America,* ed. Richard D. Hefner (New York: New American Library, 1956), bk. 3, chap. 41, 244.

29. Kerber, *Women of the Republic,* 205; Alice Rossi, *The Feminist Papers* (New York: Columbia University Press, 1973), 21.

30. Kerber, *Women of the Republic,* 282ff.

31. Cott, *The Bonds of Womanhood,* 5–18; Nancy Cott, "Passionlessness: An Interpretation of Victorian Sexual Ideology, 1790–1850," *Signs* 4 (Winter 1978): 219–36.

32. Cott, *The Bonds of Womanhood,* 5–18. See for example, Daniel Scott Smith, "Family Limitation, Sexual Control, and Domestic Feminism in Victorian America" in Mary Hartman and Lois Banner, eds., *Clio's Consciousness Raised: New Perspectives on the History of Women* (New York: Harper & Row, 1974).

33. John Ware, *Remarks on the Employment of Females as Practitioners in Midwifery, By a Physician* (Boston, 1820). See also Manzer, "Woman's Doctors," 15–20.

34. See Donegan, *Women and Men Midwives,* 164–96.

35. Charles Meigs, *Females and Their Diseases* (Philadelphia, 1848), 19, 20–21.

36. Cott, "Passionlessness," 236. See also Charles Rosenberg and Carroll Smith-Rosenberg, "The Female Animal: Medical and Biological Views of Woman and Her Role in Nineteenth-Century America," *Journal of American History* 60 (September 1973): 332–56; Carroll Smith-Rosenberg, "The Cycle of Femininity: Puberty and Menopause in Nineteenth-Century America," *Feminist Studies* 1 (Winter 1973): 58–72. Ultimately, the increasing rigidity of this point of view provoked a rebellion from feminists. See Regina Markell Morantz, "The 'Connecting Link': The Case for the Woman Doctor in 19th-Century America," in *Sickness and Health in America,* ed., Judith Leavitt and Ronald Numbers (Madison: University of Wisconsin Press, 1978), 120–

25; and William Leach, *True Love and Perfect Union: The Feminist Reform of Sex and Society* (New York: Basic Books, 1980), 19–80.

37. Thomas Ewell, *Letters to Ladies, Detailing Important Information Concerning Themselves and Infants* (Philadelphia, 1817).

38. See, for example, Samuel Gregory, *Letters to Ladies in Favor of Female Physicians* (New York, 1850).

39. Ware, *Remarks,* 3, 16.

40. *Ibid.,* 6, 7, 9.

41. *Ibid.,* 21, 4. See also Morantz, "The 'Connecting Link,' " 117–18.

42. Ware, *Remarks,* 7.

CHAPTER 2

1. Ann Preston, "General Diagnosis," 1851; Angenette A. Hunt, "The True Physician," 1851; both theses in Medical College of Pennsylvania Archives (MCP).

2. Marie Louise Shew, *Water Cure for Ladies: A Popular Work on the Health, Diet and Regimen of Females and Children,* revised by Joel Shew, M.D. (New York: Wiley & Putnam, 1844), 20, 23.

3. Angenette Hunt, "The True Physician;" Nichols, "Woman the Physician," *Water-Cure Journal* 11 (1851): 74–75 (hereafter cited as *WCJ*).

4. Richard Shryock, *Medicine and Society in America, 1660–1860* (Ithaca: Cornell University Press, 1960), 125.

5. Martin Pernick, "Medical Profession: I: Medical Professionalism," in *Encyclopedia of Bioethics,* ed. Warren T. Reich (New York: Free Press, 1978); and Pernick, "A Calculus of Suffering: Pain, Anesthesia and Utilitarian Professionalism in 19th-Century American Medicine" (Ph.D. diss., Columbia University, 1978), Intro. and chap. 1, 1–17.

6. Jeffrey L. Berlant, *Profession and Monopoly* (Berkeley: University of California Press, 1975), quoted in Pernick, "A Calculus," 128.

7. Mary Gove Nichols, "Woman the Physician," *WCJ* 12 (1851):3.

8. See Pernick, "A Calculus," 112–71.

9. Martin Kaufman, *American Medical Education* (Westport, Conn.: Greenwood Press, 1976); Robert P. Hudson, "Abraham Flexner in Perspective: American Medical Education 1865–1910," *Bull. Hist. of Med.* 56 (November–December 1972): 545–61.

10. See Pernick, "A Calculus," 25; William B. Walker, "The Health Reform Movement in the United States, 1830–1870" (Ph.D. diss., Johns Hopkins University, 1955); Ronald Numbers, "Do It Yourself the Sectarian Way," in *Medicine Without Doctors,* ed., R. Numbers, J. Leavitt, and G. Risse (New York: Science History Publications, 1977), 49–72; Joseph Kett, *The Formation of the American Medical Profession* (New Haven,: Yale University Press, 1968), 97–164; Martin Kaufman, *Homeopathy in America* (Baltimore: Johns Hopkins University Press, 1971); James Harvey Young, *The Toadstool Millionaires: A Social History of Patent Medicines in America Before Federal Regulation* (Princeton: Princeton University Press, 1961). `

11. Megali Larson, *The Rise of Professionalism* (Berkeley: University of California Press, 1977), 133.

12. The best treatments of the health-reform movement include William B. Walker, "The Health Reform Movement in the United States, 1830–1870"; Richard Shryock, "Sylvester Graham and the Popular Health Movement, 1830–1870," in *Medicine in America, Historical Essays* (Baltimore, Johns Hopkins University Press, 1966), 111–25; John Blake, "Health Reform," in E. S. Gaustad, ed., *The Rise of Adventism: Religion and Society in Mid-Nineteenth Century America* (New York, Harper and Row, 1974), 30–49; H. E. Hoff and J. Fulton, "The Centenary of the First American Physiological Society Founded at Boston by William A. Alcott and Sylvester Graham," *Bull. Hist. of Med.* 5 (October 1937):687–734; Stephen Wilner Nissenbaum, "Careful Love: Sylvester Graham and the Emergence of Victorian Sexual Theory in America, 1830–1840" (Ph.D. diss., University of Wisconsin, 1968); James C. Whorton, "Christian Physiology: William Alcott's Prescription for the Millenium," *Bull. Hist. of Med.* 49 (Winter 1975):466–81, and *Crusaders for Fitness: A History of American Health Reformers* (Princeton: Princeton University Press, 1982). Two lively popular works are James Harvey Young, *The Toadstool Millionaires;* and Gerald Carson, *Cornflake Crusade* (New York: Rinehart and Co., 1967). The public health movement is dealt with in Charles and Carroll Smith-Rosenberg, "Pietism and the Origins of the American Public Health Movement: A Note on John H. Griscom and Robert W. Hartley," *Jour. Hist. Med.* 23 (1968): 16–35; Richard H. Shryock, "The Early American Public Health Movement," in *Medicine in America,* 126–38; John D. Davies skillfully chronicles the phrenology movement in *Phrenology: Fad and Science* (New Haven: Yale University Press, 1955). Of related interest is R. Laurence Moore, *In Search of White Crows: Spiritualism, Parapsychology and American Culture* (New York: Oxford University Press, 1977); and most of the essays in Guenter Risse, Ronald Numbers, Judith Leavitt, eds., *Medicine Without Doctors: Home Health Care in American History* (New York: Science History Publications, 1977).

13. *WCJ* 7 (1849): 18. The Seventh Day Adventist publication *The Health Reformer* claimed 11,000 subscribers in 1868. See Ronald L. Numbers, "Health Reform on the Delaware," *New Jersey History* 92 (September 1974); 7.

14. *Advocate of Moral Reform,* 15 June 1839. For the convergence of health reform with other reform movements see Robert S. Fletcher, "Bread and Doctrine at Oberlin," *Ohio State Archeological and Historical Quarterly* 49 (January 1940): 58–67. Sidonia E. Taupin, " 'Christianity in the Kitchen,' or A Moral Guide for Gourmets," *American Quarterly* 15 (1963): 85–89; Thomas H. LeDuc, "Grahamites and Garrisonites," *New York History* 20 (April 1939): 189–91; Michael Katz, *The Irony of Early School Reform* (Boston: Beacon Press, 1968). For a thoughtful and highly provocative treatment see Ronald G. Walters, "The Erotic South: Civilization and Sexuality in American Abolitionism," *American Quarterly* 25 (May 1973): 177–201; and *American Reformers 1815–1860* (New York: Hill and Wang, 1978). Also innovative is William Leach, *True Love and Perfect Union: The Feminist Reform of Sex and Society* (New York: Basic Books, 1980).

15. See Martha Verbrugge, "The Ladies' Physiological Institute: Health Reform and Women in Ante-bellum Boston" (Paper delivered at Third Annual Berkshire conference on Women's History, Bryn Mawr, June 1976). The one exception to this middle-class analysis may have been the Thomsonians, a

health-reform sect which has been tentatively linked to working-class elements. I would contend that the Thomsonians do not fall out of the mainstream of the movement because health reform could very well have played a similar role in "modernizing" American workers in the antebellum period as I will argue it played for the middle class. As Paul Faler and Alan Dawley have shown, the internalization of "modern" values often transcended class divisions. See "Working Class Culture and Politics in the Industrial Revolution: Sources of Loyalism and Rebellion," *Journal of Social History* 9 (June 1976): 466–79. I am indebted to Irene Javors of City College for discussing her preliminary findings on the Thomsonians with me. See also Brian Harrison, *Drink and the Victorians* (Pittsburgh: University of Pittsburgh Press, 1971), for a similar approach to the British working class.

16. Mary Gove Nichols, *Lecutres to Women on Anatomy and Physiology* (New York: Harper and Brothers, 1846), 20.

17. William Applegate, *A Defense of the Graham System of Living* (New York: W. Applegate, 1835), 23; Shew, *Water Cure for Ladies,* 14, 15. See also Mary Gove Nichols, *A Woman's Work in Water Cure and Sanitary Education* (London: Nichols, 1874), 80.

18. See Thomas L. Nichols, *Eating to Live: The Diet Cure* (New York: M. L. Holbrook & Co., 1881); also *WCJ* 25 (1858): 53, an article by Dr. N. Bedortha of the Saratoga Springs water cure in which this general view was somewhat modified.

19. Shew, *Water Cure for Ladies,* Preface, p. iii; Mary Gove Nichols, *Lectures to Women,* 20.

20. "Duties of Physicians," *WCJ* 21 (1856): 55–56.

21. "Old School Medical Journals," *WCJ* 9 (1850): 181; Aurelia Raymond, "Thesis on the Human Brain," 1864, MCP Archives.

22. For the influence of the Enlightenment see Alice Felt Tyler, *Freedom's Ferment* (New York: Harper & Row, 1944). For Christian perfectionism see Whorton, " 'Christian Physiology,' " 466–81. For the decline of heroic therapeutics see Shryock, *Medicine and Society,* 117–32. For antielitism see Richard Shryock, "Cults and Quackery in American Medical History," Middle States Association of History and Social Studies Teachers, *Trans.* 37 (1939): 19–30.

23. See Hebbel E. Hoff, M.D., and John F. Fulton, M.D., "The Centenary of the First American Physiological Society," *Bull. Hist. of Med.* 5 (October 1939): 687–733.

24. *Ibid.,* 701. For women's role in the health reform movement see John Blake, "Mary Gove Nichols, Prophetess of Health," in *Proceedings of the American Philosophical Society* 106 (June 1962):219–34; Ronald L. Numbers, *Prophetess of Health: Ellen G. White* (New York: Harper & Row, 1976); Regina Markell Morantz, "Nineteenth Century Health Reform and Women: A Program of Self-Help," in Risse, *Medicine Without Doctors,* and "Making Women Modern: Middle Class Women and Health Reform in 19th-century America," *Journal of Social History* 10 (June 1977): 113–20; Sarah Stage, *Female Complaints: Lydia Pinkham and the Business of Women's Medicine* (New York: W. W. Norton, 1979).

25. Rev. H. Winslow, "Domestic Education in Females," vol. 1 (1847): 259–61. The concept of the "republican mother," which was given life during the

antebellum period, gained momentum through several permutations until progressive era reformers and social workers recast it in the 20th-century notion of "educated motherhood." See Linda Kerber, "Daughters of Columbia: Educating Women for the Republic, 1787–1805," in Stanley Elkins and Eric McKitrick, *The Hofstadter Aegis* (New York: Columbia University Press, 1974), and *Women of the Republic: Intellect and Ideology in Revolutionary America* (Chapel Hill: University of North Carolina Press, 1980), *passim;* Jill Conway, "Perspectives on the History of Women's Education in the United States," *Hist. of Ed. Quart.* 14 (Spring 1974): 1–12. For the progressive period see Sheila Rothman, *Woman's Proper Place* (New York: Basic Books, 1978), 97–134. For an excellent discussion of the social and economic roots of American feminism, particularly the influence of education see Keith Melder, *Beginnings of Sisterhood: The American Women's Rights Movement, 1800–1850* (New York: Schocken, 1977).

26. Frances Dana Gage, *WCJ* 17 (1854): 35. On changes, particularly in New England, which touched the lives of many in the reform leadership see the thoughtful introduction by Michael Katz to *Early School Reform.* Also Stanley Engerman, ed., *The Reinterpretation of American Economic History* (New York, 1971); Stephen Thernstrom, *Poverty and Progress* (Cambridge: Harvard University Press, 1964); Stephen Thernstrom and Richard Sennett, eds., *Nineteenth Century Cities* (New Haven: Yale University Press, 1969). Three helpful works on the family are: Kirk Jeffrey, "The Family as a Utopian Retreat from the City," *Soundings* (Spring 1972): 21–41; Kirk Jeffrey, "Family History: The Middle-Class American Family in the Urban Context, 1830–1870" (Ph.D. diss., Stanford University, 1971); Mary P. Ryan, "American Society and the Cult of Domesticity" (Ph.D. diss., University of California at Santa Barbara, 1971). See also Bernard Wishy, *The Child and the Republic* (Philadelphia: University of Pennsylvania Press, 1968); David J. Rothman, *The Discovery of the Asylum* (Boston: Little, Brown, 1971); and finally Mary Ryan, *Cradle of the Middle Class: The Family in Oneida County New York, 1790–1865* (New York and Cambridge: Cambridge University Press, 1981).

27. *Letters to the People on Health and Happiness* (New York, 1856), 7; "Shall Our Girls Live or Die," *Laws of Life* 10 (1867): 2; "To Sick Women," *WCJ* 26 (1858): 96. See also Augustus K. Gardner, "The Physical Decline of American Women," *WCJ* 29 (1860): 21–22.

28. Striking evidence for the conviction of many women writers that their grandmothers enjoyed better health can be found in Catharine Beecher, *Housekeeper and Healthkeeper* (New York, 1873), 424–28. Another possible explanation for the increase in complaints is that women were no longer willing to tolerate their ill health. See also Carroll Smith-Rosenberg, "The Hysterical Woman: Sex Roles and Role Conflict in Nineteenth-Century America," *Social Research* 39 (Winter 1972): 652–78. A large number of well-known female activists had a variety of health problems. Lucy Stone and Alice Stone Blackwell both suffered from migraines; Angelina Grimké, Margaret Fuller, Caroline Dall, Clara Barton, Catharine Beecher, Ellen and Marian Blackwell, Harriet Beecher Stowe, and Elizabeth Oakes Smith, all complained of chronic poor health.

29. *WCJ* 15 (1854): 74, 94 (italics mine). *WCJ* 20 (1855): 74.

30. *WCJ* 15 (1853): 131. See also Harriet Austin, "Woman's Present and Future," *WCJ* 16 (1853): 57.
31. "Woman's Dress," *WCJ* 11 (1851): 30; "The New Costume," *WCJ* 12 (1851): 30; "Science and Long Skirts," *WCJ* 20 (1855): 7.
32. *WCJ* 16 (1853): 120; 11 (1851): 96, and *passim*. Most of the water-cure establishments encouraged their female patients to wear reformed dress. Almost every issue of any health reform journal had something about dress. *The Water-Cure Journal* and *The Laws of Life* showed special interest in dress reform; the *Graham Journal* and the *American Vegetarian and Health Journal* less frequently. Dress reform was also a popular topic in women's rights journals like *The Una, The Lily,* and later *The Revolution.* Many of the articles in these journals pertaining to dress were written by health reformers. See especially *WCJ* 12 (1851): 33, 58; *WCJ* 34 (1862): 1–2; *WCJ* 15 (1853): 7, 10, 32, 34, 35, 131; *WCJ* 13 (1852): 111; *The Laws of Life* 10 (1867): 93–94, 129–30, 145–46; *The Revolution* 3 (1869): 149–50; *Graham Journal* 3 (1839): 301–2.
33. Boston: G. W. Light, 1839, pp. 265–66.
34. *WCJ* 1 (1846): 29.
35. See "To Her Sick Sisters," *WCJ* 26 (1858): 96; "A Bloomer to Her Sisters," *WCJ* 15 (1853): 131. There are many examples. For a possible meaning to this sense of community see Carroll Smith-Rosenberg, "The Female World of Love and Ritual: Relations Between Women in 19th Century America," *Signs* 1 (Autumn 1975): 1–29. For Nichols's quote see *A Woman's Work in Water Cure,* 14. See also Mary Gove Nichols, "To the Women Who Read the Water Cure Journal," *WCJ* 14 (1852): 68: "We do not consider ourselves doctors in the common understanding of the word—though we shall not neglect to do the highest good in this department, but we consider ourselves educators—set apart and qualified by Providence for the work. We will educate men and women for Physicians and Teachers of health, and young women to be wise wives and mothers. We will make the most beneficial impression on the world that is possible to us."
36. *Library of Health* 2 (1838): 70, 367; 6 (1842): 156; 5 (1841): 40; Thomas L. Nichols, *Health Manual: Being Also A Memorial of the Life and Work of Mrs. Mary S. Gove Nichols* (London: Allen, 1887), 22; *WCJ* 1 (1846):93: 11 (1851): 29, 38, 93; 9 (1850): 90; 14 (1852): 56; 17 (1854): 46; 22 (1856): 131; 28 (1859): 57–58; 5 (1848): 83; *Graham Journal* 2 (1838): 37, 181, 288, 385; 3 (1839): 20, 37, 82; *The Lily* 3 (1851): 27; *The Una* 1 (1854): 206; 2 (1854): 263; *Boston Medical and Surgical Journal* 40 (1849): 107; 48 (1853): 443–44. See Martha Verbrugge, "The Ladies' Physiological Institute,". Hers is the first local study we have of the rank and file. One suspects others will yield similar conclusions.
37. Chapters on Food, Cooking, and Domestic Economy in William A. Alcott, *The Young Housekeeper* (Boston: G. W. Light, 1849); "Keep Your Children Clean," *Graham Journal* 1 (1837): 176; "Masturbation and Its Effect on Health," *Graham Journal,* 2 (1838): 23. Mary Gove Nichols, *Lectures to Women,* passim. See also advertisement in the *Graham Journal* 2 (1838): 288. For articles on fresh air and bathing, *WCJ* 3 (1847): 161–68, 177; *WCJ* 4 (1847): 193; pregnancy, exercise, and childbirth: *WCJ* 3 (1847): 145, 151, 183–84; "Our New Cookbook," "How to Can a Fruit," *Laws of Life* 10

(1867): 12: "Cleanliness and Healthfulness," *Laws of Life* 10 (1867): 16; "Teething and Its Management," "Children's Dress," *WCJ* 12 (1851): 101, 104. Martha Verbrugge has also emphasized this practical dimension of the health-reform program. She contends that the Ladies' Physiological Institute helped ordinary middle-class women adjust to the opportunities and the limitations imposed on them by modern life. Verbrugge is impressed less with the radical elements of the Boston group and more with the organization's goal of easing women into traditional role patterns potentially disturbed by changing social conditions. Her study is significant because it suggests that health reform appealed to several different types of women. She argues, for example, that only a small minority of members of the Boston society were outspoken feminists. See Verbrugge, *"The Ladies' Physiological Institute."*

38. Thomas Low Nichols, "The Curse Removed; The Efficacy of Water-Cure in the Treatment of Uterine Disease and the Removal of the Pains and Perils of Pregnancy and Childbirth" (New York, 1850), 13; Trall, "Allopathic Midwifery," *WCJ* 9 (1850): 121; Mary Gove Nichols, "Maternity and the Water Cure for Infants," *WCJ* 11 (1851): 57–59; Eliza de la Vergue, M.D., "Infants, Their Improper Nursing and Medication," *WCJ* 20 (1855): 101. See an interesting autobiographical sketch by Mrs. Mary A. Torbit, "Reasons for Becoming a Lecturer," *WCJ* 14 (1851): 91.

39. Henry C. Wright, *Marriage and Parentage* (Boston, 1855; reprint, New York: Arno, 1974), 5.

40. *Ibid.*, 91, 257. Also Orson Fowler, *Love and Parentage* (New York, 1847), 272–74, *passim*. See Linda Gordon, "Voluntary Motherhood: The Beginnings of Feminist Birth Control Ideas in the United States," in Mary Hartman and Lois Banner, eds., *Clio's Consciousness Raised: New Perspectives on the History of Women* (New York: Harper & Row, 1974), 54–71, and *Woman's Body, Woman's Right* (New York: Grossman, 1976), 95–186. Not all advisors proscribed sexual intercourse without procreation. However all agreed that coitus should be approached with caution. Mechanical means of contraception were anathema because such methods degraded women by encouraging overindulgence.

41. Wright, *Ibid.*, 5.

42. See Eliza B. Duffey, *The Relations of the Sexes* (New York, 1879), especially chapter 13, "The Limitation of Offspring." Although Carl Degler has rightly reminded us that some women did have orgasms in the nineteenth century (See Degler, "What Ought To Be and What Was: Women's Sexuality in the 19th Century," *American Historical Review*, (19 December 1974), 1467–1490.), I would suggest that female orgasm was inherently more problematical than that of the male and that the nineteenth century was generally ignorant of the more subtle nature of female sexual response. Marriage counselors in the 1920s and 1930s documented this widespread ignorance and tried to correct it. Alfred Kinsey's statistics show a gradual increase in the number of married women achieving orgasm in the years after 1900. Carroll Smith-Rosenberg has examined possible differences in male and female approaches to sexuality in the nineteenth century in greater detail in a paper, "A Gentle and A Richer Sex: Female Perspectives on Nineteenth Century Sexuality" (Third Berkshire Conference on Women's History, Bryn Mawr, June 1976). See also Regina Markell Morantz, "The Scientist as Sex Crusader: Alfred

Kinsey and the American Culture," *American Quarterly* (Fall 1977), 563–89. See Duffey, *Relations of the Sexes,* chap. 13. It should be pointed out that most health reformers were also eugenicists. See Henry C. Wright, *The Empire of the Mother Over the Character and Destiny of the Race* (Boston, 1863).

43. Moreover, social reformers of all types recognized that large families hampered upward mobility. The reputation of the Irish for their alleged indulgence of the sensual passions was widespread. They had nothing but "large," "dirty" families to show for it: "Did wealth consist in children," asserted the *Common School Journal,* "it is well known, that the Irish would be a rich people; and if the old Roman law prevailed here, which granted special privilege to every man who had more than three, this people would be elevated into an aristocracy." Quoted in Katz, *Early School Reform,* 123. Many of the early school reformers, including Horace Mann, had a lively interest in health reform. Largely because of this interest the Massachusetts legislature passed a law in 1850 requiring physiological instruction in the schools.

44. William Alcott, *The Young Wife* (Boston, 1837), 87–89; *The Lily* 1 (1849): 52; Nichols, *Lectures to Women,* 212, and "Woman the Physician," *WCJ* 12 (1851): 75; Jackson, "The Women of the United States," *WCJ* 26 (1858): 3, and "Women's Rights," *WCJ* 31 (1861): 61. For an excellent summary of hereditarian views in this period see Charles Rosenberg, "The Bitter Fruit: Heredity, Disease, and Social Thought in Nineteenth Century America," *Perspectives in American History* 7 (1974): 189–238.

45. *WCJ* 1 (1846): 29.

46. For accounts of this "modern" personality type see Peter Cominos, "Late Victorian Respectability and the Social System,": *Int. Rev. of Soc. Hist.* 8 (1963): 18–48, 216–50; Herbert Gutman, "Work, Culture, and Society in Industrializing America," *AHR* 78 (June 1973): 531–87; Michael Katz, *Early School Reform;* Alan Dawley and Paul Faler, "Working Class Culture and Politics in the Industrial Revolution: Sources of Loyalty and Rebellion," *Journal of Social History* 9 (June 1976): 466–79; James T. Fawcett, "Modernization, Individual Modernity, and Fertility," in J. T. Fawcett, ed., *Studies in the Psychology of Population* (New York, 1973); Alex Inkeles, "The modernization of man," in *Modernization, the Dynamics of Growth* (New York, 1966), 138–50, "Making Men Modern: on the Causes and Consequences of Individual Change in Six Developing Countries," *Am. Jour. of Soc.* 75 (1969): 208–25, and *Becoming Modern* (Cambridge: Harvard University Press), 1974. Also Richard D. Brown, "Modernization and the Modern Personality in America, 1600–1865," *Jour. of Interdisc. Hist.* 2 (Winter 1972): 201–27. "Looking . . . at the social habits of the working people in some of our densely populated districts, it does indeed appear a hopeless effort to attack their vices, unless one could at the same time pull down their houses, and build them others adapted to a more perfect state of bodily and mental health," "Sanitary and Social Reform Coeval," by Mrs. Ellis in *Practical Educator and Journal of Health* 1 (1847): 354–55. Charles Rosenberg has made this same point in connection with 19th-century prescriptions for male sexual purity. See "Sexuality, Class, Role," *American Quarterly* 25 (May 1973): 131–53; also William Coleman, "Health and Hygiene in the Encyclopedie: A Medical Doctrine for the Bourgeoisie," *Jour. Hist. Med.* 29 (October 1974): 339–412, applies a similar argument to the French bourgeoisie.

See S. Weir Mitchell, "So great is my reverence for supreme wholesomeness, that I should almost be tempted to assert that perfect health is virtue." *Address on Opening of the Institute of Hygiene of the University of Pennsylvania* (Philadelphia, 1982), 4. A few health reformers merged the moral injunction to "guard the health of the race" with overt nativism. "Already," warned James C. Jackson,

> the decay of our women and the delicate constitutions of our young men are forcing the latter to seek revitalization by intermarriage with immigrant women from Europe. What with the decline of the Puritan and Cavalier stock on the one hand, and the great influx of foreign born on the other, it is not difficult to predict *our future.* In less than fifty years the New England type of manhood will have ceased to govern this Republic, and when once it ceases to govern it will cease to exist. . . . *Nothing but a bold and faithful advocacy of the laws of health can stop this ebbtide of human life.*

See *WCJ* 26 (1858): 4.

47. See Regina Markell Morantz, "Making Women Modern: Middle Class Women and Health Reform in 19th-Century America," *Journal of Social History* 10 (June 1977): 113–20 for a fuller discussion of this point.

48. See Alice Kessler-Harris, "Stratifying by Sex: Understanding the History of Working Women," *Labor Market Segmentation,* ed. Richard Edwards et al. (Lexington, Mass.: D.C. Heath, 1975), 217–42. I am indebted to my colleague David Katzman for the information about servants. For a stimulating discussion of the middle-class English woman's involvement in health reform see Patricia Branca, *Silent Sisterhood, Middle Class Women in the Victorian Home* (Pittsburgh: University of Pittsburgh Press, 1976), especially parts 2 and 3. Branca argues that middle-class Victorian women were the first large group to establish a modern outlook toward life and death.

49. William Leach has argued that some feminists even viewed natural rights exclusively in hygienic terms and relied heavily on ideological tools derived from science and hygiene rather than abstract principles of justice in their arguments for female equality. *True Love and Perfect Union,* 21.

50. Ellen Dubois, *Feminism and Suffrage, The Emergence of an Independent Women's Movement in America, 1848–1869* (Ithaca: Cornell University Press, 1980), 17; Carl Degler, *At Odds* (New York: Oxford University Press, 1980).

51. See for example Wright, *Marriage and Parentage,* 261–63.

52. *WCJ* 22 (1856):40; Orson Fowler, *Sexual Science, or Manhood and Womanhood* (Boston, 1869), 15. Russell Trall, founder of the Hygeio-Therapeutic College in New York, encouraged fraternization between the sexes at his school and often announced the marriages of graduates in the pages of the *Water-Cure Journal.* Several water-cure establishments were opened by couples, who graduated from the College. Trall kept track of the activities of these special students and heartily approved of their functioning as cooperative domestic and professional units. See *WCJ* 26 (1858):26, 27; *WCJ* 27 (1859):10. See also articles on "Man and Woman" in *The Una,* July, August, and September 1855, pp. 101, 118–19, 133–34.

53. See *WCJ* 21 (1856): 23; *WCJ* 20 (1855): 95; *WCJ* 17 (1854): 11; *WCJ* 26 (1856): 96.

54. "Woman's Tenderness and Love," *WCJ* 5 (1848): 95; William M. Cornell, M.D., "Woman the True Physician," *WCJ* 46 (1853): 82; *WCJ* 12 (1851): 73–

75; M. G. Nichols, "Woman, the Physician," *WCJ* 12 (1851): 73–75; "Female Physicians," *The Lily* 1 (1849): 94; and 2 (1850): 39, 70, 77; "Female Physicians," *WCJ* 31 (1861): 84; Augusta R. Montgomery, "The Medical Education of Women," 1853, thesis, MCP Archives; *Godey's Lady's Book* 44 (1852): 185–89; 61 (1860): 270–71; 54 (1857): 371; 49 (1854): 80, 368, 456; *The Revolution* 1 (1868): 170, 201, 339; 3 (1870): 252; *WCJ* 13 (1852): 34–35, 86–87; 29 (1860): 2–3, 45; 31 (1861): 42; 28 (1859): 84. Report of the Ohio Female Medical Loan Fund Assocation, *The Una,* April 1855, p. 61.

CHAPTER 3

1. Stephen Smith, M.D., "A Woman Student in a Medical College," *In Memory of Dr. Elizabeth Blackwell and Dr. Emily Blackwell* (New York: Academy of Medicine, 1911), 3–19.

2. James J. Walsh, "Women in the Medical World," *New York Medical Journal* 96 (1912):1324–28; Regina Markell Morantz, "The 'Connecting Link': The Case for the Woman Doctor in 19th-Century America," in Judith Leavitt and Ronald Numbers, eds., *Sickness and Health in America: Essays in the History of Health Care* (Madison: University of Wisconsin Press, 1978), 117–28.

3. The five "regular" schools were the Woman's Medical College of Pennsylvania (1850 to the present); New England Female Medical College (1856–1873), which merged with the homeopathic Boston University; Woman's Medical College of the New York Infirmary (1868–1899); Woman's Hospital Medical College of Chicago, later Woman's Medical College of Northwestern University (1870–1902); and Woman's Medical College of Baltimore (1882–1909). See Morantz, " 'Connecting Link,' " 117. The last statistic is taken from a survey done by W. C. Hunt, statistician, of Washington, D.C., reprinted in H. Scott Turner, "History of women in medicine," *Los Angeles J. Eclectic Med.,* 2 (1905): 125. Hunt claimed there were 7,387 women doctors in 1900. The number of male physicians in the United States in 1900 is in dispute. Census records set the figure at 132,002, the AMA at 119,749. See U.S. Bureau of the Census, *Historical Statistics of the United States: Colonial Times to 1970* (Washington, D.C., 1975), part 1, pp. 75–76.

4. W. W. Parker, M.D., "Women's Place in the Christian World: Superior Morally, Inferior Mentally to Man—Not Qualified for Medicine or Law—the Contrariety and Harmony of the Sexes," *Tr. Med. Soc. St. Va.,* 1892, pp. 86–107.

5. Paul de Lacy Baker, "Shall Women be Admitted into the Medical Profession?" *Tr. Med. Assn. St. Ala.* 33 (1880):191–206. See also Julien Picot, "Shall Women Practice Medicine?" *North Carolina Med. J.* 16 (1885):10–21; N. Williams, "A Dissertation on Female Physicians," read before the Clay, Lysander and Schroeppel (N.Y.) Medical Association, *Boston Med. & Surg. J.* 43 (1850):69–75; J. F. Ziegler, "Woman's Sphere," Presidential address to the Medical Society of Pennsylvania, *Tr. Med. Soc. St. Penn.* 14 (1882):25–38; Joseph Spaeth, "The Study of Medicine by Women," *Richmond & Louisville Med. J.* 16 (1873):40–56; *Men and Women Medical Students and the Woman Movement* (Philadelphia, 1869), *passim.*

6. J. S. Weatherly, "Woman: Her Rights, and Her Wrongs," *Tr. Med. Assn. St. Ala.* 24 (1872):63–80. For a reversal of the argument, defending female medi-

cal education as a step *up* from primitive brutality, see Edwin Fussell, *Valedictory Address to the Students of the Female Medical College of Pennsylvania* (Philadelphia, 1857), 5–6.

7. Reynell Coates, *Introductory Lecture to the Class of the Female Medical College of Pennsylvania* (Philadelphia, 1861), 3–4. See also articles cited in n. 4 and n. 5. "Female Physicians," *Boston Med. & Surg. J.* 54 (1856):169–74; and "Female Practitioners of Medicine," *Boston Med. & Surg. J.* 76 (1867): 272–74.

8. Medical women, of course, claimed just the reverse. See Weatherly, "Woman: Her Rights," 76; Sophia Jex-Blake, *Medical Women: Two Essays* (Edinburgh, 1872), 36; J. P. Chesney, "Woman as a Physician," *Richmond & Louisville Med. J.* 11 (1871):6.

9. Elizabeth Blackwell, *Pioneer Work in Opening the Medical Profession to Women* (New York, 1895): 27.

10. See, for example, Elizabeth Blackwell, *Address on the Medical Education of Women* (New York, 1856), and Elizabeth and Emily Blackwell, *Medicine as a Profession for Women* (New York, 1860).

11. Weatherly, "Woman: Her Rights," 75.

12. Edmund Andrews, M.D., "The Surgeon," *Chicago Medical Examiner* 2 (1861): 587–98, quoted in Martin Pernick, "A Calculus of Suffering: Pain, Anesthesia and Utilitarian Professionalism in 19th Century American Medicine" (Ph.D. diss., Columbia University, 1978), 131; Newspaper clipping, n.d., Chadwick Scrapbook, Countway Library, Boston, cited in Mary Walsh, *"Doctors Wanted: No Women Need Apply": Sexual Barriers in the Medical Profession, 1835–1975* (New Haven: Yale University Press, 1977), 139. For a good discussion of doctors' fears of feminization see Pernick, "A Calculus," *passim,* and Walsh, *Doctors Wanted: No Women Need Apply,* 135–46.

13. Martin Kaufman, "The Admission of Women to 19th-Century American Medical Societies," *Bull. Hist. of Med.* 50 (Summer 1976):251–59.

14. *Boston Med. & Surg. J.* 111 (1884):90; 40 (1849):505; 89 (1873):23; "The Practice of Midwifery by Females—By One of the Class," *Boston Med. & Surg. J.* 41 (1849):59–61; Coates, *Introductory Lecture,* 3–4; D. W. Graham, "The Demand for Medically Educated Women," *JAMA* 6 (1886):479.

15. E. H. Clarke, *Sex in Education: A Fair Chance for Girls* (Boston, 1983), 23; also Horatio Storer, "Letter of Resignation," *Boston Medical and Surgical Journal* 75 (1866):191–92.

16. Clarke, *Sex in Education,* 41.

17. Carroll Smith-Rosenberg, "Puberty to Menopause: The Cycle of Femininity," in *Clio's Consciousness Raised: New Perspectives on the History of Women,* ed. Mary Hartman and Lois Banner (New York: Harper & Row, 1974), 1–22. The debate over premenstrual tension and the related effects of ·woman's cycle on her psyche still goes on in medical circles. See K. J. and R. J. Lennane, "Alleged Psychogenic Disorders in Women—a Possible Manifestation of Sexual Prejudice," *New Eng. J. Med.* 290 (Feb. 8, 1973): 288–92.

18. "Female Physicians," 169; Horatio Storer, "The Fitness of Women to Practice Medicine," *J. Gynec. Soc. Boston* 2 (1870):266–67; and *ibid.,* "Female Practitioners of Medicine," 272–74; Lawrence Irwell, "The Competition of the Sexes and its Results," read before the American Association for the Advancement of Science, August 1896, *Am. Medico-Surg. Bull.* 10

(1896):316–20; A. Lapthorn Smith, "Higher Education of Women and Race Suicide," *Popular Science Monthly* 66 (1905):466–73; A. Lapthorn Smith, "What Civilization is Doing for the Human Female," *Tr. Southern Surg. & Gynec. Assn.* 2 (1889):352–60; F. W. Van Dyke, "Higher Education as the Cause of Physical Decay in Women," *Med. Rec.* 67 (1905):296–98; William Goodell, R. Gaillard Thomas, M. Allen Starr, J. J. Putnam, "Symposium on the Co-Education of the Sexes," *Med. News, N.Y.* 55 (1889): 667–72; J. T. Clegg, "Some of the Ailments of Woman Due to Her Higher Development in the Scale of Evolution, *Texas Hlth. J.* 3 (1890–1892):57–59; A. J. C. Skene, *Education and Culture as Related to the Health and Diseases of Women* (Detroit, 1889), 39.

19. M. Carey Thomas, "Present Tendencies in Women's College and University Education," *Educational Review* 25 (1908): 58.

20. Mary Putnam Jacobi, *The Question of Rest for Women During Menstruation* (New York, 1877), 227. See also C. Alice Baker to Mary Putnam Jacobi, 7 November 1874, Jacobi MSS, Schlesinger Library, Radcliffe.

21. Emily F. Pope, M.D., Augusta C. Pope, M.D., and Emma Call, M.D., *The Practice of Medicine by Women in the United States* (Boston, 1881), 7.

22. See, for example, Elizabeth C. Underhill, M.D., "The Effect of College Life on the Health of Women Students," *Woman's Medical Journal (WMJ)* 22 (February 1912): 31–33; Mary E. B. Ritter, M.D., "Health of University Girls," *California State Medical Journal* 1 (1902–3): 259–64; Clelia Mosher, M.D., "Some of the Causal Factors in the Increased Height of College Women," *Journal of the American Medical Association* 81 (August 1923): 535–38; and "Normal Menstruation and Some Factors Modifying It," *Johns Hopkins Hosp. Bull.* .12 (1901):178–79; Elizabeth R. Thelburg, "College Education a Factor in the Physical Life of Women," *WMCP Alumnae Transactions,* 1899, p. 73–87. See also Virginia Drachman, "Women Doctors and the Women's Medical Movement: Feminism and Medicine, 1850–1895," (Ph.D. diss., State University of New York at Buffalo, 1976) for a somewhat different perspective.

23. See Joseph Longshore, *Valedictory Address* (Philadelphia: Penn Medical College, 1857), 20; Ann Preston, *Valedictory Address, March 12, 1870* (Philadelphia: Women's Medical College of Pennsylvania, 1870), 5–7; "Appeal of the Corporators," Eighth Annual Announcement of the Woman's Medical College of Pennsylvania (Philadelphia, Deacon & Peterson, 1857), 16; Elizabeth and Emily Blackwell, *Medicine as a Profession,* 4; Henry Hartshorne, *Valedictory Address to the Graduating Class of the Woman's Medical College of Pennsylvania* (Philadelphia, 1872), 13–14; Louise Fiske-Byron, "Woman and Nature," *N.Y. Med. J.* 66 (1887):627–28. For Ruffin Coleman's remark see "Woman's Relation to Higher Education and the Professions as Viewed from Physiological and Other Stand Points," *Tr. Med. Assn. St. Ala.* 42 (1889): 233–47.

24. Emily Blackwell made this argument even before social Darwinism came into vogue: "Mankind," she confided to her diary, "will never be what they should be until women are nobler." Diary, 4 June 1852, p. 83, Blackwell MSS, Columbia University. See also *J. Hyg. & Herald Hlth.* 44 (1894):236; J. G. Kiernan, "Mental Advance in Woman and Race Suicide," *Alienist and Neurologist* 30 (1910): 594–99; Elizabeth Blackwell, *Pioneer Work,* 253;

Agnes Johnson, "Maternal Influence," 1868, Thesis in the Medical College of Pennsylvania Archives.

25. 23 May 1855, Hunt-Grimké Correspondence, William L. Clements Library, University of Michigan.

26. There are hundreds like G. Fenning, *Every Mother's Book: or the Child's Best Doctor, Being a Complete Course of Directions for the Medical Management of Mothers and Children* (New York, n.d.); or D. Wark, *The Practical Home Doctor for Women* (New York, 1882).

27. Chesney, "Woman as a physician," 4; Harriot Hunt address at the Worcester Women's Rights Convention, 1850, in *Proceedings of the Worcester Women's Rights Convention* (Boston: Prentiss & Sawyer, 1851), 46–47; Emmeline Cleveland, *Introductory Lecture to the Class of the Female Medical College of Pennsylvania* (Philadelphia, 1859), 7.

28. Elizabeth Blackwell, "Criticism of Gronlund's Co-operative Commonwealth; Chapter X—Woman," given before the Fellowship of New Life, n.d., 9–10; *The Influence of Women in the Profession of Medicine* (London, 1889), 11; "Anatomy," Lecture Notes, n.d., all in Blackwell MSS, Library of Congress; Grimké to Hunt, 23 May 1855, Hunt-Grimké Correspondence, William L. Clements Library, University of Michigan.

29. Joseph Longshore, *Introductory Lecture to the Class of the Female Medical College of Pennsylvania* (Philadelphia, 1859), 11; Joseph Longshore, *The Practical Importance of Female Medical Education* (Philadelphia, 1853), 6; Female Medical College of Pennsylvania, "Appeal to the Corporators," MCP Archives; Ann Preston, *Valedictory Address to the Graduating Class of the Female Medical College of Pennsylvania* (Philadelphia, 1858), 9–10.

30. Elizabeth and Emily Blackwell, *Medicine as a Profession for Women* (New York, 1860), 8–9; "Appeal to the Corporators," MCP Archives.

31. Georgiana Glenn, "Are Women as Capable of Becoming Physicians as Men," *The Clinic* 9 (1875):243–45; Jacobi, "Inaugural Address," Women's Medical College of the New York Infirmary, *Chicago Med. J. & Exam.* 42, (1881):580.

32. Samuel Gregory, "Female Physicians," *The Living Age,* 1862, pp. 73, 243–49; Ann Preston, *Introductory Lecture to the Course of Instruction in the Female Medical College of Pennsylvania* (Philadelphia, 1855), 12.

33. Longshore MSS, MCP Archives, 106.

34. Marie Zakrzewska to Elizabeth Blackwell, 21 March 1891, Blackwell MSS, Schlesinger Library.

35. Blackwell, *Pioneer Work,* 253; Emmeline Cleveland, *Valedictory Address to the Graduating Class of the Woman's Medical College of Pennsylvania* (Philadelphia, 1874), 3; Eliza Mosher, "The Value of Organization—What it Has Done for Women," *WMJ* 26 (1916): 1–4; James J. Walsh, "Women in the Medical World," *N.Y. Med. J.* 96 (1912): 1324–28.

36. Commencement of the Women's Medical College of the New York Infirmary, 25 May 1899, printed in *Final Catalogue* (New York, 1899). Also Emily Blackwell, Diary, October 1851, p. 47, Special Collections, Columbia University. Rarely until after 1900 does one come across the argument that medicine is enriching from the standpoint of personal development. It is primarily society which is to benefit; individuals gain *because* they are aiding society.

37. For use of the argument see J. Stainbeck Wilson, "Female Medical Educa-

tion," *Southern Med. & Surg. J.* 10 (1854): 1–17; Emmeline Cleveland, *Valedictory Address to the Graduating Class of the Female Medical College of
Pennsylvania* (Philadelphia, 1858), 10; Margaret Vaupel Clark, "Medical
Women's Contribution to the Education of Mothers," *WMJ* 25 (1915), 126–
28; Harriet Williams, "Women in Medicine," *Texas Med. News* 12 (1903):
613–15.

38. See Jacobi, "Inaugural Address," 561–85.

39. Frances Emily White, "The American Medical Woman," *Med. News,* N.Y.
67 (1895):123–28.

40. An interesting example of how conservative this type of argument can be is
provided by the situation in India, Pakistan, and Iran, where the seclusion of
women has existed for so long. Similar arguments for training a core of
professional women to administer to an exclusively female clientele are extremely popular. See Hanna Papenek, "Purdah in Pakistan: Seclusion and
Modern Occupations for Women," *Journal of Marriage and the Family* (August 1971), 517–30.

41. Helen Watterson, "Woman's Excitement over 'Woman'," *Forum* 16 (1893):
75–85; Mary Putnam Jacobi, "An Address Delivered at the Commencement
of the Women's Medical College of the New York Infirmary, May 30, 1883,"
Arch. Med. 10 (1883):59–71; Marie Zakrzewska, *Introductory Lecture Before
the New England Medical College* (Boston, 1859), 3–26; C. L. Franklin,
"Women and Medicine," *The Nation* 52 (1891): 131.

42. Jacobi, "Commencement Address," 70.

CHAPTER 4

1. Virginia Penny, *The Employments of Women: A Cyclopedia of Women's
Work* (Boston: Walker & Wise Co., 1863), 29.

2. Jacobi later described the school in Philadelphia as full of "much zeal but
little knowledge," in "Woman in Medicine," Annie Nathan Meyer, ed.,
Women's Work in America (New York: Henry Holt, 1891), 157.

3. Roy Lubove, "Mary Putnam Jacobi," in *Notable American Women,* vol. 2,
ed. Janet and Edward James (Cambridge: Harvard University Press, 1973),
263–65.

4. Patricia Spain Ward, "Emmeline Horton Cleveland," in *Notable American
Women,* vol. 1, p. 349–50; Jacobi, "Woman in Medicine," 157.

5. *Records of the Commissioner of Education,* 1893 (Washington, D.C.: Government Printing Office, 1895).

6. From notes "On the Education of Women Physicians," n.d. but internal
evidence suggests 1860, Blackwell MSS, Library of Congress. See also remarks of Blackwell's friend and admirer, Dr. Eliza Mosher. "Educated medical women touch humanity in a manner different than men; by virtue of their
womanhood, their interest in children, in girls and young women, both moral
and otherwise, in homes and in society." "The Value of Organization—What
it Has Done for Women," *Woman's Medical Journal,* June 1916 (reprint in
Archives of Medical College of Pennsylvania).

7. For a number of reasons, my analysis of the attitudes of the leaders of the
movement to educate women in medicine will be confined to "regular" physi-

cians. Though there were more medical sectarians among female practitioners than among males, regular physicians still accounted for 75 percent of late 19th-century women doctors, and, of course, spokespersons from this group were the only individuals who commanded much respect from the orthodox professionals, who were, by the 1880s, rapidly gaining ascendancy. Estimates regarding the distribution of women physicians are drawn from the *Records of the Commissioner of Education,* 1889–1890, 1892–1893, 1895–1896, 1898–1899, 1903 (Washington, D.C.: Government Printing Office, 1891, 1894, 1897, 1899, 1904).

8. See Annie Sturgis Daniel, M.D., "A Cautious Experiment: The History of the New York Infirmary for Women and Children and the Woman's Medical College of the New York Infirmary," *Medical Woman's Journal* 47 (February 1940); 40.

9. Blackwell, *Pioneer Work in Opening the Medical Profession to Women* (New York, 1895), 227–38.

10. Jacobi, "Woman in Medicine," 176. For a discussion of Marie Zakrzewska's similar views including an address on the subject to the New England Women's Club see Agnes Vietor, *A Woman's Quest* (New York: D. Appleton, 1924), 373–87, 398–411. Also Sarah Hackett Stevenson, "Coeducation of the Sexes in Medicine," in *Physiology of Woman* (Chicago: Fairbanks & Palmer, 1882), 143–70.

11. *Dr. Owens-Adair: Some of Her Life Experiences* (Portland, 1905), 90–91. A number of women, like Jacobi and Owens-Adair, after having received a degree from a woman's school, attended a coeducational college for a second degree. Amanda Sanford, for example, who became a well-known general practitioner in upstate New York in the 1880s also attended the University of Michigan after spending time at the Woman's Medical College of Pennsylvania and apprenticing at the New England Hospital. Kate Campbell Hurd-Mead, *Medical Women of America* (New York: Froben Press, 1933), 48.

12. See Jacobi, "Woman in Medicine," 171; Elizabeth Blackwell, *Address on the Medical Education of Women* (New York, 1863), 8–9.

13. For Jacobi's remark see "Inaugural Address to the Woman's Medical College of the New York Infirmary, 1880," *Chicago Medical Journal and Examiner* 42 (1881): 561–85.

14. For a survey of American medical education in the 19th century see Martin Kaufman, *American Medical Education* (Westport, Conn.: 1976). Also helpful is Frederick Norwood, *Medical Education in the United States before the Civil War* (Philadelphia: University of Pennsylvania Press 1944). For Baldwin's remarks see Kaufman, *Medical Education,* 111. Finally, see Steven Smith, *In Memory of Dr. Elizabeth and Dr. Emily Blackwell* (New York: New York Infirmary, 1911), 3–4.

15. For Trall see *Water-Cure Journal* 26 (1858): 26, 27; 27 (1859): 10, and letter dated 7 August 1869 to *The Revolution* 1 (August 1869): 98; and Ronald Numbers, "Health Reform on the Delaware," *New Jersey History* 42 (September 1974): 5—12. Also Frederick C. Waite, "Medical Education of Women at the Penn Medical University," *Medical Review of Reviews* 39 (June 1933): 255–60; and "American Sectarian Medical Colleges before the Civil War," *Bull. Hist. of Med.* 19 (February 1946): 148–66.

16. Kaufman, *Medical Education,* 102.

17. Kaufman, *Medical Education,* 94, 110. See also E. Ingals, M.D., "A Review of the Progress of Medical Education in Chicago, with Some Suggestions for its Advancement," *Chicago Medical Journal and Examiner* 42 (February 1881): 136–47; Thomas N. Bonner, "Dr. Nathan Smith Davis and the Growth of Chicago Medicine, 1850–1900," *Bull. Hist. of Med.* 26 (July–August 1952): 360–74.

18. Martin Kaufman, "The Admission of Women to 19th-Century Medical Societies," *Bull. Hist. of Med.* 50 (Summer 1976): 251–59.

19. See Blackwell, *Pioneer Work,* 237–38; Henry I. Bowditch, "The Medical Education of Women," *Boston Medical and Surgical Journal* 101 (10 July 1879): 67–69; "The Admission of Women to Harvard University," *Boston Medical and Surgical Journal* 100 (5 June 1879): 789–91; "The Admission of Women to Harvard Medical School," *Boston Medical and Surgical Journal* 99 (4 July 1878): 30–31. For barring women from urology clinics at Johns Hopkins see Regina Markell Morantz, "Oral Interview with Dr. Louise de Schweinitz," p. 27, Woman in Medicine Oral History Project, Medical College of Pennsylvania Archives (hereafter cited as MCP).

20. Zakrzewska to Dall, 20 and 26 October 1867, Dall MSS, Mass. Hist. Soc. See also Mary Frame Thomas, "The Influence of the Medical Colleges of the Regular School of Indianapolis on the Medical Education of Women of the State," Indiana State Medical Society, *Transactions* 33 (1883): 228–38.

21. "The Admission of Women to Harvard University," *Boston Medical and Surgical Journal* 23 (5 June 1879): 789–91; "Harvard Medical School and Women," *Boston Medical and Surgical Journal* 21 (22 May 1879) 727–28. In the 1870s it was the supporters of women physicians who defended the quality of their training. When the Philadelphia Medical Society debated the admission of women in 1870, Dr. Atlee commented, "These women's colleges stand in many respects better than many of the colleges represented in the association; they give obstetrical and clinical instruction, as is not given in a majority of the colleges represented here. . . . By the rules of our medical association, I dare not consult with the most highly educated female physician, and yet I may consult with the most ignorant masculine ass in the medical profession." Jacobi, "Woman in Medicine," 181.

22. See a history of the school with excerpts from Annual Reports and other primary material in Annie Sturgis Daniel, "A Cautious Experiment," *MWJ* 46 (August 1939): 231; 46 (October 1939): 298; 47 (February 1940): 40. See also Blackwell, *Pioneer Work,* 227–37; and Vietor, *A Woman's Quest,* 209–42.

23. See Daniel, "A Cautious Experiment," *MWJ* 46 (August 1939): 231, for excerpts for 1858 Annual Report.

24. Vietor, *A Woman's Quest,* 229.

25. The evolution of Blackwell's thought on medical education for women, as well as her strong hostility to sectarians like Lozier can be traced in the following letters to her friend Barbara Bodichon: Jan. 14, 1861; June 9, 1863; January 18, 1865; May 23, 1865; October 28, 1868; June 23, 1868; and a letter addressed "To the Reform Firm" June 3, 1858. Blackwell MSS, Columbia University. In a letter to James Chadwick, probably May 31, 1879, Mary Putnam Jacobi labeled Lozier a "celebrated charlatan," Chadwick MSS, Countway Library. For the barring of homeopathic women from the New

England Hospital see NEH Physicians Minutes, 30 September 1877, Sophia Smith Collection.

26. Daniel, "A Cautious Experiment," *MWJ* 46 (February 1940): 40.
27. Blackwell, *Pioneer Work,* 237.
28. Daniel, "A Cautious Experiment," *passim;* Kaufman, *Medical Education,* 130; George W. Corner, *Two Centuries of Medicine: A History of the School of Medicine, University of Pennsylvania, passim.* For a detailed description of the curriculum see the New York Infirmary's *Annual Announcements* by year, National Library of Medicine.
29. See Faculty Minutes, for November 1888 in Daniel, "A Cautious Experiment," *MWJ* 47 (September 1941): 272–88.
30. Kaufman, *Medical Education,* 130. It could be argued that women students had less choice in attending medical school and therefore the women's schools were not plagued with a potential loss of students every time they raised their standards. But there were a number of coeducational sectarian schools with lower standards, and Lozier's homeopathic woman's medical college competed with the New York Infirmary in New York City. Some women deliberately returned to a regular school after receiving a sectarian degree. See "Autobiography of Elizabeth Cushier," in Hurd-Mead, *Medical Women,* Appendix, 86–87. Cushier left Lozier's New York Medical College to attend the New York Infirmary.
31. See text of Blackwell's 1868 address to the Trustees in Daniel, "A Cautious Experiment," *MWJ* 47 (May 1940): 138. See Smith's comments on the examining board in *In Memory of Dr. Elizabeth and Dr. Emily Blackwell,* 15.
32. S. Josephine Baker, *Fighting for Life,* (New York: Macmillan, 1939), 33–34.
33. Sarah Adamson (Dolley), the niece of Hiram Corson, impatiently left Philadelphia to attend the new eclectic Medical College at Syracuse a year before the school in Philadelphia was founded. She and her classmate Lydia Folger Fowler (the wife of the phrenologist Lorenzo Fowler) became the second and third women respectively to receive medical degrees in the United States. See Genevieve Miller, "Sarah Adamson Dolley," *Notable American Women,* vol. 1, p. 497–99. For a history of the Philadelphia school see Guilielma Fell Alsop, *History of the Woman's Medical College* (Philadelphia: Lippincott, 1950).
34. Jacobi, "Woman in Medicine," 183.
35. Clara Marshall, *The Woman's Medical College of Pennsylvania, An Historical Outline* (Philadelphia: P. Blakiston & Son, 1897), 12.
36. Alsop, *Woman's Medical College,* 49.
37. See Frances Emily White, "The American Medical Woman," *Medical News* (3 August 1895): 12, reprint in MCP Archives. See also Annual Announcements of the Woman's Medical College of Pennsylvania, 1867–1868, 1869–1870, 1880–1881, 1888–1889, 1890–1891, MCP Archives. See Jacobi's comments about the first three decades of the school's history see "Woman in Medicine," 161–63, 170. Kaufman, *Medical Education,* 127–43.
38. Marshall, *Woman's Medical College,* 61. See letters in Bodley and Marshall Correspondence, 12 November 1888; 25 February and 20 April 1889; 5 April 1889; 16 October 1890, MCP Archives.
39. Marshall to Brown, 5 June 1890, Marshall Correspondence, MCP Archives.
40. Marshall, *Woman's Medical College,* 17.

41. Hurd-Mead, *Medical Women of America*, 30, 69; and New York Infirmary Faculty Minutes, in Daniel, "A Cautious Experiment," *Medical Woman's Journal* 48 (September 1941): 274. For a recent history of the teaching of obstetrics and gynecology see Lawrence Longo, M.D., "The Teaching of Obstetrics and Gynecology" (Unpublished paper, 1978). There is good evidence that many physicians were aware of this superior training. See Dr. Atlee's comments cited in n. 21.

42. Thomas N. Bonner, "Mary Harris Thompson," in *Notable American Women*, vol. 3, p. 454–55. Also *The Woman's Medical School of Northwestern University: The Institution and its Founders* (Chicago: H. G. Cutler, 1896), esp. 39–53.

43. *The Woman's Medical School of Northwestern University: The Institution and Its Founders*, includes partial excerpts from the annual announcements. The *Annual Announcements of the Woman's Medical College of Chicago, 1870–1892* can also be found in the National Library of Medicine.

44. See also Arthur Herbert Wilde, *Northwestern University: A History, 1855–1905* (New York, 1905), 367–89; Charles Warrington Earle, M.D., *The Demand for a Woman's Medical College in the West* (Waukegan, Ill., 1879); Helga M. Ruud, M.D., "The Woman's Medical College of Chicago," *MWJ* 53 (June 1946): 41–46; and Eliza Root, "Northwestern University Women's Medical School," Woman's Medical College of Pennsylvania Alumnae *Transactions*, 1900, p. 84–91 (hereafter cited as WMCP *Alumnae Transactions*).

45. *The Announcement of the Woman's Medical College of Baltimore* (Baltimore, 1882), 5; *ibid.*, 1888, p. 6. The National Library of Medicine has an incomplete but adequate collection of the *Catalogues and Annual Announcements* from 1882–1909.

46. Abraham Flexner, *Medical Education in the United States and Canada* (New York, 1910), 237; Lillian Welsh, M.D., *Reminiscences of Thirty Years in Baltimore* (Baltimore, 1925), 37. See also Claribel Cone, M.D., "Report of the Woman's Medical College of Baltimore," WMCP *Alumnae Transactions*, 1900, p. 95–97; and Elizabeth Mason-Hohl, M.D., "Woman's Medical College of Baltimore," *MWJ* 53 (December 1946): 58–63.

47. See Samuel Gregory, *Man Midwifery Exposed and Corrected* (Boston: George Gregory, 1848), and *Letters to Ladies in Favor of Female Physicians* (Boston: American Medical Education Society, 1850). See also George Gregory, *Medical Morals* (New York: George Gregory, 1853); and Frederick C. Waite, *History of the New England Female Medical College, 1848–1874* (Boston: Boston University School of Medicine, 1950).

48. Vietor, *A Woman's Quest*, 235–59.

49. Mary Roth Walsh, *Doctors Wanted: No Women Need Apply: Sexual Barriers in the Medical Profession, 1835–1975* (New Haven: Yale University Press, 1977), 71; Waite, *History of the New England Female Medical College*, passim. Also Helen M. Gassett, *Categorical Account of the Female Medical College, to the People of the New England States* (Boston, 1855). See also the Trustees Minutes, Faculty Minutes and Minutes of the Board of Lady Managers in the New England Female Medical College Archives, Boston University Library. Finally, see scrapbook entitled "Historical Incidents of the New

England Female Medical College," uncatalogued, Countway Library, Harvard Medical School.

50. Catalogues can be found in the New England Female Medical College Archives, Boston University Library.

51. Vietor, *A Woman's Quest,* 251; James Cassedy, "The Microscope in American Medical Science, 1840–1860," *Isis* 67 (March 1976): 76–97.

52. Vietor, *A Woman's Quest,* 250; Jacobi, "Woman in Medicine," 145.

53. Vietor, *A Woman's Quest,* 272.

54. *Ibid.,* 272–74.

55. See Virginia Drachman, *Hospital with a Heart: Women Doctors and the Paradox of Separatism at the New England Hospital, 1862–1969* (Ithaca: Cornell University Press, 1984).

56. Vietor, *A Woman's Quest,* 282–83.

57. *Ibid.*

58. Jacobi, "Woman in Medicine," 145; Vietor, *A Woman's Quest,* 272, 282. Frances Emily White on the faculty of the Woman's Medical College of Pennsylvania wrote that the New England College "forfeited its claim on the regular profession by selling its birthright for a mess of homeopathic pottage." "The American Medical Woman," *Med. News, N.Y.* 67 (1895): 123–28.

59. It is significant that Pennsylvania lacked even one medical school open to women in the 19th century.

60. Donald Fleming, *William Welch and the Rise of Modern Medicine* (Boston: Little, Brown, 1954), 77–118, is an excellent source for the study of Johns Hopkins hospital and medical school.

61. Fleming, *William Welch,* 96–99. Members of the committee included Mrs. Louis Agassiz, Mrs. S. Weir Mitchell, Mrs. Benjamin Harrison, Mrs. Alexander Graham Bell, Mrs. W. C. McCormick, Mrs. Grover Cleveland, Alice Freeman Palmer, Sarah Orne Jewett, Julia Ward Howe, Dr. Emily Blackwell, Mary Putnam Jacobi, Mrs. William Osler, Mrs. Leland Stanford, Mrs. James G. Blaine, as well as a smattering of Biddles, Drexels, Adamses, and Wideners. See pamphlet "The Women's Medical Fund and the Opening of the Johns Hopkins School of Medicine," from an exhibit prepared by the Alan M. Chesney Medical Archives, Johns Hopkins, 1979. See also Allan M. Chesney, *The Johns Hopkins Hospital and the Johns Hopkins University School of Medicine, A Chronicle,* vol. 1 (Baltimore: Johns Hopkins Press, 1943), 193–222; and Caroline Bedell Thomas, M.D., "How Women Medical Students First Came to Hopkins: A Chronicle," *Johns Hopkins Hospital Staff Newsletter,* February 1975.

62. Fleming, *William Welch,* 100.

63. For enthusiasm for coeducation among women physicians see Sarah Hackett Stevenson, "Coeducation of the Sexes in Medicine," in *Physiology of Woman* (Chicago, 1882); S. Josephine Baker, *Fighting for Life* (New York: Macmillan, 1939), 25; Emily Dunning Barringer, *From Bowery to Bellevue* (New York, 1950), 57; Mary F. Thomas, "The Influence of the Medical College on the Medical Education of the Women of the State," Indiana State Medical Society, *Transactions,* 1883, pp. 33, 228–38.

64. Blackwell to Barbara Bodichon, n.d. 1860s, Blackwell MSS, Columbia University.

CHAPTER 5

1. *Transactions of the Alumnae Association of the Woman's Medical College of Pennsylvania* (hereafter cited as WMCP *Alumnae Transactions*), Philadelphia, 1900, p. 145; Rachel L. Bodley, *The College Story: Valedictory Address to the Twenty-Ninth Graduating Class of the Woman's Medical College of Pennsylvania* (Philadelphia: Grant, Faires & Rodgers, 1881), 4–10. See also Emily F. and Augusta C. Pope and Emma L. Call, *The Practice of Medicine by Women in the United States* (Boston: Wright & Potter, 1881).

2. See WMCP *Alumnae Transactions,* 1876–1910, *passim;* and Alumnae letters in papers of Woman's Medical College of Northwestern University, Medical College of Pennsylvania Archives (MCP). Also class histories in *Woman's Medical School Northwestern University* (*Woman's Medical College of Chicago*). *The Institution and its Founders* (Chicago, H. G. Cutler, 1896); *Report of the Alumnae Association of the Woman's Medical College of the New York Infirmary* (New York, 1892), has accounts of each graduate since the first class.

3. WMCP *Alumnae Transactions,* 1901, p. 25ff.

4. For Barker and Cleveland see Alumna files, MCP Archives. See also Patricia Spain Ward, "Emmeline Cleveland," and Joan M. Jensen, "Charlotte Blake Brown," in Edward T. and Janet Wilson James, eds., *Notable American Women,* vol. 1 (Cambridge: Belknap Press, 1971), 349–50, 251–53; Marion Hunt, "Woman's Place in Medicine: The Career of Dr. Mary Hancock McLean," Mo. Hist. Soc. *Bull.,* 36 (July 1980): 255–63; see also Alumnae Records, MCP and WMCP *Alumnae Transactions,* passim.

5. Necrology Report, WMCP *Alumnae Transactions,* 1902–1903, p. 31–32; and Elizabeth Putnam Gordon, *The Story of the Life and Work of Cordelia A. Greene, M.D.* (Castile, New York, 1925), 9.

6. Hunt, "Woman's Place"; WMCP *Alumnae Transactions,* 1896, p. 23–24; Gloria Melnick Moldow, "Promise and Disillusionment: Women Doctors and the Emergence of the Professional Middle Class, 1870–1900" (Ph.D. diss., University of Maryland, 1980), 54, 62, 76, 104; WMCP *Alumnae Transactions,* 1925, p. 19–20 on Eleanor Jones, whose mother graduated in 1856.

7. Farrington to Amanda Blake, 24 July 1872, Charlotte Blake Brown MSS, San Francisco Historical Society.

8. Mary McKibben Harper, "Anna E. Broomall," *Med. Rev. of Reviews* 29 (March 1933): 132–40.

9. Moldow, "Promise and Disillusionment," iii–iv; Kahn-Binswanger file, MCP Archives; "Vivian Shirley Hears Way Woman Doctor Crashed Gate," 1923 newspaper clipping on Mary Hood, American Medical Women's Association Collection (hereafter cited as AMWA), Box 12, Folder 18, Cornell University Archives.

10. James Butler to Maggie Butler, 1 October 1896, Butler file, MCP Archives.

11. See Sarah Ernestine Howard MSS, especially for the years 1913–1918, Schlesinger Library.

12. Uncle Albert to Sabin, 29 September 1907, Sabin MSS, Smith College.

13. See Ruth Putnam, ed., *Life and Letters of Mary Putnam Jacobi* (New York: Putnam, 1925), especially letters dated 1 February 1867, p. 110; 13 January 1870, p. 233; 17 August 1869, p. 216; Undated, 1863, p. 67; 22 April 1867, p. 125; 29 May 1867, p. 141.

14. Martha May Eliot to parents, 14 July 1918, Eliot MSS, Schlesinger Library.
15. Fifty years later women were having the same financial difficulties. Rosalie Slaughter Morton commented in her autobiography, *A Woman Surgeon* (New York: Frederick A. Stokes, 1937), 23,

> Often I have been asked whether I would advise a girl with no income to study medicine. If she is being educated for missionary work, yes. If after proper scholastic education she can borrow enough to see her through four years of medical school, two years of hospital experience and one year of getting established, with the understanding that she will not be expected to pay interest until she has been in practice for three years, nor begin to repay capital for five years, yes. Otherwise, no. Had I not had a small income . . . I could not have ignored the inevitable difficulties.

16. Cost estimate from Virginia Penny, *Employments of Women: A Cyclopedia of Women's Work* (Boston, Walker Wise & Co., 1863), 25, 28. Women doctors were not the only ones to use teaching as a stepping stone to a different career. In her study of fifty-one feminist-abolitionists, Blanche Hersh found that at least half of them worked as teachers for some part of their lives. Usually it was on completion of their education and before they married, but they often used teaching to finance further education as well. Most feminists gave up because they found teaching narrow, low-paying, and unsatisfying. Sheila Rothman has pointed out that states so encouraged women in the 1850s and 1860s to become teachers and attend newly created normal schools that by the late 1880s there was a glut of teachers on the market and competition for jobs was severe. Women tended to move from teaching to reform activity or to other work still considered mainly in the female domain. See Hersh, " 'The Slavery of Sex': Feminist-Abolitionists in Nineteenth Century America" (Ph.D. diss., University of Illinois, Chicago Circle, 1975), 287. See also Richard M. Bernard and Maris A. Vinovskis, "The Female School Teacher in Ante-Bellum Massachusetts," *Journal of Social History* 10 (June 1977): 332–45; Keith Melder, "Woman's High Calling: The Teaching Profession in America, 1830–1860," *American Studies* 13 (Fall 1972): 19–32; Rothman, *Woman's Proper Place* (New York: Basic Books, 1978), 60. Whatever the variety of individual motivation, the number of female medical graduates who began their professional careers as teachers remains striking. See for example the careers of the following graduates of the WMCP: Annette C. Buckel (1858), Susan Hayhurst (1857), Phoebe Oliver Briggs (1870), Eliza Judson (1872), Hannah Jackson Price (1881), Eliza Norton Lawrence (1887), Mary Erdman Greenwald (1892), Inez C. Philbrick (1891), Lillian Welsh (1889). This list is by no means exhaustive, nor must it be confined only to the graduates of one school. See alumnae folders and WMCP *Alumnae Transactions*. See also *The Woman's Medical School of Northwestern University*, 90–157, for information on the graduates of that school, and *Report of the Alumnae Association of the Woman's Medical College of the New York Infirmary*, 1892, p. 17–33.
17. 29 October 1881, Chadwick Notebook, uncatalogued, Countway Library, Harvard Medical School. See the letters written to Clara Marshall, Marshall MSS, *passim*, but especially letters of Lillian Phlegan, 17 February 1891; Marcia P. Rogers, 7 April 1890; Mary E. Hoyt, 24 January 1891.
18. See the alumnae folders of Annette Buckel (1858), Martha E. Lovell (1899), Em-

ma M. Richardson (1898), Alice M. Seabrook (1895), Margaret Cleaver-Parrott (1895), Olive Steinmetz (1900). See also the letters of inquiry from nurses in the Clara Marshall MSS, especially Emily W. Owen to Marshall, 17 September 1890; Ellen Wagner to Marshall, 18 August 1890; Mary G. Fowler to Marshall, 8 May 1891. See WMCP *Alumnae Transations,* 1929, p. 19, for necrology report on Mary Evelyn Brydon. Jane E. Robbins's parents (New York Infirmary, 1890) preferred that she study medicine to becoming a nurse. "Memoirs of Student Days," AMWA Collection, Box 12, Folder 26, Cornell University.

19. "Woman in Medicine," in Annie Nathan Meyer, ed., *Woman's Work in America* (New York: Henry Holt, 1891), 199.

20. Long to Marshall, 13 August 1890, Marshall MSS; Dean to Marshall, 17 June 1890. See others, Marshall MSS, *passim,* MCP Archives.

21. Thompson to Marshall, 19 February 1897, Marshall MSS, MCP Archives.

22. *Godey's Lady's Book* 44 (1852): 185–190, 288; 46 (1853): 551–53; 49 (1854): 80, 368, 458; 54 (1857): 371; 61 (1860): 270–71.

23. Agnes Vietor, ed., *A Woman's Quest, The Life of Marie Zakrzewska, M.D.* (New York: D. Appleton, 1924), 124–25, 137, 203, 206–7, 210. Elizabeth Blackwell, *Pioneer Work in Opening the Medical Profession to Women* (London: Longmans, Green, 1895; reprint, New York: Schocken, 1977), 194–96.

24. See article on Mosher "The Oldest Woman Doctor Diagnoses Life," in *New York Times,* 29 March 1925.

25. Anne Walter Fearn, *My Days of Strength* (New York: Harper Bros, 1939), 11.

26. Bertha Van Hoosen, *Petticoat Surgeon* (Chicago: Pellegrini & Cudahy, 1947), 56.

27. Rosalie Slaughter Morton, *A Woman Surgeon* (New York: Frederick A. Stokes Company, 1937), 17. For Mendenhall see Mendenhall Manuscript Autobiography in Sophia Smith Collection, Smith College.

28. Mary Bennett Ritter, *More Than Gold in California, 1849–1933* (Berkeley: Professional Press, 1933), 155; Fearn, *My Days of Strength,* 12.

29. This calculation was made from charts constructed from the available information on alumna at the WMCP. Gloria Moldow found the average age at graduation of women physicians in Washington, D.C. to be thirty-five years. Moldow, "Promise and Disillusionment," 39.

30. See Longshore MSS, MCP Archives; on Wanzer see *Bull. of the San Francisco County Medical Society* 3 (November 1930): 19; on Higgins see Claire Still, "The Medical School's First Alumna" in *Stanford, M.D.* 15 (Spring 1976): 27–28; for Price see oral recollections of her daughter, Katharine Price Hubbell in Alger MSS, Schlesinger Library. For Binswanger-Kahn see biographical sketch in her file written by her sister Fanny, MCP Archives.

31. "The Oldest Woman Doctor Diagnoses Life," *New York Times,* 29 March 1925.

32. Mary Maples Dunn, "Saints and Sisters: Congregational and Quaker Women in the Early Colonial Period," *American Quarterly* 30 (Winter 1978): 582–601.

33. Nancy Cott, "Young Women in the Second Great Awakening in New England," *Feminist Studies* 3 (Fall 1975): 14–29; and Mary Ryan, "A Woman's Awakening: Evangelical Religion and the Families of Utica, New York, 1800–1840," *American Quarterly* 30 (Winter 1978): 602–23.

34. Mary Ryan's contention that women, "in addition to constituting the majority of revival converts, were also instrumental in a host of other conversions among their kind of both sexes," seems to be borne out, at least in part, by the religious events of Cordelia Greene's adolescence. See Ryan, "A Woman's Awakening," 604, and Gordon, *Cordelia A. Greene,* 6–7.

35. M. S. Legan, "Hydropathy in America," *Bull. Hist. of Med.* 45 (May 1971): 267–80.

36. Gordon, *Cordelia A. Greene,* 12.

37. *Ibid.,* 16–17, 44–45.

38. *Ibid.,* 87, 177.

39. I am indebted to Joyce Antler for helping me clarify this point. See the files of Ida Richardson, Elizabeth D. Kane, Sara C. Seward, and the numerous medical missionaries at the Woman's Medical College of Pennsylvania. Alumnae files, MCP Archives. See also the biographical sketches of the many women physicians listed in Francis Willard and Mary Livermore, eds., *American Women: 1500 Biographies* (New York: Mast, Crowell & Kirkpatrick, 1897), *passim;* Harriet Hunt's autobiography, *Glances and Glimpses* (Boston: Jewett and Co., 1856), 109; and Olive Floyd, *Doctora in Mexico* (New York: G. P. Putnam, 1944), the story of an 1897 graduate of the WMCP who spent most of her time practicing in Mexico, where her husband and she were missionaries.

40. Ronald Hogeland, "Coeducation of the Sexes at Oberlin College: A Study of Social Ideas in Mid-19th century America," *Journal of Social History* (Winter 1972): 160–76 and 164. Also Robert S. Fletcher, *A History of Oberlin College* (Oberlin: Oberlin University Press, 1943), 640ff.; and Fletcher, "Oberlin and Coeducation," *Ohio State Archeological and Historical Quarterly,* January 1938, pp. 1–19.

41. Hogeland, "Coeducation," 166; Fletcher, *A History,* 291, 382.

42. Rachel Bodley, *Memoir of Emmeline Horton Cleveland* (Philadelphia: 1979), 6.

43. See WMCP *Alumnae Transactions,* 1900, p. 203. Jacobi wrote of Cleveland that she was "a woman of real ability, and would have done justice to a much larger sphere than that to which fate condemned her." She was "possessed of much personal beauty," Jacobi recalled, but was "compelled by the slender resources of the college to unite the duties of housekeeper and superintendent to those of professor. She not unfrequently passed from the lecture room to the kitchen to make the bread for the students who boarded at the institution." "Woman in Medicine," Annie Nathan Meyer, ed., *Women's Work in America* (New York: Henry Holt, 1891), 158.

44. Religious women physicians like Emma Walker, Mary Wood-Allen, and Valeria Parker became lecturers for the American Social Hygiene Association in the 1920s. 13 January 1870, in *Life and Letters of Mary Putnam Jacobi,* ed. Ruth Putnam (New York: Putnam, 1925) 233; Belcher to Eliza Johnson, 1 December 1878, 16 September 1883, Belcher letters, in private possession of her grandniece, S. Alice McCone.

45. Blackwell, *Pioneer Work,* 27; Mosher Diary, Eliza Mosher MSS, Michigan Historical Collections; Hunt, *Glances,* 110, 126.

46. Emily Dunning Barringer, *Bowery to Bellevue* (New York: W. W. Norton, 1950), 28.

47. Manuscript Autobiography, chap. 1, p. 35, Anna Wessel Williams MSS, Schlesinger Library.
48. Davis file, MCP Archives.
49. Clipping from New Orleans *Picayune,* 22 February 1920, entitled "Woman Doctor Celebrates her 100th Birthday," in Ellen Taft Grimes file, MCP Archives.
50. WMCP *Alumnae Transactions* 1890, p. 27.
51. See for McCarn-Craig, WMPC *Alumnae Transactions* 1906, p. 29. For Winslow see Moldow, "Promise and Disillusionment," 274; Cleaves, *Biographical Cyclopedia of Homeopathic Physicians and Surgeons* (Philadelphia, 1873), 264–65; *Woman's Journal* 10 (December 1982): 404. For Stinson, WMCP *Alumnae Transactions,* 1889, p. 27. Mary Bennet Ritter also suffered from ill health, Ritter, *More Than Gold,* 169–70, as did Caroline Smith (see folder, MCP Archives) and many early health reformers, including Mary Gove Nichols and Paulina Wright Davis. Stinson graduated from the WMCP in 1869.
52. *Petticoat Surgeon,* 54–55.
53. Williams, Typescript Autobiography, chap. 2, p. 39, Schlesinger Library.
54. McGee to father, 7 June 1884; "Woman" Idea Book, December 1894; Notes, Anita Newcomb Mcgee MSS, Library of Congress. See Belva Lockwood, "My Life as a Lawyer," in *Lippincott's* (June 1888), 215–29, cited in Moldow, "Promise and Disillusionment," 2, who makes exactly this point.
55. Faculty Minutes, 1876, MCP Archives.
56. *Petticoat Surgeon,* 63.
57. *More Than Gold,* 156.
58. WMCP *Alumnae Transactions,* 1890, p. 32.
59. Florence Hazzard, "Heart of the Oak," Typescript Biography of Eliza Mosher in Mosher MSS, Michigan Historical Collections, chap. 3, p. 10.
60. It was quite common for women doctors to treat family members and women friends. See Bertha Van Hoosen's dramatic story of the delivery of her niece in *Petticoat Surgeon,* 100–102. See also Helen Morton MSS, Schlesinger Library, *passim;* Harriet Belcher Letters, (in private hands), *passim.*
61. "A Woman Doctor Who Stuck it Out," *Literary Digest,* 4 April 1925, p. 66, 67, 69.
62. Typescript Autobiography, chap. 3, p. 5. See also Jane E. Robbins (New York Infirmary, 1890), "Memoirs of Student Days," AMWA Collection, Box 12, Folder 26, Cornell University.
63. Letter from Preston to ? dated 22 January 1854, Preston, MSS, MCP Archives.
64. See various anecdotes about Cleveland in Bodley, *Memoir of Emmeline Horton Cleveland,* passim; Typescript from memorial meeting in Broomall's behalf, Broomall file; MCP Archives.
65. Letter dated 28 February 1938 to Dean Tracy, Rita S. Finkler File; Oral interview conducted by author with Katherine Boucot Sturgis, 11 July 1977, p. 31; *Women in Medicine Oral History Project;* all in MCP Archives.
66. Williams, Typescript Autobiography, chap. 5, p. 8.
67. Belcher to Eliza Johnson, 1 December 1878, Belcher Letters; Dorothy McGuigan, *A Dangerous Experiment, 100 Years of Women at the University of Michigan* (Ann Arbor: University of Michigan, 1970), 32 and chap. 7; Alumnae Questionnaire, Mosher MSS, Michigan Historical Collections. For

Van Hoosen remark see Hazzard, "Heart of the Oak," chap. 3, p. 28, Mosher MSS, Michigan Historical Collections.

68. Mendenhall Manuscript Autobiography, 10, Smith College.
69. Mendenhall Manuscript Autobiography, 8, Smith College.
70. Letters dated 16 October 1871, 6 January 1872. See also *Petticoat Surgeon,* 66.
71. John B. Gabel, ed., "Medical Education in the 1890's: An Ohio Woman's Memories," *Ohio History* 87 (Winter 1978): 61.
72. Mendenhall Manuscript Autobiography 2–21, Smith College.
73. *Ibid.,* 22.
74. Corner to Eleanor Bleumel, 19 September 1955, Box 30, Sabin MSS, Smith College.
75. 3 February 1915, Howard MSS, Schlesinger Library.
76. *More Than Gold,* 161.
77. Mosher Alumnae Questionnaire, Mosher MSS, Michigan Historical Collections.
78. Hazzard "Heart of the Oak," chap. 3, p. 27, Mosher MSS, Michigan Historical Collections.
79. Dr. Alice Ballou Eliot to Elinor Bleumel, 20 September 1955. See also Dr. Josephine Hunt to Bleumel, 25 September 1955; Dr. Ellen Finley Kiser to Bleumel, n.d., Box 30, Sabin MSS, Smith College.
80. WMCP *Alumnae Transactions,* 1905, p. 36. In 1923 Potter was appointed by Governor Gifford Pinchot the Secretary of Welfare of the State of Pennsylvania and became the first woman state cabinet officer. Pinchot enjoyed calling her the "best man in my cabinet." See brief Biographical Notes by Catharine Macfarlane, Potter MSS, MCP Archives.
81. Martha May Eliot to Papa, 11 October 1919; Howard to parents, 6 February 1915; both in Eliot MSS, Howard MSS, Schlesinger Library.
82. October 1913, Howard MSS, Schlesinger Library.
83. *Bowery to Bellevue,* 99.
84. *Fighting For Life* (New York: MacMillan, 1939), 64.
85. Gabel, ed., "Medical Education," 59, 58.
86. 26 September 1880. See also her letters home in the early years of practice, 25 July and 12 August 1893, 14 September 1894; Van Hoosen MSS, Michigan Historical Collections.
87. Gabel, ed., "Medical Education," 65.
88. See WMCP *Alumnae Transactions,* 1895, p. 124.
89. 16 July 1893, Hamilton MSS, Schlesinger Library.
90. WMCP *Alumnae Transactions,* 1900, p. 98. See also statement by Alice Higgins, WMCP *Alumnae Transactions,* 1890, p. 27. The question of confidence is complicated, however, because women's schools also seemed to suffer from a sense of inferiority.
91. Letter to family, 1 December 1872. See also letters, 1872–1875, *passim.*
92. Manuscript Autobiography, 31, Mendenhall MSS, Smith College.
93. 12 November 1916, Eliot MSS, Schlesinger Library.
94. 12 February 1916, Eliot MSS, Schlesinger Library.
95. Wherry to Elinor Bleumel, 17 September 1955; Herrinton to Bleumel, 26 October 1956; both in Box 30, Sabin MSS, Smith College. See also the letters

of Sarah Ernestine Howard and Martha May Eliot, and Mendenhall's Manuscript Autobiography for continual references to relationships between the
women students.

96. To Elinor Bleumel, 25 September 1955, Box 30, Sabin MSS, Smith College.
97. To mother, 2 May 1915, Eliot MSS, Schlesinger Library; Mendenhall Manuscript Autobiography, n.p., Smith College.
98. Mendenhall, Manuscript Autobiography, 13.
99. *Ibid.,* 15.
100. Genevieve Garcelon to Bleumel, 16 September 1955, Sabin MSS, Smith
College.
101. Mendenhall Manuscript Autobiography, section F, 1–10. Smith College.
102. Alan M. Chesney, M.D., *The Johns Hopkins Hospital and the Johns Hopkins School of Medicine, a Chronicle,* vol. 1 (Baltimore: Johns Hopkins
University Press, 1943), 10.
103. Elinor Bleumel, *Florence Sabin, Colorado Woman of the Century* (Boulder:
University of Colorado Press, 1959), 62.
104. 18 February 1916; 11 March 1916; both in Howard MSS, Schlesinger Library.
105. Dorothea Rhodes Lummis Moore, MSS, Huntington Library, San Marino,
California.
106. Blackwell, *Pioneer Work,* 28; Williams, Typescript Autobiography, chap. 2,
p. 36. Also scattered notes, n.p., *passim;* Williams MSS, Schlesinger Library.
107. 25 January 1916; 13 February 1914, Howard MSS, Schlesinger Library.
108. 13 February 1915, Howard MSS, Schlesinger Library. Neither Howard nor
Eliot ever married.
109. Hazzard, "Heart of the Oak," chap. 3, p. 15.
110. *Bowery to Bellevue,* 57.
111. Alumnae Questionnaire in Mosher MSS, Michigan Historical Collections.
112. Caroline H. Dall, ed., *A Practical Illustration of Woman's Right to Labor*
(Boston: Walker, Wise and Co., 1860), 2.
113. 11 December 1854 to "Very dear friend," Woman Physicians File, Smith
College.
114. Gertrude Baillie, M.D., "Should Professional Women Marry?" *Woman's
Medical Journal* 2 (February 1894): 33–35.
115. *Marie Elizabeth Zakrzewska: A Memoir* (Boston, The New England Hospital for Women and Children, 1903), 22; Elizabeth Cady Stanton, *Eighty
Years and More* (New York: Schocken, 1971), 172; Harriet Belcher to Eliza,
5 February 1879, Belcher Letters, in private hands; 9 April 1916, Howard
MSS, Schlesinger Library.
116. Notes, Folder 61, Williams MSS, Schlesinger Library.
117. Notes, Clelia Mosher MSS, Stanford University Library. For a wonderful
example of how real these conflicts were for women physicians see the short
story by Rosalie Slaughter (Morton), "One Short Hour," written for *Daughters of Aesculapius* (Philadelphia: George Jacobs & Co., 1897), 66–79, a
collection of fiction and non-fiction written by students and faculty of the
Woman's Medical College of Pennsylvania. In this revealing narrative, a
woman medical student in love is confronted by her fiancé with the choice
between marriage and medicine. Shocked and disappointed in her lover, the
woman rises to her full height, crushing "the rose in her hand," a gift from her

betrothed, and as "its petals fell among the cups," declares, "I have chosen, Howard,—farewell!" 79.

118. Harriet Belcher to Eliza Johnson, 18 February 1977, 10 August 1978, Belcher Letters, in private hands.

119. See *Cordelia Greene,* 20–21.

120. 15 August 1885, Mosher MSS, Michigan Historical Collections.

121. Letters not dated, but between 1871–1876, Helen Morton Papers, Schlesinger Library.

122. Carroll Smith-Rosenberg, "The Female World of Love and Ritual: Relations between Women in Nineteenth-Century America," *Signs* 1 (Autumn 1975): 1–20; Nancy Sahli, "Smashing: Women's Relationships Before the Fall," *Chrysalis* 2 (Summer 1979): 17–27. See, in the Ada Pierce McCormick, MSS, MCP Archives, Musson to Ada Pierce, undated, 1910, and Clark to Ada, 6 January 1914. Among the better known women physicians for the nineteenth and early twentieth century, the Pope sisters lived together, Elizabeth Keller lived with Lucy Sewall, Martha Tracy, dean of WMCP, lived with her dear friend Ellen Potter, also on the faculty, and Ethel Dunham lived with Martha May Eliot.

123. *Marie Elizabeth Zakrzewska, A Memoir,* 29.

124. Mendenhall Manuscript Autobiography, 18, Smith College.

125. See the alumnae folders of Edith Schad (1890), Mary G. Erdman (1892), Lorilla F. Bullard Tower (1894), May Sibley-Lee (1884), Eliza M. Lawrence (1887), Mary L. McLean (1887), Julia Wyant Perry (1891), Martha Pike Sanborn (1893), Mararet Cleaver Parrot (1895), Rachel Stieren (1898), Caroline A. Stevens Frizzel (1875). See also WMCP *Alumnae Transactions,* 1906, p. 32, for information on Tyson.

126. "Inaugural Address at the Opening of Woman's Medical College of the New York Infirmary," October 1880, reprinted in the Women's Medical Association of New York City, ed., *Mary Putnam Jacobi: Pathfinder in Medicine* (New York: G. P. Putnam, 1925), 390. For hints as to the tension in Jacobi's marriage see a letter from her husband, Abraham Jacobi, to her dated simply "21 March." Jacobi MSS, Schlesinger Library.

127. See Bodley's survey, *The College Story* which indicates 27 percent, and Pope, Pope and Call, *The Practice of Medicine,* whose figure is 15 percent. My own calculations with the alumnae of the Woman's Medical College of Pennsylvania show that approximately 337 out of 937 graduates in the years 1852–1900 married (about 35 percent). My suspicion is that marriage became slightly more common in the last two decades of the century, when the percentage of graduates who married rises from 33 percent (1852–1879) to 36 percent (1880–1900). Information was gleaned from the alumnae records and class lists printed in the *Register of the Alumnae Association,* Philadelphia, 1970. I included in the married group all hyphenated last names plus those few I knew to be married from other sources. Thus the list is conservative. For missionary couples see the WMCP alumnae files of Anna Jones Thoburn (1882), Margaret Cleaver Parrot (1895), Jenny Tylor Gordon (1892), Laura Hyde Roote (1883), Marion Fairweather Sterling (1885), Mary Le Burnham Ancell (1896). See also the obituary of Lucilla Green Cheney (1875) in WMCP *Alumnae Transactions,* 1879, p. 12. The Woman's Medical

College of Chicago also trained a number of missionary couples. See *The Woman's Medical School of Northwestern University,* 90ff., and 57. As for women who married doctors, calculations both from the WMCP alumnae files and the information in the WMCP *Alumnae Transactions,* revealed that approximately one-third (29) of the 86 women for whom there is complete information married doctors (34 percent). See the letters of inquiry both from doctors and doctors' wives seeking information about matriculating at the school in the Clara Marshall Papers: Charles T. Watkins to Marshall, 31 March 1891; Clara E. Jones to Marshall, 2 February 1891; Thomas P. Carracott to Marshall, 27 August 1891; Alice A. Hungerford to Marshall, 31 October 1890; Mary A. Nutting to Marshall, 13 July 1888. On Longshore and Brown see *Notable American Women* and the manuscript biography of his wife by Thomas Longshore in the MCP Archives. For other women who attended medical school after marriage see news of Alice Higgins, Florence Preston Stubbs, and Gertrude M. Streeper, WMCP *Alumnae Transactions,* 1890, p. 26–27.

128. For 1900 see *Statistics of Women at Work, Based on unpublished information derived from the schedules of the Twelfth Census, 1900* (Washington: Government Printing Office, 1907). For 1910 and 1920, *Fourteenth Census of the United States,* vol. 4: "Population, 1920: Occupations" (Washington: Government Printing, Office, 1923). For 1930, *Fifteenth Census of the United States,* vol. 5 (Washington: Government Printing Office, 1933). For 1940, *Sixteenth Census of the United States,* vol. 3 (Washington: Government Printing Office, 1943). For 1950, *U.S. Census of Population, 1950,* Special Reports: "Occupational Characteristics" (Washington: Government Printing Office, 1956).

129. See the round-robin letter in Mary Loog and Frances Ancell files dated 2 December 1945. See also files of Julia March Baird (1896), Orie Moon Andrews (1857), Elinor Galt-Simmons (1879), Katherine Brandt de Wolfe (1887). Also letters from Mary Beard to Kate Campbell Hurd-Mead referring to Mead's husband suggests that Mead's marriage too was both happy and productive. Mead MSS, all in MCP Archives. See finally, Rosalie Slaughter Morton, *A Woman Surgeon,* 142ff., for a description of her own marriage.

130. See the Thomas Longshore Manuscript Biography and Notes from interview with Longshore's daughter, Mrs. Lucretia Blankenburg, Longshore MSS, MCP Archives; Oral Interview in 1979 with Mr. Stacy May. I am grateful to Ruth Abram for sharing this interview with me.

131. See WMCP *Alumnae Transactions,* 1890, p. 26–27.

132. *Memorial Addresses on the Life and Character of Dr. Esther Hawkes* (Lynn, Mass.: Boy's Club Press, 1906), 15.

133. *More Than Gold,* 238.

134. These dual career marriages included that of Drs. Charlotte and Fred Baker. Charlotte Johnson Baker had been inspired by Eliza Mosher to study medicine at Vassar when the latter served a term as resident physician there. Later Baker assisted Mosher at the Woman's Reformatory Prison at Sherborn before attending the Michigan University Medical School. Baker practiced with her husband and had two children. See Willard and Livermore, *American Women,* vol. 1, p. 46.

135. *Bowery to Bellevue,* 67.
136. Yarros to Margaret Craighill, dean of WMCP, 6 March 1943, Yarros File, MCP Archives.
137. From newspaper clipping (name of paper and date missing) in Maria Homet file, MCP Archives.
138. WMCP *Alumnae Transactions,* 1892, p. 24.
139. Lillian Welsh, *Reminiscenses of Thirty Years in Baltimore* (Baltimore: Norman, Remington, 1925) 44–45.
140. *Ibid.*

CHAPTER 6

1. For an overview of these changes see William G. Rothstein, *American Physicians in the Nineteenth Century, From Sects to Science* (Baltimore: Johns Hopkins University Press, 1972); James G. Burrow, *The American Medical Association: Voice of American Medicine* (Baltimore: Johns Hopkins Press, 1973); Rosemary Stevens, *American Medicine and the Public Interest* (New Haven: Yale University Press, 1971); L. James O'Hara, "An Emerging Profession: Philadelphia Medicine, 1860–1900" (Ph.D. diss., University of Pennsylvania, 1976); Morris Vogel and Charles Rosenberg, eds., *The Therapeutic Revolution* (Philadelphia: University of Pennsylvania Press, 1980); George Rosen, *The Structure of American Medical Practice, 1875–1941* (Philadelphia: University of Pennsylvania, 1983).
2. O'Hara, "An Emerging Profession," 30; Megali Larson, *The Rise of Professionalism* (Berkeley; University of California Press, 1977), chap. 2.
3. Avery to Dall, 25 May 1862, 13 July 1862, Caroline Dall MSS, Massachusetts Historical Society.
4. Emily F. and Augusta Pope, and Emma L. Call, *The Practice of Medicine by Women in the United States* (Boston, 1881).
5. *Transactions of the Alumnae Association of the Woman's Medical College of Pennsylvania,* 1906, p. 32, and 1907, p. 25 (hereafter cited as WMCP *Alumnae Transactions*).
6. See Mary R. Dearing, "Anita Newcomb McGee," in Edward T. and Janet James, eds., *Notable American Women* (Cambridge: Harvard University Press, 1975), 464–66; and Anita Newcomb McGee and Simon Newcomb MSS, Library of Congress; Rosalie Slaughter Morton, *A Woman Surgeon* (New York: Frederick A. Stokes, 1937), 23.
7. Van Hoosen to sister, 22 July 1890, 26 October 1892, 2 November 1892; Van Hoosen to parents, 10 April 1893, 9 July 1893, 28 July 1893; and to sister 9 February 1899; all in Van Hoosen MSS, Michigan Historical Collections.
8. Belcher to Eliza, 10 August 1878, 5 February 1879, Belcher Letters, in private hands.
9. Belcher to Eliza, 13 July 1879, 16 November 1879, 1 and 9 February 1880, 11 July 1880, 6 March 1881, Belcher Letters, in private hands.
10. 2 February 1882, 30 November 1882, 20 January 1884, 15 March 1885, 4 October 1885, Belcher Letters, in private hands.
11. From 1938 (no other date) clipping from Philadelphia *Daily Ledger,* in Reel Folder, Alumna Files, Medical College of Pennsylvania Archives (MCP Ar-

chives), WMCP *Alumnae Transactions,* 1888, p. 16–17; *Annual Report of the New England Hospital,* 1875, p. 17.

12. WMCP *Alumnae Transactions,* 1894, p. 52, and 1892, p. 22; *The Woman's Medical School: Northwestern University, The Institution and its Founders, Class Histories, 1870–1896* (Chicago: H. G. Cutler, 1896), 98–100, 103.

13. 7 January 1910, New England Hospital Collection (NEH), Box 16, Smith College.

14. WMCP *Alumnae Transactions,* 1886, p. 14–15.

15. Elizabeth Blackwell, *Pioneer Work in Opening the Medical Profession to Women* (London: Longmans, Green, 1895), 193, 194; WMCP *Alumnae Transactions,* 1876–1900, *passim;* Letter from Dr. R. M. DeHart to Zakrzewska on her own hygiene lecturing, *Annual Report of the New England Hospital for Women and Children* (Boston, 1875), 16–17.

16. Josephine Baker, *Fighting for Life* (New York: Macmillan, 1939), 51–53; Mary Putnam Jacobi, "Woman in Medicine," in Annie Nathan Meyer, ed., *Woman's Work in America* (New York: Henry Holt, 1891), 201. It was assumed that women did much better in small towns. See Eliza H. Root, "The Distribution of Medical Women in the State of Illinois," *Woman's Medical Journal (WMJ)* 14 (May 1904): 100–101.

17. 22 May 1887, Eliza Mosher MSS, Michigan Historical Collections; WMCP *Alumnae Transactions,* 1880, p. 14; "The Woman Physician in the Country," *WMJ* 12 (January 1902); 4.

18. Interview with Dr. Pauline Stitt, 9 December 1977, p. 11–12, Women in Medicine Oral History Project, MCP Archives.

19. D. W. Cathell, *The Physician Himself, And Things That Concern His Reputation and Success* (Philadelphia: F. A. Davis, 1890), 99.

20. Elizabeth Putnam Gordon, *The Story of the Life and Work of Cordelia A. Greene, M.D.* (Castile, New York: The Castilian, 1925); Kathryn K. Sklar, *Catharine Beecher* (New Haven: Yale University Press, 1973), 214–15; Regina Markell Morantz, "Making Women Modern: Middle Class Women and Health Reform in 19th Century America," *Journal Social History* 10 (June 1977): 103–20; William Leach, *True Love and Perfect Union: The Feminist Reform of Sex and Society* (New York: Basic Books, 1980), *passim.*

21. Gordon, *Cordelia Greene,* 12.

22. Marshall S. Legan, "Hydropathy in America: A Nineteenth Century Panacea," *Bull. Hist. of Med.* 45 (May 1971): 267–80; Harry B. Weiss and Howard R. Kimbel, *The Great American Water-Cure Craze* (Trenton: The Past Times Press, 1967); Samuel A. Cloyes, *The Healer: The Story of Dr. Samantha S. Nivinson and Dryden Springs, 1820–1915* (Ithaca, N.Y.: DeWitt, 1969); Cordelia Greene, M.D., *The Art of Keeping Well* (New York: Dodd, Mead, 1905); Rachel Brooks Gleason, M.D., *Talks to My Patients* (New York: M. L. Holbrook, 1895).

23. For an excellent article concerning this kind of work for women physicians see Constance McGovern, " 'Doctors or Ladies?' Women Physicians in Psychiatric Institutions, 1872–1900," *Bull. Hist. of Med.* 55 (Spring 1981): 88–107.

24. "Women's Work in the Care of the Insane," WMCP *Alumnae Transactions,* 1900, p. 38.

25. McGovern, " 'Doctors or Ladies,' " 103.

26. "The Woman Physician and a Vast Field of Usefulness Unrecognized by Her," WMCP *Alumnae Transactions,* 1903, pp. 72–81, 73.

27. McGovern, " 'Doctors or Ladies,' " 105–7.

28. WMCP *Alumnae Transactions,* 1892, p. 47.

29. Dorothy McGuigan, *A Dangerous Experiment, One Hundred Years of Women at the University of Michigan* (Ann Arbor, University of Michigan Press 1970), 64–68.

30. See Vaughan's letter to Mosher, 17 October 1895, Mosher MSS, Michigan Historical Collections. See "Reports from Various Parts of the United States," in WMCP *Alumnae Transactions, 1900,* pp. 120–36.

31. See members of the University of Michigan League to Mosher, 7 March 1896; L. H. Stone on behalf of Michigan State Federation of Women's Club's to Mosher, 29 January 1896; both in Mosher MSS, Michigan Historical Collections.

32. See Caroline L. Hunt, *The Life of Ellen H. Richards: 1842–1911* (Washington: American Home Economics Assn., 1942); Emma S. Weigley, "It Might Have Been Euthenics: The Lake Placid Conferences and the Home Economics Movement," *American Quarterly* 26 (March 1974): 79–96. See also Margaret Rossiter, *Women Scientists in America* (Baltimore: Johns Hopkins Press, 1982), 70. Rossiter is incorrect in crediting male physicians with originating hygiene courses.

33. Lillian Welsh, *Reminiscences of Thirty Years in Baltimore* (Baltimore: Norman, Remington, 1925), 115.

34. McGuigan, *A Dangerous Experiment,* 64–68.

35. McGuigan, *A Dangerous Experiment,* 64–68. See also the comments about a similar aversion on the part of the coeds at Stanford University in the early 20th century to Mosher's cousin, Dr. Clelia Mosher. Regina Markell Morantz, Esther Bridgeman Clarke, Oral History, 19 December 1977, pp. 12–15, MCP Archives. Mary Bennett Ritter was much better liked at Berkeley. See her autobiography, *More than Gold in California* (Berkeley: Professional Press, 1933), 201–17.

36. Welsh *Reminiscences,* 5; McGuigan, *A Dangerous Experiment,* 67.

37. McGuigan, *A Dangerous Experiment,* 67.

38. Estelle Freedman, "Separatism as Strategy: Female Institution Building and American Feminism, 1870–1930," *Feminist Studies* 5 (Fall 1979): 512–39; Kathryn Kish Sklar, "Florence Kelly: Resources and Achievements" (Paper given at Fifth Berkshire Conference on the History of Women, Vassar College, June 1981).

39. See report by Marion M. Grady, WMCP *Alumnae Transactions,* 1900, p. 144; and Eliza Root, "The Medical Woman as Teacher in Medical Schools," *WMJ* 11 (September 1901): 325–33.

40. Elizabeth D. Robinton, "Anna Wessel Williams," in Barbara Sicherman and Carol Hurd Green, eds., *Notable American Women: The Modern Period* (Cambridge: Belknap Press, 1980), 737–39. See also "Women Physicians in Medical Research Work," *WMJ* 19 (January 1909): 9.

41. *An Atlas of the Medulla and Midbrain* (Baltimore: Friedenwald, 1901). For information on Mall and Sabin see Donald Fleming, *William H. Welch and the Rise of Modern Medicine* (Boston: Little, Brown, 1954), 164–76; 100–104; Elinor Bluemel, *Florence Sabin: Colorado Woman of the Century* (Boulder:

University of Colorado Press, 1959), 49–52; Vincent Andriole, "Florence Rena Sabin—Teacher, Scientist, Citizen," *Jour. Hist. Med. and Allied Sciences* 14 (July 1959): 320–50, 323–24; Florence Sabin, *Franklin P. Mall, The Story of a Mind* (Baltimore: Johns Hopkins, 1934).

42. See Eliza Root, "The Woman as Teacher in Medical Schools." See also Dean Martha Tracy's assessment of the problem after the first decade of the 20th century, "The Woman's Medical College of Pennsylvania," *WMJ* 29 (October 1919): 202–8.

43. Alice Hamilton, *Exploring the Dangerous Trades* (Boston: Little Brown, 1943), 97.

44. Andriole, "Florence Rena Sabin," 325.

45. For an interesting point of view, see Miriam Slater and Penina Glazer, "Women Research Scientists: Few Professional Progenitors, Fewer Professional Progeny," unpublished paper which is part of a larger project on women professionals.

46. Andriole, "Florence Rena Sabin," 325.

47. Bluemel, *Florence Sabin,* 84; Louise de Schweinitz to Elinor Bluemel, 25 September 1955, Sabin MSS, Box 30, Smith College.

48. Bluemel, *Florence Sabin,* 87; Mendenhall, Manuscript Autobiography, n.p.; and Dr. Esther Richards to Elinor Bluemel, 19 September 1955, Sabin MSS, Box 30, both at Smith College.

49. Bluemel, *Florence Sabin,* 62.

50. See the warm correspondence between Welsh, Sherwood, and Sabin, especially the collection of letters in November 1924, Sabin, MSS, American Philosophical Society; Bluemel, *Florence Sabin,* 65. Also Sabin's remarks about Welsh in *A Tribute to Lilian Welsh* (Baltimore: Goucher College, 1938), 9–17. For Sabin's opinion of women's abilities, Bluemel, *Florence Sabin,* 124.

51. Philadelphia *Evening Bulletin,* 8 November 1869.

52. See Bio. Sketch and Clippings from Syracuse Sunday *Herald,* 23 February 1903, Anna Manning Comfort Papers, Box 12, Syracuse University; Jacobi, "Woman in Medicine," 189–90; S. Penfield to Kate Campbell Hurd-Mead, 13 April 1934 in Lozier file, MCP Archives; and Mendenhall, Manuscript Autobiography, 134–35, Smith College.

53. Jacobi, "Woman in Medicine," 190.

54. In 1932, for example, a study by the AMA noted that 99 out of the 696 hospitals approved for internship by the Council on Medical Education were open to women interns. Kate Campbell Hurd-Mead, *Medical Women of America* (New York: Froben Press, 1933), 50.

55. Emily Dunning Barringer, *Bowery to Bellevue* (New York: W. W. Norton, 1950), 68.

56. Jacobi, "Woman in Medicine," 191; Barringer, *Bowery to Bellevue,* 87–96; Mendenhall, Manuscript Autobiography, 63, Smith College.

57. 12 February 1916, Martha May Eliot MSS. See also Eliot to her parents, 25 January 1917, 13 June 1920, 11 July 1920; and Ernestine Howard to her parents, 4 June 1918 and 27 October 1916; all in Ernestine Howard MSS. Schlesinger Library.

58. Jacobi, "Woman in Medicine," 192; Jacobi to James R. Chadwick, 12 February and 31 May 1979; Anna Broomall to Chadwick, 17 March and 10 Novem-

ber 1879; Mary Thompson to Chadwick, 4 June 1879; all in Chadwick MSS, Countway Library, Harvard Univeresity Medical School.

59. Barringer, *Bowery to Bellevue* 116, 133–34, 175–207. For the more good-natured hazing of Mary Bates, first female intern at Cook County Hospital in Chicago see Bertha Van Hoosen, "Opportunities for Medical Women Interns," *MWJ* 33 (1926): 282, and letter from Bates to Dr. Elizabeth Mason-Hohl, n.d. (after 1900), in AMWA Collection, Box 12, Folder 25, Cornell University. For Van Hoosen's own experience with hazing at Kalamazoo St. Hospital see her autobiography, *Petticoat Surgeon* (Chicago: Pellegrini & Cudahy, 1947), 83, 14–143, 127–28.

60. Mendenhall, Manuscript Autobiography, n.p., Smith College.

61. Charles Rosenberg, "Social Class and Medical Care in Nineteenth Century America: The Rise and Fall of the Dispensary," *Jour. Hist. Med.* 29 (January 1974): 32–54.

62. The number of women reported in the WMCP *Alumnae Transactions* who managed to go to Europe is really quite striking. Also see Hurd-Mead, *Medical Women of America*, 33; Emmeline Cleveland, Anna Broomall, and Frances Emily White folders in the Alumnae File, MCP Archives; for Welsh and Williams see their respective biographies in *Notable American Women;* for Angell, WMCP *Alumnae Transactions,* 1907, p. 25. Also Anna M. Fullerton, "Women Students in Vienna," Philadelphia *Medical Times* 15 (1884–1885): 356; Morton, *A Woman Surgeon,* 105ff.; Lucy Sewall to Caroline Dall, 1 February 1863, Dall MSS, Mass. Historical Society; Susan Dimock to Dr. H. Cabot, 9 October and 17 October 1873, 25 October 1868, 8 February 1869, Box 1, New England Hospital Papers, Smith College.

63. Hurd-Mead, *Medical Women of America,* 34. Alice Bigelow, who interned at the NEH in 1905, had similar things to say about her mentors. Bigelow, "Medical Memoranda," New England Hospital Papers, Box 7, Smith College.

64. Barringer, *Bowery to Bellevue,* 81.

65. Florence Hazzard, "Heart of the Oak," typescript biography of Eliza Mosher in Mosher MSS, Michigan Historical Collections, 4. It is important to note that few men were getting similar obstetrical training during this period.

66. Mary McKibben Harper, "Anna E. Broomall, M.D.," *The Medical Review of Reviews* 39 (March 1933): 132–39, 137. For an example of the pride women physicians took in their surgical accomplishments see Dr. Keller's report on the NEH in WMCP *Alumnae Transactions,* 1892, p. 83. Rachelle Yarros, who worked closely for a number of years with Hull House in Chicago, wrote similarly of Broomall's extraordinary training, which was "one of the greatest assets in my work." Yarros, "From Obstetrics to Social Hygiene," *MWJ* 33 (November 1926): 306.

67. Ritter, *More Than Gold,* 171; Ritter to Hurd-Mead, 9 February 1935, AMWA Collection, Van Hoosen Papers, Uncat., MCP Archives; Charlotte Blake Brown, "Obstetric Practice Among the Chinese in San Francisco," *Pacific Med. and Surg. Jour.* 26 (1883–1884): 15–21; Joan M. Jensen, "Charlotte Blake Brown," in Janet and Edward James, eds., *Notable American Women* (Cambridge: Harvard University Press, 1973), vol. 1, pp. 251–53.

68. Clipping in Chadwick Scrapbook, 20 September 1882, Chadwick MSS, Countway Library, Harvard Medical School.

69. See Anna Wessel Williams's comments about Daniel in her Typescript Auto-

biography, chap. 5, p. 3, in Williams MSS, Schlesinger Library; Josephine Baker, "Annie Sturgis Daniel, M.D., 1858–1944," *MWJ* 51 (September 1944): 34–35; "Editorial," MWJ *Ibid.*, 36; Roy Lubove, "Annie Sturgis Daniel," in Janet and Edward James, eds., *Notable American Women*, vol. 1, pp. 429–30.

70. *Report of Out-Practice* (New York, 1891), 2–3, in N.Y. Academy of Medicine; Belcher to Eliza, 20 January 1878, Belcher Letters, in private hands.

71. Williams, Typescript Autobiography, chap. 5, p. 10. See also Josephine Baker, *Fighting for Life*, 48–49; Alice Hamilton to Agnes, 27 November 1893, Mendenhall, Manuscript Autobiography, 43–45.

72. Daniel, *Report*, 10–11.

73. WMCP *Alumnae Transactions*, 1892, p. 97.

74. *Ibid.*, 82, 97.

75. See Florence Sabin's comments in Sabin, *A Tribute to Lilian Welsh*, 14–17. In 1883 the Woman's Dispensary was founded in Washington, D.C., by Annie Rice and Jeannette Sumner, two graduates of the WMCP.

76. Jacobi, "Woman in Medicine," 189, 176.

77. Italics mine. Editorial in *JAMA* 35 (August 1900): 501, quoted in David Rosner and Gerald Markowitz, "Doctors in Crisis: Medical Education and Medical Reform in the Progressive Era, 1895–1915," *American Quarterly* 25 (March 1973): 83–107.

78. Gulielma Fell Alsop, *History of the Woman's Medical College Philadelphia, Pennsylvania, 1850–1950* (Philadelphia: J.B. Lippincott, 1950), 160–61; WMCP *Alumnae Transactions*, 1907, pp. 46–51, and 1908, pp. 26–27.

79. Letter to Interns, 30 March 1883, Box 27, New England Hospital Papers, Smith College. Virginia Drachman chronicles these clashes in *Hospital With a Heart* (Ithaca: Cornell University Press, 1984), 110–21.

80. Letter of Resignation, 1892, New England Hospital Papers, Smith College.

81. Response to Interns, 30 October 1891, New England Hospital Papers, Smith College.

82. Hurd-Mead, *Medical Women of America*, 34.

83. Mary Hobart, Paper Relating to Work of Young Doctors, 1 November 1895, Box 7, Folder 5, New England Hospital Papers, Smith College.

84. Italics mine. Hamilton to Agnes, 26 October 1893, Hamilton MSS, Schlesinger Library.

85. Hamilton to Agnes, 26 October, 19 November, 5 December 1893, 4 April 1894, Hamilton MSS, Schlesinger Library.

86. *Fighting for Life*, 46.

87. Kleinert to Macfarlane, 10 March 1962; Kleinert Folder, Alumnae File, MCP Archives; Alice Bigelow, "Medical Memoranda," New England Hospital Papers, Smith College.

88. See *The Story of the Children's Hospital*, (San Francisco, 1974); WMCP *Alumnae Transactions*, 1900, p. 120; Ishbel Ross, *The New York Infirmary: A Century of Devoted Service, 1854–1954* (New York, 1954).

89. Clara Marshall, *Valedictory Address*, 13 March 1879 (Philadelphia, 1879), 6–7; Martin Kaufman, "The Admission of Women to 19th-Century Medical Societies," *Bull. Hist. of Med.* 50 (Summer 1976): 251–60. Two good accounts of discrimination are Mary Roth Walsh, "*Doctors Wanted: No Women Need Apply*": *Sexual Barriers in the Medical Profession, 1835–1975* (New

Haven: Yale University Press, 1977), and Gloria Melnick Moldow, "The Gilded Age: Promise and Disillusionment: Women Doctors and the Emergence of the Professional Middle Class, Washington, D.C., 1870–1900" (Ph.D. diss., University of Maryland, 1980).

90. Belcher to Eliza, 9 February 1880, Belcher Letters, in private hands. This low participation may have been more apparent than real. Cora Marrett suggests that in many cities the comparative percentage of female affiliation paralleled that of men. See "On the Evolution of the Women's Medical Societies," *Bull. Hist. of Med.* 53 (Fall 1979): 434–48.

91. WMCP *Alumnae Transactions,* 1900, p. 124.

92. "The women physicians of the West," *Colorado Med. Jour.* 6 (1900): 302; Quoted in Marrett, "Evolution," 439.

93. Mary Stark quoted in Florence Cooksley, "History of Medicine in Monroe County," *N.Y. St. Jour. Med* 37 (1937): 88. Quoted by Marrett, "Evolution," 447.

94. *WMJ* 12 (July 1902): 223.

95. *WMJ* 11 (July 1901): 254, 270.

96. *WMJ* 12 (July 1902): 170–71.

97. Clipping, Philadelphia Ledger, 1938, Reel Folder, Alumnae Files, MCP Archives; Harper, "Anna E. Broomall," 137.

98. Beula Sundell questionnaire, Beula Sundell Folder, Alumnae Files, MCP Archives.

CHAPTER 7

1. "The Influence of Women in the Profession of Medicine," in *Essays in Medical Sociology,* 2 vols. (London: Ernest Bell, 1902, reprint, New York: Arno, 1972), vol. 2, pp. 5–6, 12.

2. *Pathfinders in Medicine* (New York: Medical Life Press, 1929), 673–74.

3. Jacobi to Blackwell, 25 December 1888, Blackwell MSS, Library of Congress.

4. See René Dubos, *Mirage of Health* (New York: Harper & Row, 1959), 117–18.

5. See Barbara Rosenkrantz, *Public Health and the State* (Cambridge: Harvard University Press, 1972), 74–96, 177–85; Charles Rosenberg, *The Cholera Years* (Chicago: University of Chicago Press, 1962), *passim,* and "Florence Nightingale on Contagion: The Hospital as a Moral Universe," in Charles Rosenberg, ed., *Healing and History; Essays for George Rosen* (New York: Neale Watson, 1979), 116–36.

6. For a fascinating view of the effects of Blackwell's family life on her psychology see Margo Horn, "The Effect of Family Life on Women's Role Choices: The Case of the Blackwell Women" (Paper delivered at the Fourth Berkshire Conference on the History of Women, Mount Holyoke College, 23–25 August 1978); *Pioneer Work in Opening the Medical Profession to Women* (London: Longmans, Green, 1895; reprint New York: Schocken, 1977) 27. See also Nancy Sahli, "Elizabeth Blackwell, M.D. (1821–1910): A Biography" (Ph.D. diss., University of Pennsylvania, 1974).

7. *Pioneer Work,* 28.

8. *Pioneer Work,* 35.

9. Lloyd Stevenson, "Science Down the Drain, On the Hostility of Certain Sanitarians to Animal Experimentation, Bacteriology and Immunology," *Bull. Hist. of Med.* 29 (January–February 1955): 1–26; Charles and Carroll Smith-Rosenberg, "Pietism and the Origins of the American Public Health Movement: A Note on John H. Griscom and Robert M. Hartley," *Jour. Hist. Med.* 23 (Spring 1968): 16–35.

10. "The Influence of Women," 26–27.

11. "Why Hygienic Congresses Fail," in *Essays on Medical Sociology*, vol. 2, p. 73.

12. "The Influence of Women," 5–6. See also "The Human Element in Sex," in *Essays in Medical Sociology*, vol. 1, p. 69.

13. "The Influence of Women," 10, 13, 21. Also "Why Hygienic Congresses Fail," *passim*. On antivivisection see Richard D. French, *Antivivisection and Medical Science in Victorian Society* (Princeton: Princeton University Press, 1975); James Turner, *Reckoning with the Beast: Animals, Pain, and Humanity in the Victorian Mind* (Baltimore: Johns Hopkins Press, 1980).

14. "Scientific Method in Biology," in *Essays in Medical Sociology*, vol. 2, pp. 90, 119.

15. 17 August 1869, in *Life and Letters of Mary Putnam Jacobi*, ed. Ruth Putnam (New York: Putnam, 1925), 216.

16. Undated, 1863, *Life and Letters*, 67.

17. 1 February 1867, *Life and Letters*, 110.

18. 11 March 1871, Jacobi MSS, Schlesinger Library.

19. 22 April 1867, 13 January 1870, *Life and Letters*, 125, 233–34.

20. Jacobi to her mother, 22 December 1867, 13 November 1866, *Life and Letters*, 100–101, 157.

21. Dr. Allan Wyeth, quoted in *Life and Letters*, 325.

22. 29 May 1867, *Life and Letters*, 141.

23. Indeed, Dr. Herbert C. Miller in his 1981 Abraham Jacobi lecture to the American Academy of Pediatrics has called Mary Putnam Jacobi the "mother of American pediatrics." See "Intrauterine Growth Retardation: An Unmet Challenge," presented in April 1981, Washington, D.C., reprints available at the Department of Pediatrics, University of Kansas Medical Center.

24. "Shall Women Practice Medicine?" reprinted from *North American Review*, 1881, in The Women's Medical Association of New York City, eds., *Mary Putnam Jacobi, Pathfinder in Medicine* (New York, G.P. Putnam, 1925), 390.

25. Italics mine. Jacobi to Blackwell, 25 December 1888.

26. "Specialism in Medicine," *Arch. Med.* 7 (1882), reprinted in *Mary Putnam Jacobi, Pathfinder in Medicine*, 358; "Inaugural Address at the Opening of the Woman's Medical College of the New York Infirmary, October 1, 1880," *ibid.*, 334; "Annual Address Delivered at the Commencement of the Woman's Medical College of the New York Infirmary, May 30, 1883," *ibid.*, pp. 293; "Shall Women Practice Medicine?" *ibid.*, 373.

27. See Notes, "On the Education of Women Physicians," Blackwell MSS, Library of Congress; "The Influence of Women," 19–20, 27–29, especially where she denounces the "narrow and superficial materialism which prevails so widely amongst scientific men."

28. "Specialism in Medicine," 358; "Shall Women Practice Medicine?" 373; "Commencement Address, 1883," 392.

29. "Female Physicians for Insane Women," *Med. Rec.* 37 (10 May 1890): 543, "Woman in Medicine," in Annie Nathan Meyer, ed., *Woman's Work in America* (New York: Henry Holt, 1891), 177.
30. "Inaugural Address," 1880, pp. 348, 352, 354.
31. "Commencement Address," 1883, pp. 392–93, 397, 400.
32. Jacobi to Blackwell, 25 December 1888; "Commencement Address," 401; "Shall Women Practice Medicine?" 390.
33. Mary Putnam Jacobi, "Social Aspects of the Readmission of Women into the Medical Profession," in *Papers and Letters Presented at the First Woman's Congress of the Association for the Advancement of Women, October, 1873* (New York, 1874), 134; Elizabeth Blackwell, Letter to the Editor of *The Philanthropist*, February 1889, reprint in Blackwell MSS, Schlesinger Library.
34. Jacobi to Mother, 13 January 1870; Blackwell, "The Influence of Women," 5, Jacobi, "Social Aspects," 173.
35. Blackwell to Lady Byron, 5 August 1852, Blackwell MSS, Library of Congress.

CHAPTER 8

1. See Ann Douglas (Wood), " 'The Fashionable Diseases': Women's Complaints and Their Treatment in Nineteenth-Century America," *Jour. of Interdisc. Hist.* 4 (Summer 1973): 25–52; Charles Rosenberg and Carroll Smith-Rosenberg, "The Female Animal: Medical and Biological Views of Woman and Her Role in Nineteenth-Century America," *Journal of American History* 60 (September 1973): 332–56; Carroll Smith-Rosenberg, "The Cycle of Femininity: Puberty and Menopause in 19th-Century America," *Feminist Studies* 1 (Winter 1973): 58–72; Carroll Smith-Rosenberg, "The Hysterical Woman: Sex Roles and Role Conflict in 19th-Century America," *Social Research* 39 (Winter 1972): 652–78; G. J. Barker-Benfield, *The Horrors of the Half-Known Life: Male Attitudes Toward Women and Sexuality in Nineteenth-Century America* (New York: Harper & Row, 1976); and Sarah Stage, *Female Complaints: Lydia Pinkham and the Business of Women's Medicine* (New York: W. W. Norton, 1979), 74–75.
2. For the medicalization of childbirth, see Jane Bauer Donegan, *Women and Men Midwives* (Westport, Conn.: Greenwood Press, 1978); Catherine Scholten, " 'On the Importance of the Obstetrick Art': Changing Customs of Childbirth in America, 1760–1825," *William and Mary Quarterly* 34 (July 1977): 426–45; Richard W. Wertz and Dorothy C. Wertz, *Lying-In: A History of Childbirth in America* (New York: Free Press, 1977). For a more extreme view of doctors' culpability, see Mary Roth Walsh, "*Doctors Wanted: No Women Need Apply*": *Sexual Barriers in the Medical Profession, 1835–1975* (New Haven: Yale University Press, 1977), 76–105; Virginia Drachman, "Women Doctors and the Women's Medical Movement: Feminism and Medicine, 1850–1895" (Ph.D. diss., State University of New York at Buffalo, 1976); and Patricia Branca, *Silent Sisterhood: Middle-Class Women in the Victorian Home* (Pittsburgh: Carnegie Mellon Press, 1975), 62–73; and Laurie Crumpacker, "Female Patients in Four Boston Hospitals of the 1890s" (Paper delivered at the Third Annual Berkshire Conference on the History of Women, October 1974), copy on deposit at the Schlesinger Library, Cam-

bridge, Mass. In some cases historians have merely assumed the accuracy of nineteenth-century statements when critics of male midwifery insisted that women were more willing to "wait on nature." For an example of the contention that men interfered more than women, see Samuel Gregory, *Man-Midwifery Exposed and Corrected* (Boston, 1848), 12–13. Because midwives did not use instruments and rarely administered drugs, contemporaries mistakenly assumed that women physicians would follow suit. Here they underestimated the impact of professional training, a matter about which historians of female professionalism are still in conflict. For the differences in practice between physicians and midwives at parturition see Janet Bogdan, "Care or Cure?: Childbirth Practices in Nineteenth-Century America," *Feminist Studies* 4 (June 1978): 92–99.

3. Douglas (Wood), " 'The Fashionable Diseases,' " 13. See also Drachman, "Women Doctors," 121–26; Walsh, *"Doctors Wanted,"* 76–105; Branca, *Silent Sisterhood,* 62–73; Crumpacker, "Female Patients," *passim.*

4. Charles Rosenberg, "The Bitter Fruit: Heredity, Disease and Social Thought," in Rosenberg, ed., *No Other Gods, On Science and American Social Thought* (Baltimore: Johns Hopkins Press, 1976), 25–53; Richard Hofstadter, *Social Darwinism in American Thought* (1944; reprinted by Beacon Press, New York, 1955).

5. Clarke, *Sex in Education,* (Boston: Osgood and Co., 1874), 133. See also Elizabeth Fee, "The Sexual Politics of Victorian Anthropology," *Feminist Studies* 1 (Winter-Spring 1973): 23–39.

6. All quoted in Charles and Carroll Smith-Rosenberg, "The Female Animal," 56, 57.

7. Although Benfield's portrait of 19th-century male physicians is quite overdrawn, he has asked some interesting questions. See my review of *The Horrors of the Half-Known Life* in *Bull. Hist. of Med.* 51 (Summer 1977): 307–10.

8. In this regard see Mary Ryan, "The Power of Women's Networks: A Case Study of Female Moral Reform in Antebellum America," *Feminist Studies* 5 (Spring 1979): 66–86.

9. H. Tristam Englehardt, Jr., "The Disease of Masturbation: Values and the Concept of Disease," *Bull. Hist. of Med.* 48 (Summer 1974): 234–48.

10. George J. Munroe, "A Case in Practice," *Alabama Medical and Surgical Age* 2 (1889/1890): 213–14.

11. Christopher Lasch, *Haven in a Heartless World, The Family Besieged* (New York: Basic Books, 1977), 17–18; Jacques Donzelot, *The Policing of Families* (New York: Random House, 1979).

12. A look at the case studies published in the Alumnae *Transactions* of the Woman's Medical College of Pennsylvania (hereafter cited as WMCP *Alumnae Transactions*) suggests a patient population almost exclusively female. See also the *Woman's Medical Journal* (*WMJ*), which comments in an article on Sarah C. Hall, a pioneer woman doctor, "Like every other woman in the profession Dr. Hall's practise is largely limited to that of women and children." *WMJ* 4 (February 1895): 236–37. Indeed, many male physicians had cordial relationships with their professional sisters and sent them female patients who either requested a woman doctor or who they themselves determined needed to be under the care of a woman. Eliza Mosher's surgery

professor at Michigan, Dr. Corrydon L. Ford, sent his daughter to live with her for a while to allow Mosher to build up her health. A. J. Skene, the well-known Brooklyn gynecologist, also sent a number of patients to Mosher. See Mosher to sister, 22 May 1887; Frank Rockwell, M.D., to Mosher, 24 April 1889; Mosher to Clelia Mosher, 23 November 1903, "Dr. McCorkle sends me all his young girls and young women." All in Mosher MSS, University of Michigan. See also Anna Manning Comfort, casebooks, Syracuse University; Elizabeth Blackwell MSS Library of Congress, *passim;* Bertha Van Hoosen MSS, University of Michigan, *passim.*

13. Ella Ridgeway, "The Causes of Uterine Diseases" (M.D. thesis, Woman's Medical College of Pennsylvania, 1873). All Woman's Medical College theses may be found in the Medical College of Pennsylvania Archives (MCP), Philadelphia. Anna Longshore-Potts, *Discourses to Women on Medical Subjects* (San Diego, 1897), 122; Rosalie Slaughter Morton, *A Woman Surgeon* (New York: Frederick A. Stokes, 1937), 86; "Phimosis in the Female" *WMJ* 16 (May 1906): 76–77.

14. Sarah Adamson Dolley, *Closing Address* (Philadelphia: Woman's Medical College of Pennsylvania, 1874), 3; Clara Marshall, *Valedictory Address* (Philadelphia: Woman's Medical College of Pennsylvania), 7; Comment about Dimock quoted in speech by Joseph Lowell reprinted in pamphlet "The Opening of Johns Hopkins Medical School of Women," a reprint from *The Century Magazine,* 1891, in box labeled "Physicians, U.S.," Smith College; Morton, *A Woman Surgeon,* vii.

15. *Maryland Medical Journal* 10 (1883): 424.

16. W. S. Brown, M.D., *The Capacity of Women to Practice the Healing Art,* Lecture delivered 9 November 1859, Boston, 1859, p. 8; C. L. Franklin, "Woman and Medicine," *The Nation* 52 (February 1891): 131; Effa Davis, "Obstetric Complications From a Preventive Point of View," *WMJ* 20 (July 1910): 139–45; Elizabeth and Emily Blackwell, *Medicine as a Profession for Women* (New York, 1860), 10–11; Amanda C. Price, "The Necessity for Women Physicians" Thesis, 1871, MCP Archives.

17. Arthur Ames Bliss, *Blockley Days: Memories and Impressions of a Resident Physician, 1883–1884* (Philadelphia: Printed for private circulation, 1813), 14; quoted in Leo James O'Hara "An Emerging Profession, Philadelphia Medicine 1860–1900" (Ph.D. diss., University of Pennsylvania, 1976), 225.

18. Belcher to Eliza Johnson, 23 September 1877, Belcher Letters, in private hands.

19. Elizabeth L. Peck, "Presidential Address," WMCP *Alumnae Transactions,* 1901, p. 42; Lena V. Ingraham, *ibid.,* 1887, p. 43; Sarah R. Munro, *ibid.,* 1884, p. 27; Bertha R. Lewis, *ibid.,* 1895, p. 130.

20. Bigelow, "Medical Memoranda," New England Hospital Papers, Box 7, Smith College; Mary Bates, "Report of the 13th Annual meeting of the Western Surgical & Gynecological Association," *WMJ* 14 (January 1904): 9; Belcher to Eliza Johnson, 22 October 1875, Belcher Letters, in private hands.

21. See S. Weir Mitchell, *Fat and Blood* (Philadelphia: B. Lippincott & Co., 1902); Anna Robeson Burr, ed., *Weir Mitchell: His Life and Letters* (New York: Duffield & Co., 1929). For differing interpretations of Mitchell see Ann Douglas (Wood), " 'The Fashionable Diseases' "; and Regina Markell Morantz, "The Lady and Her Physician," in Lois Banner and Mary Hartman,

eds., *Clio's Consciousness Raised, New Perspectives on the History of Women* (New York: Harper & Row, 1974), 1–22, 38–53. For Jane Addams's experience with Mitchell, which was similarly unhelpful, see Allen F. Davis, *American Heroine, The Life and Legend of Jane Addams* (New York: Oxford University Press, 1973), 27–29.

22. For information on Gilman's breakdown, see her autobiography, *The Living of Charlotte Perkins Gilman* (New York, 1935; reprint, New York: Harper & Row, 1975), 90–106; see also Mary Hill, *Charlotte Perkins Gilman, The Making of a Radical Feminist, 1860–1896* (Philadelphia: Temple University Press, 1980); and Carl Degler, "Charlotte Perkins Gilman," in Janet and Edward James, eds., *Notable American Women* (Cambridge: Harvard University Press, 1971), vol. 2, pp. 39–42. For Gilman's reminiscences about Jacobi see WMCP *Alumnae Transactions,* 1907, p. 66.

23. 21 March 1891, Blackwell MSS, Schlesinger Library.

24. Comfort MSS, Case Book for 1868, pp. 49, 45, 43 (Box 14), Syracuse University. See Clara Swain, "Endometritis" Thesis, 1869 MCP Archives, a typical example. For Jacobi's case see WMCP *Alumnae Transactions,* Philadelphia, 1889, p. 66; Regina Markell Morantz and Sue Zschoche, "Professionalism, Feminism, and Gender Roles: A Comparative Study of Nineteenth-Century Medical Therapeutics," *Journal of American History* 62 (December 1980): 568–88.

25. "The Therapeutic Revolution: Medicine, Meaning and Social Change in Nineteenth Century America," in Charles Rosenberg and Morris Vogel, eds., *The Therapeutic Revolution* (Philadelphia: University of Pennsylvania Press, 1979), 3–26.

26. 27 November 1853, Blackwell MSS, Library of Congress.

27. 21 March 1891, Blackwell MSS, Schlesinger Library.

28. Dolley to Elijah Pennybacker, 3 February 1858, MCP Archives. See flier on lecture to ladies by Ann Preston, MCP Archives; Elizabeth Blackwell, *Pioneer Work in Opening the Medical Profession to Women* (London: Longmans, Green, 1895; reprint, New York: Schocken, 1977), 193–94; Caroline B. Mitchell to Blackwell regarding agenda for her talk to a mothers' meeting, 22 May 1889, Blackwell MSS, Library of Congress; Eliza Mosher to sister, 11 August 1889, Mosher MSS, Michigan Historical Collections; Clelia Mosher MSS, Stanford University, *passim,* and *Health and the Woman Movement,* (New York: YWCA, 1916); Anna Galbraith, *Personal Hygiene and Physical Training for Women* (Philadelphia: W. B. Saunders, 1913); Rose Wood-Allen Chapman, *Dr. Mary Wood-Allen, A Life Sketch* (Chicago: Ruby Gilbert, 1908); Charlotte Blake-Brown, "The Health of Our Girls," *Transactions* of the Medical Society of California 26 (1896): 193–202; Blackwell to Barbara Bodichon, 2, 3, and 4 November 1867, on appointment of "one of our Young infirmary Dr.s. Professor of Hygiene" at Vassar, Blackwell MSS, Columbia University; Alida C. Avery, "On Vassar College," in Anna C. Brackett, ed., *The Education of American Girls* (New York, G. P. Putnam, 1874), 346–61. See also Prudence Saur, *Maternity: A Book for Every Wife and Mother* (Chicago, L. P. Miller, 1889), iii; Anna Longshore-Potts, *Love, Courtship and Marriage* (San Diego: by author, 1891), and *Discourses to Women on Medical Subjects* (San Diego: by author, 1897), x; Rachel Brooks Gleason, *Talks to My Patients, Hints on Getting Well and Keeping Well* (M. L. Holbrook,

London, 1895), vi; Sarah Hackett Stevenson, *Physiology of Women* (Chicago: Fairbanks, Palmer, 1882), 16, 25; and the numerous books and pamphlets by Elizabeth Blackwell.

29. Annie Sturgis Daniel, "A Cautious Experiment: The History of the New York Infirmary for Women and Children and the Woman's Medical College of the New York Infirmary," *MWJ* 47 (July 1940): 301. Also Blackwell in *Pioneer Work,* 277: "An intelligent young coloured physician, Dr. Cole, who was one of our resident assistants, carried on this work with tact and care."

30. "Pioneer Medical Women of Cleveland," *Journal of the American Medical Women's Association* 6 (May 1951): 186–89; Pamphlet by Edna H. Nelson, Superintendant, "The Women and Children's Hospital," reprint from *Hospital Council Bull.,* January 1941, p. 10, Schlesinger Library. See also Lilian Welsh, *Reminiscences,* for a description of the medical social work carried out by the women physicians at the Evening Dispensary for Working Women in Baltimore, chap. 4, pp. 48–61. For the Philadelphia Woman's Hospital see report by Mary Griscom, WMCP *Alumnae Transactions,* 1896, p. 37.

31. "The Opening of Johns Hopkins Medical School to Women," n.p.

32. WMCP *Alumnae Transactions,* 1880, p. 18–19.

32. Anna Fullerton, "Report From the Woman's Hospital of Philadelphia," WMCP *Alumnae Transactions,* 1890, p. 76; Grace Upson, "Report," *ibid.,* 1887, p. 5–157; Carolyn C. Ladd, "Physical Training in its Relation to the Health and Education of Women," *ibid.,* 1890, p. 42; Esther Parker, M.D., "Facts Concerning Physical Conditions of Women During College Life," *WMJ* 22 (August 1912): 171–73.

34. Mosher, "The Aetiology, Prophylaxis and Early Treatment of Pelvic Disorders in Girls and Young Women," *WMJ* 19 (May 1909): 87–91; and Reminiscences, Mosher MSS, Michigan Historical Collections; Whetmore, "The Better Preparation of our Women for Maternity," *WMJ* 12 (September 1902): 205–8. See also Sarah Hackett Stevenson, chapter entitled "The Happiness of True Motherhood," in *Physiology of Woman,* 91; and comments of Helen Putnam and Emma Culbertson after an American Academy of Medicine Symposium, "The Place of Women in the Modern Business World" *Bull. Amer. Acad. of Med.* 9 (October 1908): 379–80.

35. Wood-Allen, *Marriage, Its Duties and Privileges* (Chicago: Fleming H. Revell, 1901), 17, 57, 72. See also Rose Wood-Allen Chapman, *Dr. Mary Wood-Allen, passim;* Davis, "The Determination of Sex at Will," WMCP *Alumnae Transactions,* 1899, p. 149; Childs, "College Women and Motherhood," *WMJ* 23 (February 1913): 40. See also Sophie M. Hartley, M.D., "The Influence of Higher Education Upon Woman with Reference to Her Ability to Propagate the Species," *WMJ* 4 (January 1895): 319–21.

36. Rachel Brooks Gleason, *Talks To My Patients,* 299ff.; Stevenson, "Coeducation of the Sexes," in *Physiology of Women,* 74–75, 160; also Mary Putnam Jacobi, "Menstrual Activity and Physical Health," in Brackett, *The Education of American Girls,* 279.

37. "The Importance of Teaching the Conservation of Nervous Energy to Our Advanced Women Students," *WMJ* 23 (October 1913): 217–20.

38. Margaret Colby, "Presidential Address," *WMJ* 12 (July 1902): 154; "Athletics in Our Schools and Colleges," *WMJ* 20 (September 1910): 181–82; Wood-

Allen, *Marriage,* 117; Anna Manning Comfort, Thesis on Menstruation, n.d. Box 14, Comfort MSS, Syracuse University.

39. "Address to Obstricians," *WMJ* 15 (October 1905): 196–97. Also Prudence Saur, *Maternity,* 156, 170–72; Stevenson, *Physiology of Women,* 21; Wood-Allen, *Marriage,* 135–41.

40. From Clipping on Mosher in Mosher MSS, *New York Times,* n.d., 1925. See *New York Times,* clipping, 1925 and clipping from Brooklyn *Eagle,* 4 June 1915, Mosher MSS, Michigan Historical Collections; T. Bannon, "Modern Motherhood" in *American Journal of Surgery and Gynecology* 12 (1899): 146; Sarah Hall, "The Physical and Moral Effects of Abortion," (1869–1870); Charlotte Whitehead Ross, "Abortion" (1874–1875): Annetta Kratz, "An Essay on Criminal Abortion," (1870–1871), all Theses in MCP Archives; Mary J. Safford Blake, *Prenatal Influence* (Boston, 1878); Saur, *Maternity,* 150; Mary A. Dixon-Jones, "Abortion: Its Evils and Its Sad Consequences," *WMJ* 3 (August 1894): 31.

41. In the nineteenth century those with highly conservative attitudes toward sex favored the spacing of children through abstinence, other women physicians through some variation on the rhythm method. Only when one progresses into the twentieth century do women like Dr. Rachelle Yarros appear, who favor mechanical methods. See Maude Glasgow's critique of the views of the liberal sexologist William J. Robinson, M.D., "Sexual Morality—Another Point of View," in *Med. Rev. of Rev.* 18 (1912): 319–22; Anna Fullerton "The Health of the Woman of the Period," *WMJ* 1 (1893): 2–23, about the evils of sexual excess. Sarah Hackett Stevenson quote, Stevenson, *Physiology of Women,* 91. See also Wood-Allen, *Marriage,* 103–4, 184; Emma Drake, M.D., *What a Young Wife Ought to Know* (Chicago: John C. Winton, 1901), 79–96; On Menopause see Anna Galbraith, "Are the Dangers of the Menopause Natural or Acquired?—A Physiological Study," *American Gynecological and Obstetrical Journal* 15 (October 1899) 291–314; Wood-Allen, *Marriage,* 216; Emma F. Drake, *What Every Woman of Forty-Five Ought to Know* (Philadelphia: Vir Publishing, 1902); Kate Campbell Hurd-Mead, "The Middle-Aged Woman: What Can Be Done To Increase Her Efficiency," WMCP *Alumnae Transactions,* 1913, p. 98–114; Gleason, *Talks to My Patients,* 216–24; Stevenson, *Physiology of Women,* 136–39; Sara E. Greenfield, M.D., "The Dangers of Menopause," *WMJ* 12 (August 1902): 183–85. This list of citations is by no means exhaustive and is a mere sampling.

42. "Woman in Medicine," *WMJ* 3 (July 1894): 15–16.

43. Anna McFarland, "The Relation of Operative Gynecology to Insanity," *WMJ* 2 (February 1894): 40–41; Luther, "Woman's Work in the Care of the Insane," WMCP *Alumnae Transactions,* 1900, p. 38; "Comments on Psychiatry and the Woman Doctor," *ibid.,* 1903, p. 78; Mary Rushmore, "Factors For and Against Gynecological Operations," *WMJ* 21 (May 1911): 957; Flora L. Aldrich, "Another Consideration of Some Criticisms," *WMJ* 2 (May 1894): 106; Mary E. Bates, "Report of the 13th Annual Meeting of the Western Surgical and Gynecological Association," E. M. Roys-Gavitt, "Extraction of the Ovaries for the Cure of Insanity," *WMJ* 1 (1893): 123–24; Mary A. Spink, "The Relation of Female Sexual Organs to Mental Disease," *WMJ* 1 (1893): 59–63; Mary A. Dixon-Jones, "Oophorectomy in Diseases of

the Nervous System," *WMJ* 4 (1895): 1–5, 30–39, and Letter to the Editor
from Eliza Y. Burnside, *ibid.,* 47.

44. McGee comment in Idea Book, 1892, McGee MSS, Library of Congress;
Elizabeth Keller, "A Case of Laparatomy," WMCP *Alumnae Transactions,*
1887, p. 61–65; Mary A. D. Jones, "Seven Cases of Tait's Operation," *ibid.,*
1886, p. 33; Anita Tyng, "A Case of Clitoridectomy" *ibid.,* 1878, p. 25. (This
procedure was performed not for masturbation but for disease of the organ
itself, though in discussing the history of the procedure Tyng makes no criticism of the use of the operation for masturbation and is well aware that such
use has, on occasion, taken place.) Anita Tyng "Case of Removal of Both
Ovaries" ("Battey's Operation"), *ibid.,* 1880, p. 27; Charlotte Blake Brown,
"Ovariotomy," *ibid.,* p. 30. "Tait's" operation included the removal of the
fallopian tubes. See Lawrence D. Longo, "The Rise and Fall of Battey's
Operation: A Fashion in Surgery," *Bull. Hist. of Med.* 53 (Summer 1979):
244–67.

45. Emily Dunning Barringer, *Bowery to Bellevue,* (New York: W. W. Norton,
1950), 217; Morton, *A Woman Surgeon,* 131. See Mary Putnam Jacobi,
"Woman in Medicine," in Annie Nathan Meyer, ed., *Woman's Work in
America* (New York, 1891), 203; Lilian Welsh, *Reminiscences of Thirty Years
in Baltimore* (Baltimore: Norman, Remington, 1925), 42; Anna Fullerton,
"Surgery or Electricity in Gynecology and Pedaetry," *WMJ* 1 (1893): 118–21.
Ironically male physicians were not the only ones to be accused of irresponsi-
bility in surgery. In 1892 Dr. Caroline S. Pease of the Hudson River State
Hospital wrote a letter of inquiry to Clara Marshall, dean of her alma mater,
the Woman's Medical College of Pennsylvania. Pease had been asked to
testify in a libel suit brought against the Brooklyn *Eagle* by Dr. Mary Dixon-
Jones, another alumna of the school. It seems that in 1889 the *Eagle* ran a
long series of articles over the course of several months accusing Dixon-Jones
of irregularities in the organization and financing of a Brooklyn woman's
hospital which she and her son owned and operated as a private institution.
The articles became more and more lurid as the *Eagle* claimed to uncover
gross malpractice, which included misinforming patients of their condition in
order to do unnecessary operations. Dr. Dixon-Jones was finally tried for
manslaughter but was ultimately acquitted. Dr. Pease had been called to
testify on behalf of the *Eagle.* She wrote that "of course," she had a low
opinion of Dixon-Jones, but she hesitated to testify because "the publicity
such women received invariably caused injury to every respectable woman
practitioner." She believed the *Eagle* was sincerely friendly to women physicians and committed to the "larger cause." Although we do not know
whether or not Pease herself testified against Dixon-Jones, other prominent
men and women physicians in Brooklyn did. Though Dixon-Jones did not win
her case, she remained visible in her profession, building her reputation as a
surgeon with the publication of over thirty papers, and the associate editorship for a short while of two medical journals—the *Woman's Medical Journal*
and the *Philadelphia Times and Register.* Because of her achievements in
pathology, Kelly and Burrage saw fit to include her in their classic biographical guide to well-known 19th-century physicians. See Howard A. Kelley and
Walter Burrage, eds., *American Medical Biographies* (Baltimore, 1920), 677;
Caroline S. Pease to Clara Marshall, 18 January 1892; Marshall to Pease, 20

January 1892, Marshall MSS, MCP Archives; Dixon-Jones's story can be followed almost daily from April to June 1889 in the Brooklyn *Eagle* and sporadically thereafter until the denouement, 31 December 1889.

46. Scott to Blackwell, 13 May 1896, Blackwell MSS, Library of Congress; Kelly, "Conservatism in Ovariotomy," *JAMA* 26 (26 February 1896) 249–50; I. N. Love, "Meddlesome Gynecology," published in the *Medical Mirror*, June 1903, reprinted in WMJ 3 (June 1903): 121. See also the following for similar protests from other male physicians: Ely Van De Warker, "The Fetich of the Ovary," *Am. J. of Obs. and the Diseases of Women and Children* 54 (July–December 1906): 366–73; M. Yarnall, "Too Much Surgery," *Texas Health Jour.* 3 (1891): 351–52; I. L. Watkins, "Letter" *Alabama Med. & Surg. Age.* 2 (1888/90): 188–90; William Goodell, "The Abuse of Uterine Treatment Through Mistaken Diagnosis," *Medical News* 55 (December 1889): 621–25; "Symposium on the Therapeutics of Diseases of Women," *Transactions of the Colorado State Medical Society*, 1891–1892, pp. 21–22, 332–48.

47. A. F. A. King, "The Physiological Argument in Obstetric Studies and Practice," *Am. J. of Obs. and Diseases of Women and Children*, 21 (April 1888): 372; Henry T. Byford, "The So-called Physiological Argument in Obstetrics," *ibid.*, 21 (September 1888): 889. See also H. M. Cutts, "The Necessity of Preparatory Treatment for Child-Bed," *ibid.*, 19 (August 1886): 796–801; T. P. White, "The Normal Puerperal State," *ibid.*, 19 (November 1886): 1191–1205; Thomas Opie, "Is the Frequent Use of Forceps Abusive?" *ibid.*, 21 (October 1888), 1088–92.

48. Jane S. Heald, "Obstetrics" 1855; Phoebe Wilson, "Disquisition on Parturition" 1857. Both theses in MCP Archives. For a general overview, see Wertz and Wertz, *Lying-In*.

49. Phoebe Oliver, "Eclampsia" 1869; Katharine D. Perry, "Puerperal Troubles" 1887; Louis Schneider, "Anaesthesia in Natural Labor" 1859; all Theses in MCP Archives.

50. Lucy R. Weaver, "Symptoms of Puerperal Peritonitis" 1879; Mary Jordan Finley, "On Vesico Vaginal Fistula" 1880; See also Margaret Hoeflich, "Eclampsia" 1872–1873; Laura V. Gustin, "A Thesis on Interference in Natural Labor" 1873, all Theses in MCP Archives.

51. Maria E. Zakrzewska, "Report of One Hundred and Eighty-Seven Cases of Midwifery in Private Practice," *Boston Medical and Surgical Journal* 121 (December 1889): 557–60. See also Frances Rutherford, "The Perineum and Its Care during Parturition," WMJ 2 (February 1894): 29–33; Mary Wherry, "The Prevention of Lacerations of the Perineum," *ibid.*, 13 (January 1903): 5–6; Agnes Eichelberger, "Prophylaxis in Obstetrics," *ibid.*, 11 (July 1901): 255–58; Eliza Root, "The Study and Teaching of Obstetrics," *ibid.*, 9 (October 1899): 324–28; Saur, *Maternity*, 218–20; Stevenson, *Physiology of Woman*, 91.

52. Root, "Study and Teaching of Obstetrics," 324–28; Anna E. Broomall, "The Operation of Episiotomy as a Prevention of Perineal Ruptures during Labor," *Am. J. of Obs. and Diseases of Women and Children* 11 (July 1878): 517–27.

53. See Gloria Melnick Moldow, "Promise and Disillusionment: Women Doctors and the Emergence of the Professional Middle Class, 1879–1900" (Ph.D. diss., University of Maryland, 1980), 107.

54. See Wertz and Wertz, *Lying-In*, 150–54, 164–73; and Judith Walzer Leavitt,

"Birthing and Anesthesia: The Debate over Twilight Sleep," *Signs* 6 (Autumn 1980): 147–64.

55. In 1980 I published a longer version of the study to follow. I have uncovered no new evidence to contradict those conclusions. Four years ago I made the point that gender had only a very slight effect on the choice of therapy, but a palpable effect on the experience of the patient. Since that conclusion has been misinterpreted by some readers I wish to reiterate it now; indeed, I would emphasize it even more strongly. See Morantz and Zschoche, "Professionalism, Feminism, and Gender Roles," 584.

56. Case records are available only after 1887 for Boston Lying-In Hospital. Please refer to Appendix for a detailed explanation of the methodology used for these hospital studies.

57. Charles E. Rosenberg, "And Heal the Sick: The Hospital and the Patient in 19th-Century America," *Journal of Social History* 10 (June 1977): 428–47.

58. Emma L. Call, "The Evolution of Modern Maternity Technic," *Am. J. of Obs. and Diseases of Women and Children* 58 (September 1908): 392–404. For an explicit statement of Marie Zakrzewska's philosophy concerning the hospital's admission practices, see her comments in New England Hospital, Annual Report, 1868, pp. 9–21, New England Hospital Papers, Smith College. Virtually every New England Hospital annual report contains rather self-conscious testimony concerning the advantages of the hospital's Christian atmosphere. For example, see New England Hospital, Annual Report, 1873, pp. 5–7; *ibid.*, 1880, pp. 5–9. See also Grace E. Rochford, "The New England Hospital for Women and Children," *JAMWA* 5 (December 1950): 497–99; *Memoir of Susan Dimock* (Boston, 1875), 37–39.

59. See Boston Lying-In Hospital inpatient and outpatient records and New England Hospital Obstetrical Records, Countway Library, Harvard Medical School.

60. See Appendix for an explanation of how this information was determined.

61. See Walsh, *"Doctors Wanted,"* 93–95; Branca, *Silent Sisterhood*, 86–90; and Crumpacker, "Female Patients."

62. The choice of statistical methods was dictated to some degree by the relative paucity of data on the Boston Lying-In case records. Direct comparisons between hospitals were limited to tests for significant differences in the frequency of occurrence for which chi square tests of independence were used. For analyses of data within each hospital, a variety of methods was used in all instances where a significant difference is either claimed or rejected, a probability level of .05 was the minimum level accepted. See Appendix.

63. Crumpacker, "Female Patients."

64. Morantz and Zschoche, "Professionalism, Feminism, and Gender Roles," 481–83.

CHAPTER 9

1. "Can Men and Women Doctors Be a Help to Each Other?" *Woman's Medical Journal* 15 (February 1905): 30–32; U.S. Department of the Interior, *Report of the Commissioner of Education*, 1889–1890, 1895–1896, 1898–1899, 1903 (Washington, D.C.: U.S. Government Printing Office); *Alumnae Cata-*

logue of the University of Michigan, 1837–1921 (Ann Arbor: University of Michigan Press, 1923).

2. The notorious exceptions were the Massachusetts Medical Society and the Montgomery County Medical Society in Pennsylvania, both of which put up dramatic rear-guard actions, only to succumb in the 1880s. See Mary Roth Walsh. *"Doctors Wanted: No Women Need Apply": Sexual Barriers in the Medical Profession 1835–1975* (New Haven: Yale University Press, 1977), 159–65; and Mary Putnam Jacobi, "Woman in Medicine," in Annie Nathan Meyer, ed., *Woman's Work in America* (New York, 1891), 205.

3. Jacobi, "Woman in Medicine," 202–4; Clara Marshall, *The Woman's Medical College of Pennsylvania: An Historical Outline* (Philadelphia, 1897), 89–142 has a list of publications. Also the *Woman's Medical Journal* published a monthly bibliography after 1911. See *WMJ* 21 (January 1911): 8.

4. *WMJ* 18 (April 1908): 86.

5. Cora B. Marrett, "On the Evolution of Women's Medical Societies," *Bull. Hist. of Med.* 53 (Fall 1979): 434–38. Also *Transactions* of the Alumnae Association of the Woman's Medical College of Pennsylvania (hereafter cited as WMCP *Alumnae Transactions*), Philadelphia, 1875–1921, *passim.*

6. The association was originally titled the Medical Women's National Association. See Regina Markell Morantz, "Bertha Van Hoosen," in *Notable American Women: The Modern Period,* ed. Barbara Sicherman and Carol Hurd Green (Cambridge, Mass.: Harvard University Press, 1980), 706–7. For news of other women's medical societies see *WMJ* 18 (April 1908): 63 and *WMJ, passim,* 1900–1920.

7. Walsh, *"Doctors Wanted,"* 178–267; "Medical Education Numbers," *JAMA,* 1910–1930; William Chafe, *The American Woman* (New York: Oxford University Press, 1972), 89–112; Barbara Harris, *Beyond Her Sphere, Woman and the Professions in American History* (Westport, Conn.: Greenwood Press, 1978), 95–126.

8. Charles Rosenberg, "The Therapeutic Revolution: Medicine, Meaning and Social Change in Nineteenth-Century America," in Morris J. Vogel and Charles Rosenberg, eds., *The Therapeutic Revolution: Essays in the Social History of American Medicine,* 18.

9. See Edmund D. Pellegrino, "The Sociocultural Impact of Twentieth-Century Therapeutics," in Rosenberg and Vogel, eds., *The Therapeutic Revolution,* 245–66; Richard Shryock, *Medicine and Society in America, 1660–1860* (Ithaca: Cornell University Press, 1960), 117–66; William G. Rothstein, *American Physicians in the Nineteenth Century* (Baltimore: Johns Hopkins University Press, 1972), 261–81; Rosemary Stevens, *American Medicine and the Public Interest* (New Haven: Yale University Press, 1971), 38–39.

10. Stevens, *American Medicine,* 39.

11. Quoted in Donald Fleming, *William Welch and the Rise of Modern Medicine* (Boston: Little, Brown, 1954), 104.

12. Both physicians's comments quoted in Rosenberg, "The Therapeutic Revolution," 20. See also Gerald Geison, "Divided We Stand: Physiologists and Clinicians in the American Context," and Russ Maulitz, "Physician versus Bacteriologist": The Ideology of Science in Clinical Medicine," both in Rosenberg and Vogel, eds., *The Therapeutic Revolution.*

13. Fleming, *William Welch,* 104–5; Maulitz, "Physician versus Bacteriologist,"

91–98; Robert E. Kohler, "Medical Reform and Biomedical Science: Biochemistry—A Case Study," in Rosenberg and Vogel, eds., *The Therapeutic Revolution,* 27–35.

14. See Morris Vogel, *The Invention of the Modern Hospital: Boston, 1870–1930* (Chicago: University of Chicago Press, 1980); and "The Transformation of the American Hospital, 1850–1920," in Susan Reverby and David Rosner, eds., *Health Care in America* (Philadelphia: Temple University Press, 1979), 105–16; David Rosner, *A Once Charitable Enterprise, Hospitals & Health Care in Brooklyn & New York, 1885–1915* (New York: Cambridge University Press), 1982.

15. "The Human in Medicine, Surgery and Nursing," *MWJ* 32 (May 1925): 117–19. See also Emily Dunning Barringer, *Bowery to Bellevue: The Story of New York's First Woman Ambulance Surgeon* (New York: W. W. Norton, 1950), 244; and Josephine Baker, *Fighting for Life* (New York: Macmillan, 1939), 248, for other responses similar to Mosher's.

16. Elizabeth Peck, M.D., "Presidential Address," WMCP *Alumnae Transactions,* 1901, p. 42ff.; Harding to Van Hoosen, 6 May 1936, Van Hoosen MSS, Medical College of Pennsylvania Archives (MCP); Baker, *Fighting for Life,* 248; Barringer, *Bowery to Bellevue,* 244.

17. Robert Wiebe, *The Search for Order, 1877–1920* (New York: Hill and Wang, 1967), 295. See also Samuel P. Hays, "Political Parties and the Community-Society Continuum," in William N. Chambers and Walter D. Burnham, eds., *The American Party Systems* (New York: Oxford University Press, 1967); and Rowland Berthoff, "The American Social Order, A Conservative Hypothesis," *American Historical Review* 65 (April 1960): 495–514.

18. Wiebe, *Search for Order* 113–16; See also Burton Bledstein, *The Culture of Professionalism* (New York: W. W. Norton, 1976), *passim;* E. Richard Brown, *Rockefeller Medicine Men* (Berkeley: University of California Press, 1979); Paul Starr, *The Social Transformation of American Medicine* (New York: Basic Books, 1982); Robert E. Kohler, "Medical Reform," 27–66.

19. *JAMA* 37 (September 1901): 145–46; Also Kohler, "Medical Reform," 34.

20. Kohler, "Medical Reform," 34; Maulitz, "Physician versus Bacteriologist," *passim.*

21. Stevens, *American Medicine and the Public Interest,* 58–59, 69; Kohler, "Medical Reform," 30–31.

22. Editorial in *JAMA* 35 (August 1900): 501, quoted in David Rosner and Gerald Markowitz, "Doctors in Crisis: Medical Education and Medical Reform During the Progressive Era, 1895–1915," *American Quarterly* 25 (March 1973): 83–107.

23. Stevens, *American Medicine and the Public Interest,* 68; Robert Hudson, "Abraham Flexner in Perspective: American Medical Education, 1865–1910," *Bull. Hist. of Med.* 56 (November–December 1972), 545–61.

24. Report of the Dean of the Woman's Medical College, Northwestern University, President's Report, 1897–1898, 41, Northwestern University Archives (NU).

25. See Address delivered by Dr. Emily Blackwell at the 31st Annual Commencement, 25 May 1899, Woman's Medical College of the New York Infirmary, *Final Catalogue,* June 1899, p. 9–19.

26. See Blackwell's Address, *Final Catalogue,* and also her remarks in the

WMCP Alumnae *Transactions,* 1899, p. 76–80. Also Clara Marshall, "Our Point of View," *Bulletin of the Woman's Medical College of Pennsylvania* 66 (December 1915): 12.

27. *Twenty-third Annual Announcement of the Northwestern University Woman's Medical School, 1891–92,* (Chicago: 1892), 5.

28. *Northwestern University, A History, 1855–1905* (New York: 1905), 381; President's Report, 1891–1892, Frank B. Crandon Papers, 23, NU Archives.

29. *Ibid.,* 24.

30. See Report of the Dean of the Women's Medical School in the President's Report, 1895–1896, p. 33; 1897–1898, p. 41, NU Archives.

31. President's Report for 1899–1900, 1900–1901; Board of Trustees Minutes, 1900, 1901, 1902 NU Archives; Leslie B. Arey, *Northwestern University Medical School, 1859–1959* (Evanston: Northwestern University, 1951), 118–22.

32. Erlanger Report and these replies are found in the Joseph Erlanger MSS, Washington University Medical School, St. Louis.

33. 29 December 1917, Erlanger MSS.

34. W.S. Carter to Erlanger, 26 December 1917, Erlanger MSS.

35. Both letters dated 28 December 1917, Erlanger MSS.

36. 25 December 1917.

37. 5 January 1918. See also letters from Union, 26 December 1917, and Marquette, 27 December 1917.

38. 27 December 1917; 3 January 1918.

39. 27 December 1917.

40. 26 December 1917.

41. Harvard finally admitted women in 1946, Jefferson in 1961. Columbia, Yale, and Pennsylvania had opened their doors in 1918.

42. WMCP *Alumnae Transactions,* 1917, p. 78; Clara Raven, M.D., "Bertha Van Hoosen," *Journal of the American Medical Women's Association* (*JAMWA*) 18 (July 1963): 239.

43. Purnell's comments in WMCP *Alumnae Transactions,* 1918, p. 52–53; Welsh's comments in WMCP *Alumnae Transactions,* 1912, p. 22.

44. Gulielma Fell Alsop, *A History of the Woman's Medical College* (Philadelphia: J.B. Lippincott, 1950), 155–63.

45. See "Material Received from Mr. Hay," Folders 13 and 14, which contain letters regarding this matter, MCP Archives.

46. Undated Report, Hay Box, Folder 13, MCP Archives.

47. *Ibid.*

48. "Statement of the Woman's Medical College of Pennsylvania On Support of its Application for State Aid," 1904, Martha Tracy MSS, Folder 14, MCP Archives.

49. Morris to Frances Daskam, 20 October 1960, Morris Folder, Alumnae Files, MCP Archives.

50. Abraham Flexner, *Medical Education in the United States and Canada* (New York: The Carnegie Foundation, 1910), 296.

51. WMCP *Alumnae Transactions,* 1911, p. 35–36.

52. Colwell to Dr. Annie Bosworth, Secretary to the Dean, in Clara Marshall MSS, MCP Archives; and WMCP *Alumnae Transactions,* 1913, p. 134ff.

53. 14 February 1913. See also letters dated 28 January 1913, 16 January, 18 March, 28 March, 18 July 1914, and 30 June 1916 in Clara Marshall MSS, MCP Archives.

54. See Alsop, *Woman's Medical College,* 173, WMCP *Alumnae Transactions,* 1917, p. 77; *ibid.,* p. 132.

55. Alsop, *Woman's Medical College,* 225–29. Also the American Medical Women's Association Minutes, 15–17 May 1927, p. 45–48, AMWA Collection, Cornell University.

56. See Estelle Freedman, "Separatism as Strategy: Female Institution Building and American Feminism, 1870–1930," *Feminist Studies* 5 (Fall 1979): 512–29, for an important and suggestive beginning.

57. This description of modern therapeutics relies on Edmund D. Pellegrino, M.D., "From the Rational to the Radical: The Sociocultural Impact of Modern Therapeutics," in Vogel and Rosenberg, eds., *The Therapeutic Revolution,* 253–56; and George L. Engel, "The Need for a New Medical Model: A Challenge for Medicine," *Science* 196 (April 1977): 129–35.

58. Elizabeth Gregg, "The Tuberculosis Nurse under Municipal Direction," *Public Health Nursing Quarterly* 5 (October 1913): 16. I am indebted to Dr. Barbara Bates for this citation.

59. Rosner and Markowitz, "Doctors in Crisis," 89.

60. Statistics on the numbers of women graduate students are taken from the *Records of the Commissioner of Education,* 1894–1895, 1910, 1915, 1918 (Washington, D.C.: Government Printing Office). Statistics on women welfare workers, "physicians and surgeons attendants," and "keepers of charitable and penal institutions" are taken from U.S. Bureau of Census, *U.S. Census of Population* (Washington, D.C.; U.S. Government Printing Office, 1900, 1910, 1920). See also Lois Scharf, *To Work and to Wed* (Westport, Conn.: Greenwood Press, 1980), 5–6.

61. Barbara Harris, *Beyond Her Sphere, Women and the Professions in American History,* (Westport, Conn.: Greenwood Press, 1978), 101.

62. Henry F. May, *The End of American Innocence* (New York: Knopf, 1959); William L. O'Neill, *Divorce in the Progressive Era* (New Haven, Conn.: Yale University Press, 1967); James R. McGovern, "The American Woman's Pre-World War I Freedom in Manners and Morals," *Journal of American History* 55 (September 1968): 315–33; Regina Markell Morantz, "The Scientist as Sex Crusader: Alfred Kinsey and American Culture," *American Quarterly* 29 (Winter 1977): 563–89; Sheila M. Rothman, *Women's Proper Place* (New York: Basic Books, 1978); and John Burnham, "The Progressive Era Revolution in Attitudes Toward Sex," *Journal of American History* 59 (March 1973): 885–908.

63. Harris, *Beyond Her Sphere,* 134.

64. Joyce Antler, "Feminism as Life Process: The Life and Career of Lucy Sprague Mitchell," *Feminist Studies* 7 (Spring 1981): 134–57.

65. The Council on Medical Education introduced their rating system in 1910.

66. Moses to Elinor Bleumel, 6 September 1955, Sabin MSS, Box 30, Smith College.

CHAPTER 10

1. *Woman's Medical Journal (WMJ)* 25 (December 1915): 279–80.

2. See Editorial in *WMJ* 18 (April 1898): 45; and Margaret E. Colby's presidential address to the Iowa Society of Medical Women, *WMJ* 12 (July 1902): 153–55.

3. "Medical Women and Hospital Appointments," *WMJ* 11 (August 1901): 307; "Women Physicians in Public Institutions, *WMJ* 18 (April 1908): 70; "Our Denver Letter," *WMJ* 19 (March 1909): 60–61; "Hospital Opportunities for Women" *WMJ* 20 (January 1910): 17; "Medical Women—In History and In Present Day Practice," *WMJ* 27 (April 1917): 86; Ruth W. Lathrop, "Women Physicians as Teachers," *WMJ* 18 (April 1908): 70–72; Announcements of the admission of women to Yale and Columbia, *WMJ* 26 (August 1916): 203; and *WMJ* 25 (March 1916): 70. These are a mere sampling of many articles devoted to these topics.

4. Bertha Van Hoosen, "Looking Backward," *Journal of the American Medical Women's Association* 5 (October 1950): 406–8.

5. Potter to Mrs. F. Daskam, 1 June 1950, Medical College of Pennsylvania Archives, (MCP); "The Medical Woman as Teacher in Medical Schools," *WMJ* 11 (September 1910): 325–30.

6. "Medical Opportunties for Women," *MWJ* 34 (June 1927): 173–74. The *Woman's Medical Journal* changed its name to the *Medical Woman's Journal* (*MWJ*) in 1922.

7. WMCP *Alumnae Transactions,* 1912, p. 43.

8. *Ibid.,* 44.

9. *Ibid.,* 43.

10. *Ibid.,* 77.

11. *Ibid.,* 79.

12. See the comparative study including charts and statistics published in the *Bulletin of the Woman's Medical College of Pennsylvania* 65 (March 1915): 19–21; "The Field for Women of Today in Medicine," *WMJ* 26 (February 1916): 41–44. For the publicity campaign at the Woman's Medical College see the *Bulletin of the Woman's Medical College of Pennsylvania* 66 (December 1915), and 71 (March 1921), *passim;* and the pamphlet *Natural Guardians of the Race,* 1926, published by the college. Also *Bulletin of the Woman's Medical College of Pennsylvania* 65 (June 1914), *passim;* and Ellen C. Potter's article "The Choice of a Vocation," 17–72. Also Lida Stewart-Cogill, "Deficiencies in Follow-up Methods for Mothers' Health," WMCP *Alumnae Transactions,* 1920, p. 17.

13. See for example the letters of support during the 1915–1916 endowment campaign from the Philadelphia *Evening Bulletin;* President Woodrow Wilson, William A. Welch, M.D., of Johns Hopkins; Rudolph Blankenburg, Mayor of Philadelphia; and N. P. Colwell, Secretary of the AMA Council on Medical Education, who wrote that the college was conducted with "high ideals" and that money given to continue its existence would be a "splendid investment" to "aid in the training of more thoroughly qualified women physicians, who have a distinct place in the social needs of the American people." *Bulletin of the Woman's Medical College of Pennsylvania,* 66 (March 1916): 11, and 66 (December 1916): 14–15.

14. "Suggestions as the Future Policy of the Journal," *WMJ* 19 (January 1910): 10–11; *WMJ* 20 (February 1910): 34; "Segregation" *WMJ* 21 (May 1911): 104; Luella E. Astell, M.D., "Opportunity," *WMJ* 23 (November 1913): 241–43.

15. WMCP *Alumnae Transactions,* 1892, p. 126.

16. *WMJ* 18 (April 1898): 45.

17. See Minutes of this meeting, November 1915, in American Medical Women's

Association, AMWA MSS, Box 1, Folder 3, Cornell University; see also Bertha Van Hoosen, *Petticoat Surgeon* (Chicago: Pelligrini & Cudahy, 1947), 200–215.

18. *WMJ* 26 (May 1916): 132; *WMJ* 26 (April 1916): 97–98; *WMJ* 26 (June 1916): 159; *WMJ* 27 (January 1917): 245.

19. For the position of female physicians in the profession in California see *Bulletin of the Medical Women's National Association*, July 1925, p. 19; Van Hoosen, *Petticoat Surgeon*, 203. See the brief history of the American Women's Hospitals by Nancy Hewitt in *Collections, The Newsletter of the Archives and Special Collections on Women in Medicine*, published by the Medical College of Pennsylvania, June 1982. The *Woman's Medical Journal* published periodic reports on the accomplishments of American Women's Hospitals from 1918 on.

20. See Minutes of the Board of Directors of the Medical Women's National Association, June 1924, AMWA Collection, Cornell University; Hamilton to Mary O'Malley, M.D., 27 September 1922, in National Women's Party MSS, Reel 17, Schlesinger Library. Finally Hamilton to Ann Reed Bremner of the *Survey*, 10 February 1938, in American Social Hygiene Association Archives, University of Minnesota.

21. Emily Bacon to Elinor Bleumel, 21 September 1955, Sabin MSS, Box 30, Smith College; Macfarlane to Sabin, 18 September 1936; Sabin to Macfarlane, 22 September 1936; Macfarlane to Sabin, 28 September 1936; Sabin to Macfarlane, 9 October 1936; Sabin to Mead, 9 September 1935; Sabin to Van Hoosen, 1 April 1933; Van Hoosen to Sabin, 9 January 1933, 23 August 1922, 25 April 1933, all in Sabin MSS, American Philosophical Society.

22. Walker to Van Hoosen, 6 February 1940, Van Hoosen MSS, Medical College of Pennsylvania Archives (MCP).

23. See the minutes of the Medical Women's National Association meeting for 26 June 1923, p. 15, AMWA Collection, Cornell University; Rosemary Shoemaker to Bertha Van Hoosen, 7 July 1939; Jane Sands Robb to Van Hoosen, 5 July 1935, in Van Hoosen MSS, MCP Archives. For male membership in the AMA see James G. Burrow, *AMA: Voice of American Medicine* (Baltimore: Johns Hopkins, 1963), 49–51.

24. Carol Lopate, *Women in Medicine* (Baltimore: Johns Hopkins University Press, 1968), 17.

25. *Bulletin of the Medical Women's National Association*, April 1926, p. 10.

26. *WMJ* 21 (May 1911): 105–15; Presidential Address of Eleanor C. Jones, published in *WMJ* 23 (July 1913): 159; Marion C. Potter, "Legal Medicine," *WMJ* 24 (June 1914): 114–15; Minutes of the Medical Women's National Association meeting, June 1921, especially Report of Dr. Elizabeth Bass, p. 7, AMWA Collection, Cornell University.

27. See Paul Boyer, *Urban Masses and Moral Order in America, 1820–1920* (Cambridge: Harvard University Press, 1978), especially 189–90; Robert Wiebe, *The Search for Order* (New York: Hill and Wang, 1967); and John Burnham's excellent essay in John Burnham, John D. Buenker, and Robert M. Crunden, eds., *Progressivism* (Cambridge: Schenkman Publishing Company, 1977) 3–29; quotation cited by Burnham, *Progressivism*, 6.

28. Wiebe, *Search for Order*, 169, 174; Burnham, *Progressivism*, 18–20.

29. *WMJ* 20 (August 1910): 161–64. See also Luella E. Axtell, "Presidential Ad-

dress" to Wisconsin Medical Women's Society, *WMJ* 23 (November 1913): 241–43: "The Medical Woman is a close point of contact between science and humanitarianism. Her social instincts make her a peculiarly fit tool in the fashioning of a better social order, especially in the work touching home and child life."

30. For an excellent discussion of this transition, see Barbara Rosenkrantz, "Cart Before Horse: Theory, Practice and Professional Image in American Public Health, 1810–1920," *Jour. Hist. Med* 29 (Spring 1975): 55–73.

31. For Woman's Medical College of Pennsylvania alumnae association meetings see the *Alumnae Transactions,* 1890–1920, *passim;* Miriam Bitting-Kennedy "Gonorrhoea in Women," and Caroline Purnell, "Gonorrhoea as an Etiological Factor in Pelvic Inflammation," where Purnell observed, "Just as long as physicians teach men that social conditions require or make it necessary for them to have extra-marital intercourse, and suggest methods of protection to themselves so that they can have impure intercourse, just so long will women continue to suffer from this dread disease." Both in WMCP *Alumnae Transactions,* 1898, p. 49–56; Bertha C. Downing, "The Child—Some of His Needs Which the Medical Profession Are Neglecting," *ibid.,* 1907, p. 97ff.; Jane Kimmel Garver, "A Study in Heredity," *ibid.,* 1892, p. 62ff; Frances Van Gasken, "Tenement Houses in Philadelphia," *ibid.,* 1895, p. 112; Frieda E. Lippert, "Possibilities of Medical Charity," *ibid.,* 1894, pp. 70–77; Lena Ingraham, "Preventive Medicine," *ibid.,* 1887, p. 44; Ella L. Dester, "On the Desirability of Examination of the Eyes of All School-Children," *ibid.,* 1892, p. 156. See, for example, articles on Chicago's sewage problem (a cause of typhoid), protestations against quackery, information on an outbreak of bubonic plague in San Francisco, and a report on the international prostitution problem in the *WMJ* 13 (January 1903). See also Josephine L. Peavey, M.D., "Criminal Abortion," *WMJ* 9 (June 1899): 209–16; Helen C. Putnam, "Against the Spirocheta Pallida and Diplococcus of Neisser," *WMJ* 19 (January 1909): 1–24; Evangeline W. Young, "The Conservation of Manhood and Womanhood," *WMJ* 20 (March 1910): 51–52; "Means for Securing Sex Hygiene," *WMJ* 23 (January 1913): 13; "The Tuberculosis Congress," *WMJ* 11 (August 1901): 303; Sophia Hinze Scott, "Prevention of Infant Mortality," *WMJ* 21 (July 1911): 141–44; Isabelle Thompson Smart, "Relation of Women in Industry to Child Welfare," *WMJ* 21 (March 1911): 45–49; Helen C. Putnam, "Resume of an Address Given on Efficient Teaching of Hygiene and Morals in the Public Schools," *WMJ* 19 (May 1909): 101; Emily Wright, M.D., "Duty of the Employer to Employee as Regards Recreation: Duty to the Poor," *WMJ* 16 May 1906): 69–70; "Health of Pottery Workers," "Child Labor Law in Illinois," "A Woman Health Officer," *WMJ* 13 (May 1903): 93–94; "Child Labor," *WMJ* (April 1903): 71–72; "The Need for Sex Hygiene," *WMJ* 22 (December 1912): 288; "The Ballot for Women a Great Factor in Social Reform," *WMJ* (December 1912) 289. See also Louise Fiske Bryson, M.D., "Women Physicians and Public Health," in *Woman's Cycle* 1 (9 January 1890): 3; "What Shall We Do with the Poor," *Woman's Cycle* 1 13 June 1890, p. 3–4, and "Disciplining the Machine," *ibid.,* 2 (24 July 1890): 3–4. See also Alice Hamilton, M.D., "Occupational Conditions of Tuberculosis," *The Charities & The Commons* 16 (5 May 1906): 205–7, and "The Social Settlement and Public Health, *ibid.,* 17 (9 March 1907): 1037–1040. These citations are merely for example and do not

cover in any thorough manner the vast number of articles written and published by women physicians on these various topics. For the medical profession's response to social reform see Lloyd C. Taylor, *The Medical Profession and Social Reform, 1885–1945* (New York: St. Martin's Press, 1974); James G. Burrow, *Organized Medicine in the Progressive Era* (Baltimore: Johns Hopkins University Press, 1977); Paul Starr, *The Social Transformation of American Medicine* (New York: Basic Books, 1982), 180–98, 235–89.

32. *WMJ* 15 (April 1905): 83; Morton, *A Woman Surgeon* (New York: Frederick A. Stokes, 1937), 165.

33. Morris Fishbein, *A History of the American Medical Association* (Philadelphia, 1947), 999.

34. Morton, *A Woman Surgeon,* 166–67.

35. Yarros's comments can be found in the WMCP *Alumnae Transactions,* 1913, p. 111.

36. Morton, *A Woman Surgeon,* 166–69. Also reports in the *WMJ* 11 (February 1911): 33–36; *WMJ* 6 (July 1906): 16; *WMJ* 12 (July 1912): 158–61; Rosalie Slaughter Morton, "Woman's Place in the Public Health Movement," read before the AMA Section on Preventive Medicine and Public Health," June 1911; *WMJ* 12 (May 1912): 99–102; and *WMJ* 12 (April 1912): 83–87; and Kate Campbell Hurd-Mead, "The Duty of Medical Women for Public Health Education," *WMJ* 14 (May 1914): 89–92. See also report on the formation of the committee from the New York *Herald Tribune,* 10 April 1910.

37. See for example, "Women's Clubs and Sanitary Science," *WMJ* 11 (June 1901); and "Women's Clubs and Sanitary Effort," *WMJ* 11 (July 1901): 229–93.

38. See the editorial on the importance of good housekeeping, "Housekeeping a Neglected Science and Art," *WMJ* 13 (March 1903): 51–52; and Marguerite W. Moir, "Preventive Medicine and Euthenics," *WMJ* 34 (January 1927): 7–9.

39. See the program for the lecture series at the Academy in Emma Walker MSS, Smith College; flier for Brooklyn lecture series in Clelia Mosher MSS, Stanford. Also the letter to Clelia from Eliza Mosher, 13 December 1909, in which Eliza writes, "We are all busy with our hygiene teaching under the direction of the AMA." Mosher MSS, Stanford University. See also *WMJ* 11 (January 1911): 9.

40. Annual Report of the State Chairwoman of Health of the California Federation of Women's Clubs, n.d., in Anita Newcomb McGee MSS, Library of Congress; see also Report of Dr. Belle Wood-Comstock, president of the Woman's Medical Society of Los Angeles, in the *Bulletin of the Medical Women's National Association,* July 1926, pp. 30–31.

41. Morton, *A Woman's Surgeon,* 174–75.

42. Fishbein, *A History of the American Medical Association,* 273.

43. Morton, *A Woman Surgeon,* 169; Sadler, Report of the Chairman of Public Health, June 1929, minutes of the Medical Women's National Association 1929 meeting, AMWA Collection, Cornell University.

44. See *Bulletin of the Woman's Medical College of Pennsylvania* 66 (December 1915): 24–25; *ibid.,* (March 1916): 20, and pamphlet, *Medical Women in Health Education,* n.d., but probably 1918, in MCP Archives.

45. Minutes of the Medical Women's National Association Meeting, 26 June 1923, pp. 24ff., AMWA Collection, Cornell University.

46. See MWNA Minutes, 1922, p. 5; 1923, 1925, *passim.* See also the program of the International Conference of Women Physicians, 17–24 October 1919, organized by the Social Morality Committee and the War Work Council of the YWCA (in the MCP Archives); Morton, *A Woman Surgeon,* 157; Reports of the Committee on Public Health, *Bulletin of the MWNA,* July 1925, p. 15–16; October 1925, pp. 14, 15–17; July 1926, pp. 20–21, 30–32; October 1926, pp. 17, 21.

47. *WMJ* 20 (February 1910): 44.

48. Barringer, *Bowery to Bellevue* (New York: W. W. Norton, 1950), 233.

49. *WMJ* 20 (February 1910): 37ff.

50. See Putnam, "Against the Spirocheta Pallida and Diplococcus of Neisser," *WMJ* 19 (January 1909): 1–14; "The Teaching of Hygiene in America," *WMJ* (June 1909): 11–14, and "Biologists in Public Schools, An Aid to Morals and Prosperity," *WMJ* 17 (May 1907): 273–78; also Editorial, "The Need for Sex Hygiene," *WMJ* 22 (December 1912): 288; "Means for Securing Sex Hygiene," *WMJ* 23 (January 1913): 13. For information on Putnam's career see the obituaries and other materials in her alumna file, MCP Archives.

51. WMCP *Alumnae Transactions,* 1920, p. 59.

52. See pamphlet *Medical Women in Health Education,* n.p., n.d. (but probably 1918), published by the Woman's Medical College, MCP Archives. For an extensive analysis of antivenereal disease campaigns during this period see Allan Brandt, *No Magic Bullet: A Social History of Venereal Disease in the United States Since 1880* (New York: Oxford University Press, 1985).

53. "The Social Causes of Criminal Abortion," *WMJ* 14 (October 1904): 221–25; Rosalie Slaughter Morton, "A Higher Standard of Morality," *WMJ* 21 (January 1910): 1–9; Maude Glasgow, "Side Lights on the Social Peril," *WMJ* 24 (July 1914): 139–43; Evangeline W. Young, "The Conservation of Manhood and Womanhood," *WMJ* 20 (March 1910): 51–52, and "The Early Corruption of Girls a Factor in Prostitution," *WMJ* 23 (October 1913): 225–27; Edith Spaulding, "Mental and Physical Factors in Prostitution," *WMJ* 24 (July 1914): 1–5; Lenna L. Meanes, "Presidential Address," *WMJ* 20 (August 1910): 161–64. See also Linda Gordon and Ellen Dubois, "Seeking Exstasy on the Battlefield: Danger and Pleasure in Nineteenth-Century Feminist Sexual Thought," *Feminist Studies* 9 (Spring 1983): 7–26, for an excellent discussion of changing feminist sexual ideology.

54. Kate Campbell Hurd-Mead, "The Medical Inspection of Schools from the Standpoint of the Physician," *WMJ* 22 (December 1912): 281–86; "What Is Being Done In Boston to Secure Medical Women as School Inspectors," *WMJ* 22 (February, March 1912): 61, 41; "Child Development," *WMJ* 17 (February 1907): 219–21.

55. WMCP *Alumnae Transactions,* 1917, p. 94–100.

56. *WMJ* 25 (May 1915): 97.

57. "Eugenics or Deficiency," *WMJ* 21 (October 1911): 216–19; Pauline Townsend-Hansen, "Eugenics," *WMJ* 21 (July 1911): 156–59; Minutes of the Medical Women's National Association meeting 25–26 May 1925, Cornell University; Isabelle Thompson Smart, "Some Potent Factors in the Seeming Increase in Mental Defects," *WMJ* 23 (December 1913): 264–67; Teresa Bannan, "Modern Motherhood," *WMJ* 15 (June 1905): 129–30; Edith Spaulding, "Mental and Physical Factors in Prostitution," *WMJ* 24 (July

1914): 1–5; Sophia Hinze Scott, "Prevention of Infant Mortality," *WMJ* 21 (July 1911): 141–44.

58. "The Medical Inspection of Schools from the Standpoint of the Physician," *WMJ* 22 (December 1912): 281–86; also Lenna Meanes, "Presidential Address," where she speaks of the "yellow peril," 162.

59. See "Protest Against the Teaching of Birth Control," *MWJ* 32 (December 1925): 320; also "Women Doctors and Social Morality," clipping in Eliza Mosher Papers, from *New York Times,* 1925, in which she says, "Many of the women who eagerly advocate birth control are too lazy to bear children and are fearful of endangering the beauty of their physical forms." Michigan Historical Collections. See also Teresa Bannan, "Modern Motherhood," *WMJ* 15 (June 1905): 129–30. Also see Brooklyn *Eagle* 4 June 1915, for a discussion of the signing by prominent physicians (headed by Abraham Jacobi) of a petition at the Academy of Medicine urging a state amendment that would no longer make it a crime for physicians to give out birth control information. Women doctors divided on the issue. Mosher came out against it, but Dr. Elizabeth Muncie, a Brooklyn colleague, supported it. See also Inez Philbrick, "The Social Causes of Criminal Abortion," *WMJ* 14 (October 1904) 221–25.

60. 15 February 1916, Children's Bureau Central Files, 191-4-1920, Box 22, National Archives.

61. One of the most prominent of these male clinicians was Robert Latou Dickinson, a Brooklyn gynecologist and early sex researcher, who published an important collection of case studies, *One Thousand Marriages,* in 1931. See Inez Philbrick, "Criminal Abortion." For more on Dickinson see James W. Reed, *From Private Vice to Public Virtue* (New York: Basic Books, 1978), 143–66; Regina Markell Morantz, "The Scientist as Sex Crusader: Alfred Kinsey and American Culture," *American Quarterly* 39 (Winter 1977): 563–89. For other examples of liberal clinicians see C. W. Malchow, "Unequalized Sexual Sense and Development the Great Cause of Domestic Infelicity and Nervousnesss in Women," *Northwestern Lancet* 23 (1903): 64–68; Malone Duggan, "The Instruction of Women on the Questions of Sex, Venereal Diseases and Early Detection of Cancer," *Texas State Journal of Medicine,* (March 1908), 286–87; G. H. Swayze, "Daughters of Eve," *Medical Times* 37 (1909): 298–303.

62. "Phimosis in the Female," *WMJ* (May 1906): 70–72, 76–77. Phimosis is "adhesion between the clitoris and the prepuce."

63. See the survey itself in the Mosher papers, Stanford University. Two sensitive though contrasting historical treatments are Carl Degler, "What Ought to Be and What Was," *American Historical Review* 79 (December 1974): 1467–90; and Rosalind Rosenberg, *Beyond Separate Spheres* (New Haven: Yale University Press, 1982), 178–97.

64. Italics mine; "Birth Control and Its Relation to Health and Welfare," *MWJ* 32 (November 1925): 268–70; see also *Bulletin of the Medical Women's National Association,* October 1928, p. 12–13, for a discussion of birth control by the Race Betterment Committee. See also the program of the "First Pennsylvania State Conference on Birth Control," at the Ritz Carleton Hotel, Philadelphia, 13 January 1922, sponsored by the American Birth Control League, in which Kate Baldwin, Lida Stewart-Coghill, Catherine MacFar-

lane, and other women physicians spoke. MacFarlane MSS, MCP Archives; "Birth Control and the Woman Physician," a talk given by Hannah Stone, M.D., who ran Sanger's Birth Control Clinical Research Bureau in New York, MCP Archives; letters from Margaret Sanger to Bertha Van Hoosen, 11 July 1933, and 4 February 1937; Lydia DeVilbiss to Van Hoosen, 12 October 1937, in Van Hoosen MSS, MCP Archives. See Alice Hamilton, *Exploring the Dangerous Trades* (Boston: Little, Brown, 1943), 110, where she talks about being drawn into the birth control movement by Dr. Yarros. There is still a great deal of information to be gleaned on the participation of women physicians, especially in running the birth control clinics, in the Sanger papers, Smith College. A number of women doctors served on the Council of the Voluntary Parenthood League, including Kate Baldwin, Mary Elizabeth Bates, Anna E. Blount, Lydia DeVilbiss, Antoinette Konikow, and Hilda H. Noyes. Stationery in Children's Bureau files, National Archives. See also Jim Reed, *From Private Vice to Public Virtue;* and Linda Gordon, *Woman's Body, Woman's Right* (New York: Viking Press, 1976).

65. Editorial, *WMJ* 19 (March 1909): 59.
66. Baker, *Fighting for Life* (New York: Macmillan, 1939), 64–107.
67. "The Division of Child Hygiene of the Department of Health of New York City," *WMJ* 20 (April 1910): 72–75, 76.
68. *Fighting for Life,* 113; "The Division of Child Hygiene of the Department of Health of New York City," 73. For opposition to midwives among women physicians see Margaret Colby, "Pregnancy and Parturition from a Woman's Point of View," *WMJ* 12 (December 1902): 272; Margaret Butler "Introductory Address" to the Medical Class of 1913, Woman's Medical College of Pennsylvania, 1913, Butler's Alumnae Folder, MCP Archives; and "Symposium on Midwifery," WMCP *Alumnae Transactions,* 1913, p. 69–90.
69. Baker, *Fighting for Life,* 113.
70. *Ibid.,* 115.
71. *Ibid.,* 115ff.
72. For a summary of this work see Rosalie Slaughter Morton, "Woman's Place in the Public Health Movement," *WMJ* 22 (April and May 1912): 83–87; 99–102. See Nancy Weiss, "The Children's Bureau: A Case Study in Women's Voluntary Networks" (Paper delivered at the Third Berkshire Conference on the History of Women, Bryn Mawr College, 9–11 June 1976; and *Save the Children: A History of the Children's Bureau* (Ph.D. diss., University of California, Los Angeles, 1974), 10, for an especially insightful study of the Bureau's work and significance, the study on which this discussion is based.
73. Kimball, Report, Children's Bureau Record Group, 102 Folder 4-0-1-1, quoted in Weiss, "The Children's Bureau," p. 12.
74. Mrs. P. S. to Julia Lathrop, Kansas City, Mo., 17 August 1919; Mrs. Max West to Mrs. P. S., 21 August 1919; Mrs. H. B. to Children's Bureau, 29 February 1916; Lathrop to Mrs. H. B., 2 March 1916. All in Children's Bureau Record Group 102, Folder 4-2-1-0, National Archives.
75. Mrs. F. G., Andrus, Wis., to Miss Gertrude B. Knipp, 1 October 1917; Mrs. Max West to Mrs. F. G., 6 October 1917; Children's Bureau Record Group 102, Folder 2-4-2-03. In her Manuscript Autobiography Mendenhall writes of having criticized the Bureau's prenatal care pamphlets as unrealistic for rural

mothers. See her discussion of her work for the Bureau, first in Washington, D.C., and then in Wisconsin. Mendenhall MSS, 55, Smith College.

76. 30 January 1917, Children's Bureau Record Group 102, Box 22, National Archives.

77. See Taylor, *The Medical Profession and Social Reform*, chapter 5.

78. Taylor, *The Medical Profession and Social Reform*, 107–9; Sheila Rothman, *Woman's Proper Place* (New York: Basic Books, 1978), 136–53; J. Stanley Lemons, *The Woman Citizen* (Urbana: University of Illinois Press, 1973), 153–80.

79. Baker, *Fighting for Life*, 138.

80. See "Report of the Accomplishments under the Maternity and Infancy Act," *MWJ* 32 (November 1925): 308–9; "Report of the Idaho Bureau of Child Hygiene," *MWJ* 33 (December 1926): 344–46; "Sheppard-Towner Work in Pennsylvania," *MWJ* 34 (June 1927): 16–18. These are just examples. See also the *Bulletin of the Medical Women's National Association*, July 1927, p. 21–22.

81. Minutes of the annual meeting of the Medical Women's National Association, 25–26 May 1925, n.p., AMWA Collection, Cornell University.

82. For a description of social therapeutics see Morris Vogel, "Machine Politics and Medical Care: The City Hospital at the Turn of the Century," Morris Vogel and Charles Rosenberg, *The Therapeutic Revolution*, 159–64. For excellent accounts of the defeminization of the Academy and of science itself see Rosalind Rosenberg, *Beyond Separate Spheres*, passim; and Margaret Rossiter, *Women Scientists in America* (Baltimore: Johns Hopkins University Press, 1983).

83. See, for example, Mary Lobdell, "Can Men and Women Doctors Be a Help to Each Other?" *WMJ* 15 (February 1905): 30–32, where she writes, "The woman doctor has come, and she has come to stay; though she has not, and I think never will come in alarmingly large numbers." See also Gertrude Baillie, "Should Professional Women Marry?" *WMJ* 2 (February 1894): 33–35.

84. Minutes of the Medical Woman's National Association meeting, June 1924, p. 18–19.

85. WMCP *Alumnae Transactions*, 1918, p. 39.

86. *Ibid.*, 21. Also a report on the work of the American Women's Hospitals, *Ibid.*, p. 42.

87. See Richard Cabot, "Women in Medicine," *JAMA* 65 (11 September 1915): 947–48; rejoinder by S. Adolphus Knopf, *WMJ* 25 (July 1916): 159–60; for newspaper accounts see Philadelphia *Record*, 3 June 1915; Philadelphia *Press*, 3 June 1915; Philadelphia *Record*, 4 June 1915; Philadelphia *Evening Bulletin*, 3 June 1915; Philadelphia *Public Ledger*, 3 June 1915; and Magazine Section of the *Public Ledger*, 20 June 1915.

88. *Bulletin of the Woman's Medical College of Pennsylvania*, January 1924, pp. 6–7. See also Avis Marion Saint, "Women in Public Service," *Public Personnel Studies* 8 (July, August, September 1930): 104–7, 119–22.

89. Diary, 1915, 1916. In the possession of her grand-niece Beatrice Beech Macleod.

90. For recent work on professionalization that does take women into account see Joan Jacobs Brumberg and Nancy Tomes, "Women in the Professions: A

Research Agenda for Historians," *Reviews in American History* 10 (June 1982): 275–96.

91. Sinclair Lewis, *Arrowsmith* (New York: Signet Classics, 1980), 213–15.
92. Charles Rosenberg, "Martin Arrowsmith: The Scientist as Hero," *American Quarterly* 15 (Fall 1963): 447–59.
93. See "Report from Kansas," Minutes of the Medical Women's National Association Meeting, June 1924, p. 47.
94. Tower to Bleumel, 15 December 1955, Box 30, Sabin MSS, Smith College.

CHAPTER 11

1. *New York Times,* 16 September 1921.
2. *Journal of the American Association of University Women* 15 (October 1921): 1–2.
3. Baker, *Fighting for Life* (New York: Macmillan, 1939), 190–91.
4. See Hamilton, *Exploring the Dangerous Trades* (Boston: Little, Brown, 1943), 252ff. Helen Taussig, another medical "star," had a similar experience with the Harvard School of Public Health. See A. McGee Harvey, *Adventures in Medical Research* (Baltimore: Johns Hopkins University Press, 1974), 232–33.
5. See tables in Appendix of Patricia M. Hummer, *The Decade of Elusive Promise, Professional Women in the United States, 1920–1930* (Ann Arbor: Research Press, 1976), 143–48; sources: "Medical Education Numbers" by year of the *Journal of the American Medical Association,* 1910–1930; U. S. Bureau of Education, "Bienneal Survey of Education," 1920–1930. See also Hummer's discussion, 61.
6. *Women in Medicine,* October 1936, p. 14.
7. *Fighting for Life,* 201.
8. Rosalie Slaughter Morton, *A Woman Surgeon* (New York: Frederick A. Stokes, 1937), Preface, vii; Baker, *Fighting for Life,* 35.
9. Alumnae *Transactions* of the Woman's Medical College of Pennsylvania, 1917, p. 78 (hereafter cited as WMCP *Alumnae Transactions*).
10. See clipping from the *New York Times,* "Medical Profession Recognizing Women Physicians on an Equal Plane," 1929, in Connie Guion MSS, Smith College; Florence Sherbon, "Women in Medicine," *Medical Woman's Journal (MWJ)* 32 (September 1925): 240–42.
11. For Sabin's comment see Madelaine R. Brown, M.D., to Elinor Bleumel, 4 October 1955, Sabin MSS, Box 30, Smith College. For a similar account by Alice Hamilton, see a letter to her sister Edith, 25 May 1918, Hamilton MSS, Schlesinger Library. Thanks to Barbara Sicherman for this reference. Also Voorhis, "The Medical Woman of the Future," *MWJ* 36 (July 1929): 174–76; Yarros, "Medical Women of Tomorrow," *MWJ* 26 (June 1916): 147. Finally Sherbon, "Women in Medicine," p. 241–2.
12. For Van Hoosen's work see "Opportunities for Medical Women Interns," *MWJ* 33 (April 1926): 102–5; *MWJ* 33 (May 1926): 126–28; *MWJ* 33 (December 1926): 341–43; "Shall Medical Women Hold Official Positions in the A.M.A.?" *MWJ* 34 (October 1927): 287–88; "Medical Opportunities for Women" *MWJ* 34 (June 1927): 173–75; "The Woman Physician—Quo Va-

dis?" *MWJ* 36 (January 1929): 1–4. For the quotation from Van Hoosen see *Bulletin of the Medical Women's National Association,* October 1930, p. 8, and July 1925, p. 19. See also "Report of Committee on Medical Opportunities for Women," Minutes of the 1929 meeting of the Medical Women's National Association (MWNA), AMWA Collection, Cornell University, Box 1, Folder 11.

13. Inez Philbrick, "Women, Let Us Be Loyal to Women!" *MWJ* 36 (February 1929): 39–42.

14. See Lois Scharf, *To Work and to Wed: Female Employment, Feminism, and the Great Depression* (Westport, Conn.: Greenwood Press, 1980), 21; Hummer, *Elusive Promise,* 113–31; William Chafe, *The American Woman* (New York: Oxford University Press, 1972), 89–132; Carl Degler, *At Odds: Women and the Family in America from the Revolution to the Present* (New York: Oxford University Press, 1980), 395–435; Estelle B. Freedman, "The New Woman: Changing Views of Women in the 1920's," *Journal of American History* 61 (September 1974): 372–93; Frank Stricker, "Cookbooks and Law Books: The Hidden History of Career Women in Twentieth-Century America." *Journal of Social History* 10 (Fall 1976): 1–19; Winifred D. Wandersee, *Women's Work and Family Values, 1920–1940* (Cambridge: Harvard University Press, 1981), 7–84.

15. Scharf, *To Work and to Wed,* 15–16, 41; Bromley, "Feminist—New Style," *Harper's Monthly Magazine,* 155 (October 1927): 552–60.

16. Ethel Puffer Howes, "Continuity for Women," *Atlantic Monthly* 130 (December 1922): 735; Anne S. Richardson, "When Mother Goes to Business," *Woman's Home Companion* 57 (December 1930): 22; Suzanne La Follette, *Concerning Women* (New York: Albert and Charles Bond, 1926), 270; Lorinne Pruette, "The Married Woman and the Part-Time Job," *Annals of the American Academy of Political and Social Science,* 143 (May 1929): 302.

17. For early attempts to combine career and family, see Joyce Antler, "Feminism as Life Process: The Life and Career of Lucy Sprague Mitchell," *Feminist Studies* 7 (Spring 1981): 134–57. See Mary Ross, "The New State of Women in America" in S. D. Schmalhausen and V. F. Calverton, eds., *Woman's Coming of Age* (New York: Horace Liveright, 1931), 546.

18. Bromley, "Feminist—New Style," 556; Luella E. Astell, "Presidential Address," *WMJ* 23 (November 1913): 241–43.

19. "Modern Homemaking in Relation to the Liberal Arts College for Women," *Journal of the American Association of University Women* 19 (October 1925): 7–8.

20. Scharf, *To Work and to Wed,* 42, 202–27; Hummer, *Elusive Promise,* 7; Lois Banner, *Women in Modern America: A Brief History,* 2d ed. (New York: Harcourt Brace, 1984), 160; Watson's comment is reprinted in an edition of *These Modern Women,* edited by Elaine Showalter (Old Westbury: Feminist Press, 1978), 144. See also John B. Watson, *Psychological Care of Infant and Child* (New York: W. W. Norton, 1928); and U. S. Department of Labor, *Are You Training Your Child to Be Happy?* (Washington, D.C.: Children's Bureau, 1928).

21. Quoted in June Sochen, *The New Woman in Greenwich Village, 1910–1920* (New York: Quadrangle, 1972), 49–50.

22. Ross, "The New State of Women," 546; Hansl, "What About the Children?

The Question of Mothers and Careers," *Harper's Monthly Magazine* 154 (January 1927): 220–27. See Elaine Showalter's sensitive and intelligent introduction to *These Modern Women,* 7. Collier, *Marriages and Careers: A Study of One Hundred Women Who are Wives, Mothers, Homemakers and Professional Women* (New York: The Channel Bookshop, 1926). See Banner, *Women in Modern America,* 154.

23. Pruette, *Women and Leisure: A Study of Social Waste* (New York: Dutton & Co., 1924); Chafe, *The American Woman,* 102.

24. Sherbon, "Women in Medicine," 242.

25. Irma Benjamin, "Marriage and Fame," Philadelphia *Public Ledger,* 17 January 1932.

26. Connie Guion to Dean Lucy Wilson of Wellesley College, 26 September 1949, Guion MSS, Box 2, Smith College; Brown, "What Medicine Offered in 1888 and Now in 1938," reprint from *Woman's City Club Magazine,* August 1838, in "Women Physicians-U.S." Box, Smith College.

27. Interview of author with Marion Fay, 11 July 1977, p. 14–15, Women in Medicine Oral History Project. See also Interview with Dr. Katherine Sturgis, 11 and 12 July 1977, p. 32 for a similar perspective. Medical College of Pennsylvania Archives (MCP).

28. For more on Dr. Arthur E. Hertzler, Koeneke's husband, see Hertzler's autobiography, *The Horse and Buggy Doctor* (Lincoln; University of Nebraska Press, 1938); Women in Medicine Oral History Project, Introductions to oral histories of Drs. Irene Koeneke, Katherine Sturgis, Natalie Shainess, Caroline Bedell Thomas, and Louise de Schweinitz, MCP Archives. See also Sherbon, "Women in Medicine," 242.

29. Interview of author with of Louise de Schweinitz, 18 and 25 February 1977, p. 42, MCP Archives.

30. See Showalter, *These Modern Women,* Introduction, 21; all citations are taken from "Men are Queer That Way: Extracts from the Diary of An Apostate Woman Physician," *Scribner's Magazine* 93 (June 1933): 365–69.

31. Information on Ulrich's later career from Scharf, *To Work and to Wed,* 126. Interestingly, Ulrich worked in the 1920s with Dr. Valeria Parker, another social hygiene activist who explained why she never practiced: "I am a graduate physician; but because I married another graduate physician who didn't want his wife to practice, at the time when I should have been practicing, I was taking care of my babies." Minutes of the Medical Women's National Association, 1924, p. 55, AMWA Collection, Cornell University.

32. Edith Clark, "Trying to be Modern," *Nation,* 125 (1927): 153–55; Pruette, "Why Women Fail," Schmalhausen and Calverton, *Woman's Coming of Age,* 23.

33. Frank Stricker argues that jobs in these latter areas actually increased in the 1920s and that the growth demonstrated women's continued interest in work and their dissatisfaction with uninterrupted domesticity. See "Cookbooks and Lawbooks," *passim.*

34. See "Medical Education in the U.S." *JAMA* 57 (19 August 1911): 655; F. C. Zapffe, "Analysis of Entrance Credentials Presented by Freshmen Admitted in 1929," *Journal of the American Association of Medical Colleges* 5 (July 1930): 231; "Medical Education in the United States," *JAMA* 95 (16 August 1930): 504; N. P. Colwell, "Present Needs in Medical Education," *JAMA* 82

(15 March 1924): 839; Rosemary Stevens, *American Medicine and the Public Interest* (New Haven: Yale University Press, 1971), *passim*. The higher numbers of women reflected temporary increases during the World Wars. See appropriate "Medical Education in the U.S." numbers by year in *JAMA*.

35. "Women in Medicine," 240–41.

36. Oral Interview of Dr. Katherine Sturgis, 38; Oral Interview of Dr. Pauline Stitt, 9 December 1977, p. 26–32; both in MCP Archives.

37. "Self-Help for College Students," U.S. Dept. of the Interior, Bureau of Education, Bulletin no. 2, 1929, p. 58–61.

38. WMCP *Alumnae Transactions*, 1918, p. 62.

39. U.S. Dept. of Interior, Bureau of Education, "Scholarships and Fellowships: Grants Available in the United States Colleges and Universities," Bull. no. 15, 1931, p. 93–96, cited in Hummer, *Elusive Promise*, 63; Chase Going Woodhouse, "Opportunities for Women in the Medical Profession, Report of a Conference on Opportunities for Women in the Medical Profession and the Selection of Medical Students," *Bulletin of the Woman's Medical College of Pennsylvania* 88 (May 1938): 10. See also Martha Tracy's Report, WMCP *Alumnae Transactions*, 1918, p. 62.

40. See Martha Tracy, "Greetings," Conference on Opportunities for Women in the Medical Profession," *WMCP Bulletin*, 4; F. C. Zapffe, "Analysis of Entrance Credentials Presented by Freshmen Admitted in 1929," 233–34; Burton D. Meyers, "Report on Application for Matriculation in Schools of Medicine in the United States and Canada, 1929–1930," American Association of Medical Colleges *Journal* 5 (March 1930): 65–66.

41. Meyers, "Report," 87–88. For distribution of acceptances, see Education Numbers of *JAMA* for the appropriate years. See also Arthur C. Curtis, M.D., "The Woman as a Student of Medicine," *Bulletin* of the Association of American Medical Colleges (AAMC), 2 (April 1927): 140–48.

42. Elizabeth Etheridge, "Grace Goldsmith," in *Notable American Women: The Modern Period*, eds. Barbara Sicherman and Carol Hurd Green (Cambridge: Harvard University Press, 1980), 284–85; Tracy, "What Has Become of Women Graduates in Medicine," *Bulletin* of the AAMC 2 (March 1927): 53.

43. See A. C. Curtis, "The Woman as a Student of Medicine"; Van Hoosen, "Quo Vadis," 2; Brown to Sabin, 15 January 1922, Sabin MSS, American Philosophical Society; *Bulletin of the Woman's Medical College of Pennsylvania*, 73 (January 1923): 6.

44. Tracy, "Greetings," 4–5; Hummer, *Elusive Promise*, 65; Carol Lopate, *Women in Medicine* (Baltimore, Johns Hopkins, 1968), 93–94; Davis G. Johnson and Edwin B. Hutchings, "Doctor or Dropout? A Study of Medical Student Attrition," *Journal of Medical Education* 41 (1966): 1107–1204.

45. *Bulletin* of the MWNA, October 1928, p. 10; WMCP *Alumnae Transactions*, 1929, p. 27.

46. 27 September 1922, National Women's Party MSS, Reel 17, Schlesinger Library. Thanks to Barbara Sicherman for the citation.

47. On standards, see Eleanor M. Hiestand-Moore, "Reform in the Government Medical Schools" WMCP *Alumnae Transactions*, 1896, p. 65ff.; Inez C. Philbrick, "Medical Colleges and Professional Standards," *JAMA* (15 June 1901) 1700–1702; Helen MacMurchey, "Medical Women and Hospital Appointments," *WMJ* 11 (August 1901): 307; Editorial, "Hospital Opportunities for

Women," *WMJ* 20 (January 1910): 17; Mary Sutton Macy, "Medical Women—In History and Present Day Practice," *WMJ* 27 (April 1917): 86.

48. Van Hoosen, "Opportunities for Women Interns," *MWJ* 33 (March, April, May 1926): 65 and *passim,* Sturgis File, letters dated 6 July 1918, 20 July 1918, and 24 October 1918, MCP Archives.

49. Oral Interview of Louise de Schweinitz, 34–35, MCP Archives.

50. Richards to Elinor Bleumel, 10 September 1955, Box 30, Sabin MSS, Smith College.

51. Eliot to parents, 13 June 1920, Eliot MSS, Schlesinger Library.

52. Interview of author with of Alma Dea Morani, 19 and 21 January 1977, p. 34–35, MCP Archives; Van Hoosen, "Opportunities for Medical Women Interns," *MWJ* 33 (December 1926): 342.

53. Scharf, *To Work and to Wed,* 84–85, 91.

54. Interview of author with Marion Fay, Ph.D., 11 July 1977, p. 7, MCP Archives, Robert S. and Helen M. Lynd, *Middletown in Transition* (New York: Harcourt Brace, 1937), 57.

55. "President's Annual Report," *Women in Medicine,* October 1939, p. 17, 19; *ibid.,* April 1936, p. 12; July 1936, p. 13; July 1939, p. 12; January 1941, p. 8; July 1941, p. 25. See also *Bulletin of the MWNA,* July 1933, p. 16.

56. "Report of the Regional Director for New England," AMWA MSS, Box 10, Folder 4, Cornell University. See also letters to the Medical Women of Connecticut from Mead, 14 August 1930, 20 March 1930; Mead to Dr. M. May Allen, 19 November 1929; Elvenor Ernest to Louise Tayler-Jones, 23 October 1930, 21 May 1930; and to Dr. Sylvia Allen, 17 December 1931; and to Rosa Gantt, 15 April 1932, AMWA MSS, Box 10, Folder 10, and Box 4, Folder 31. See the rest of Box 10, especially folders 5, 8, 16, for other information regarding membership drives. Also see Box 12, Folder 31. All in AMWA MSS, Cornell University.

57. *Journal of the American Medical Women's Association (JAMWA)* 4 (May 1949): 198; Editorial, *JAMWA* 2 (September 1947): 410; Philbrick Questionnaire, 1944, Philbrick File; Mabel Gardner to Catherine MacFarlane, 4 February 1942, Macfarlane MSS, both in MCP Archives.

58. Interview of author with Harriet Hardy, 13 and 14 October 1977, p. 56; Interview with Harriet Dustan, 4 and 5 April 1977, p. 43–44; Interview wtih Katherine Sturgis, 77; Interview with Caroline Bedell Thomas, 71; Interview with Louise de Schweinitz, 101; Interview with Esther Bridgeman Clark, 19 December 1977, 33; Interview with Beryl Michaelson, 27 July 1977, 55. All in Women in Medicine Oral History Project, MCP Archives.

59. Editorial, *JAMWA* 1 (May 1946): 39; *JAMWA* 11 (September 1956): 323 for sample "program" for the year. See also "Message from the President," *Women in Medicine,* October 1940, p. 7; Emily Dunning Barringer, "Nineteen Forty-One and the Woman Doctor," and "Address of the Retiring President," in *Women in Medicine,* July 1941, p. 8–22, 23–27.

60. See Florence Del. Lowther and Helen R. Downes, "Women in Medicine," *JAMA* 129 (13 October 1945): 512–14; "Women in Medicine," *JAMWA* 1 (June 1946): 93–95; "Editorial," *JAMWA* 1 (October 1946): 201–2. See also Hulda Thelander, "Opportunities for Medical Women," *JAMWA* 3 (February 1948): 67.

61. "The American Woman Physician: Doorway to the Second Century,"

JAMWA 19 (January 1964): 45–49; "Symposium: Medical WomanPower—Can it be Used More Efficiently?" *JAMWA* 17 (December 1962): 973–85, see especially comments of Dr. Toby Helfand and follow-up letter to the editor and comment "More on Physician Mothers," in *JAMWA* 19 (April 1964): 311. Also the report on "Psychiatric Residency Training for Physician Mothers: A Progress Report," *JAMWA* 19 (April 1964): 311.

62. Chafe, *The American Woman*, 199–245; Barbara Easton, "Feminism and the Contemporary Family," *Socialist Review* 8 (May–June 1978): 11–36; *JAMA* 240 (22/29 December 1978): 2822–23.

63. Also interesting to note was the fact that Rose wrote about the request to Florence Sabin—a research scientist who had no connection with the obstetrical field whatsoever—presumably because Sabin was one of the few women physicians she could think of who had an honored reputation among men physicians. See Rose to Sabin, 22 December 1926. Sabin would have none of the idea, and was justifiably annoyed. Sabin to Rose, 31 December 1926, Sabin MSS, American Philosophical Society.

64. Nellie S. Noble, "A Message from the President: War Service." *Women in Medicine,* October 1939, p. 24; "Our Part in National Defense," and "Legislative," *Women in Medicine,* October 1940, p. 24–25; "Report of the Retiring President," *Women in Medicine,* July 1942, p. 17; "Report of Committee on Army Resolutions," *Women in Medicine,* July 1939, p. 18; Emily Dunning Barringer, "Nineteen Forty-One and the Woman Doctor," "Report of the Retiring President," *Women in Medicine,* July 1942, p. 17, 25; "President's Message," *ibid.,* January 1943, p. 12; "Our Cause in Congress," *ibid.,* April 1943, p. 8–9; Emily Dunning Barringer, "Commissions for Women Physicians," *ibid.,* July 1943, pp. 11–14; "Women Physicians in the Army of the United States, *ibid.,* October 1945, pp. 7–9; "Women Physicians Commissioned in the Armed Services as of September 1, 1944," *ibid.,* October 1944, p. 16; "Report by Elizabeth Mason-Hohl, *ibid.,* January 1945, p. 19.

65. Baker, "Presidential Address," *Women in Medicine,* July 1936, pp. 12–14; "New Business," *ibid.,* July 1939, p. 19; Barringer, "A Step Forward on a Difficult Quest," *ibid.,* October 1939, p. 23–24.

66. Observer status allows the representative to present reports and evaluate policy, but not to vote. Interview of author with Carol Davis-Grossman, Executive Director of AMWA, 20 April 1984.

67. *JAMWA* 19 (January 1964): 56–57; Interview with Carol Davis-Grossman.

68. For the lack of interest in AMWA of interviewees of the Women in Medicine Oral History Project who graduated from medical school during the 1950s and early 1960s see the transcripts of Frances Conley, 20 June 1977, p. 61; Ann Barnes, 29 September 1977, p. 61; Grace Holmes, 25 and 28 February 1977, p. 80; Florence Haseltine, 8 August 1977, p. 102; and Gillian Karatinos, 29 October 1977, p. 62, MCP Archives. See also Lopate, *Women in Medicine,* 17.

69. Interview of author with Dr. Clair M. Callan, presently president of AMWA, 15 January 1985; Interview with Carol Davis-Grossman.

70. See, for example, Kathleen Lusk Brooke, "Drs. Carol & Ted Nadelson on Dual-Career Marriage," *JAMWA* 37 (November 1982): 292–304; Adele N. Brodkin et al., "Parenting and Professionalism—A Medical School Elective," *JAMWA* 37 (October 1982): 227–330; Serena-Lynn Brown and Robert Klein,

"Woman-Power in the Medical Hierarchy," *JAMWA* 37 (June 1982): 155–64; Marcia Angell, "Juggling the Personal and Professional Life," *JAMWA* 37 (March 1982): 64–68; Jean Hamilton and Barbara Parry, "Sex-Related Differences in Clinical Drug Response: Implications for Women's Health," *JAMWA* 38 (September/October 1983): 126–32.

71. *Medical Education in the United States* reprint, (New York: Arno Press, 1972), 178–79.

72. For a fine account of the transformation of the hospital as an institution from a charitable to a business enterprise see David Rosner, *A Once Charitable Enterprise, Hospitals and Health Care in Brooklyn and New York* (New York: Cambridge University Press, 1983). See also Charles Rosenberg, "The Hospital in America: A Century's Perspective," in *Medicine and Society: Contemporary Medical Problems in Historical Perspective* (Philadelphia: American Philosophical Society, 1971), and "From Almshouse to Hospital: The Shaping of Philadelphia General Hospital," *Health and Society* 60 (1982): 108–54; Virginia Drachman, *Hospital With a Heart: Women Doctors and the Paradox of Separatism at the New England Hospital, 1862–1969* (Ithaca: Cornell University Press, 1984).

73. See Helena Wall, "Feminism and the New England Hospital," *American Quarterly* 32 (Fall 1980): 435–52, for an excellent analysis of this last decade. For a more detailed summary of the hospital's difficulties in the first half of the twentieth century, see Drachman, *Hospital with a Heart*, chap. 7.

74. Faxon Report, 2; NEH Trustees to Staff, Circular letter, 5 November 1951; all in Blanche Ames MSS, Schlesinger Library. cited in Wall, "Feminism," 439.

75. This was a solution which many women's hospitals eventually were forced to take. The Northwestern Hospital in Minneapolis merged with the Abbott Hospital to become the Abbott-Northwestern Hospital in 1970, and the New York Infirmary joined with Beekman Hospital in 1979.

76. Ames to Narcissa Vanderlip, 26 May 1961, Margaret Noyes Kleinert MSS, Schlesinger Library; Ames to New Corporation members, n.d. (probably October/November 1953), Blanche Ames MSS, Schlesinger Library. Wall, "Feminism," 445.

77. Nelson to Potter, 27 November 1951; Blanche Ames MSS, Schlesinger Library; Wall, "Feminism," 449.

78. "Womanly Attributes . . . Application to Medicine and the Hospital," Blanche Ames MSS, Schlesinger Library; Wall, "Feminism," 444. Drachman, *Hospital with a Heart*, 211.

79. Interview with Marion Fay, 11 July 1977; 8, 13; Interview with Katherine Sturgis, 9; Women in Medicine Oral History Project, MCP Archives. See also Ellen C. Potter, M.D., acting president, "Report to the Alumnae Association," 1941, Potter MSS, MCP Archives.

80. Lopate, *Women in Medicine,* 91; Johnson and Hutchins, "Doctor or Dropout?" 1159. The college trained roughly 25 percent of women medical graduates between 1905–1910, 20 percent between 1912–1921, and 10 percent in the 1930s. In 1964 Catherine Macfarlane estimated that 6 percent of women physicians were trained by the school. See Martha Tracy, "Women Graduates in Medicine," *passim,* and Dr. Catherine Macfarlane, "The Woman's Medi-

cal College of Pennsylvania," *Transactions & Studies of the College of Physicians of Philadelphia*, 33 (July 1965): 41.

81. Potter to Jean Strump, n.d. but ca. 1950, Potter MSS, MCP Archives. AMWA felt similarly about the New York Infirmary and other women's institutions. See Proceedings of the 13th Annual Meeting, 1927, p. 41–48, AMWA MSS, Cornell University: *Bulletin of the Medical Women's National Association*, April 1926, p. 19; Mrs. Frank Vanderlip, "Are Special Provisions Necessary for Women Physicians Today," *Women in Medicine*, July 1940, p. 8–11.

82. Margaret Craighill to Florence Sabin, 1 April 1941, Sabin MSS, American Philosophical Society. See also *Women in Medicine*, October 1936, p. 20; Emily Dunning Barringer, "Address Delivered at the Eighty-Seventh Opening of the Medical College of Pennsylvania," *Women in Medicine*, October 1937, p. 19; *ibid.*, October 1940, p. 18; *ibid.*, April 1941, p. 25.

83. Oral Interview with Marion Fay, 7, 17 MCP Archives; Craighill to Sabin, 1 April 1941, Sabin MSS, APS; Sabin to Louise Pearce, 17 March 1942; Pearce to Sabin, 18 March 1943; all in Sabin MSS, American Philosophical Society.

84. Interview with Marion Fay, 19–20, 21–22, MCP Archives.

85. *Ibid.*, 22–25. See also "Report on the Woman's Medical College of Pennsylvania," *JAMWA* 1 (June 1946): 28.

86. Interview with Marion Fay, 39; Interview with Alma Morani, 89–91; Interview with Katherine Sturgis, 72–74 MCP Archives. Catherine Macfarlane to Margaret Noyes Kleinert, 17 April 1964: "The situation is even worse now. The latest College catalogue lists 292 officers of instruction—192 men and one hundred women. What would Dr. Van Hoosen say?" Kleinert MSS, Schlesinger Library. See supportive material on file with Fay interview, MCP Archives, especially notes of my interview with Dr. Morani, 4 April 1977; and interview with Charles Glanville, vice president in charge of planning and development in the late 1960s, n.d.

87. Interview with Alma Morani, 90–92; Interview with Katherine Sturgis, 73, MCP Archives; Mary Riggs Noble to Margaret Noyes Kleinert, 15 September 1951; Catherine Macfarlane to Dr. Teresa McGovern, 10 May 1964; all in Kleinert MSS, Schlesinger Library.

88. Interview of author with Dr. Marjorie Wilson, 1 November 1977, p. 73–74, Women in Medicine Oral History Project, MCP Archives.

89. Interview with Marion Fay, 42–49; Interview with Charles Glanville, n.d., pp. 1–2, MCP Archives.

90. Information on faculty was gathered by counting female faculty listed in catalogues and announcements for appropriate years. Information on the percentage of male students was provided by the college's registrar office in June 1984.

91. Interview with Marion Fay, 49. Interview with Alma Morani, 92. MCP Archives. For alumnae responses see Margaret Noyes Kleinert to Mrs. Keiner, 3 September 1969, Kleinert MSS, Schlesinger Library; and Viola Erlanger to Mrs. Kaiser, 22 August 1961, Erlanger file, MCP Archives.

92. "Barnard Alumnae in Medicine," *Barnard Alumnae Magazine*, Fall 1977, p. 41. In addition, see my interview with Dr. Joni Magee, also one of the last to attend the school as a woman's institution, 1 April 1977, pp. 25–27, Women in Medicine Oral History Project, MCP Archives.

CHAPTER 12

1. William Chafe, *The American Woman,* (New York: Oxford University Press, 1972), 218–19; Robert W. Smuts, *Women and Work in America* (New York: Columbia University Press, 1959), 36–37, 63–64.

2. J. A. Wilson Keyes, M. P., and J. Becker, "The Forecast of Medical Education: Forecast of the Council of Deans," *Journal of Medical Education* 50 (March 1975): 319–27; Judith B. Braslow and Marilyn Heins, "Women in Medical Education, A Decade of Change," *New England Journal of Medicine* 304 (7 May 1981): 1129–35. See also Marilyn Heins, M.D. "Update: Women in Medicine," forthcoming in *JAMWA,* Fall, 1985.

3. Harry Braverman, *Labor and Monopoly Capital, The Degradation of Work in the Twentieth Century* (London: Monthly Review Press, 1974), 271–83.

4. Peter Filene, *Him/Her/Self* (New York: New American Library, 1974), 172–74; Mary Ross, "Shall We Join the Gentlemen?" *Survey* 57 (1 December 1926): 263–66; Robert S. and Helen M. Lynd, *Middletown: A Study in Contemporary American Culture* (New York: Harcourt, Brace, 1929), 83–85; Winifred Wandersee, *Women's Work and Family Values, 1929–1940* (Cambridge: Harvard University Press, 1981), especially 7–26; Lois Scharf, *To Work and to Wed: Female Employment, Feminism, and the Great Depression* (Westport, Conn.: Greenwood Press, 1980), 39–42; Valerie Kincade Oppenheimer, *The Female Labor Force in the United States* (Berkeley: University of California Press, 1970), 25–63.

5. "The New Feminists: Revolt Against 'Sexism,' " *Time* 94 (21 November 1969): 53–56; "Women's Lib: The War on 'Sexism' " *Time* 94 (31 August 1970): 71–78; Francine Klagsburn, ed., *The First MS Reader* (New York: *Ms.* Magazine, 1973), 262–72; "A Personal Report," *Ms.* 1 (July 1972).

6. For a very helpful discussion of these issues see Barbara Melosh, "*The Physician's Hand*": *Work Culture and Conflict in American Nursing* (Philadelphia: Temple University Press, 1982), 15–27. See, for example, Amitai Etzioni, ed., *The Semi-Professions and Their Organization* (New York: Free Press, 1969); William J. Goode, "Community within a Community: The Professions," *American Sociological Review* 22 (April 1957): 194–200; Ernest Greenwood, "Elements of Professionalization," in Howard Volmer and Donald Mills, eds., *Professionalization* (Englewood Cliff, N. J.: Prentice Hall, 1960); Talcott Parsons, "Professions and Social Structure," *Social Forces* 12 (May 1939): 450–62; and William J. Goode, "Encroachment, Charlatanism, and the Emerging Profession: Psychology, Medicine, and Sociology," *American Sociological Review* 25 (April 1960): 902–14.

7. See Rosner and Markowitz, "Doctors in Crisis: Medical Education and Medical Reform During the Progressive Era, 1895–1915," *American Quarterly* 25 (March 1973): 83–107; see also E. Richard Brown, *Rockefeller Medicine Men: Medicine and Capitalism in America* (Berkeley: University of California Press, 1979); Megali Larson, *The Rise of Professionalism* (Berkeley: University of California Press, 1977); Burton J. Bledstein, *The Culture of Professionalism* (New York: W. W. Norton, 1978).

8. Eliot Friedson, *Profession of Medicine* (New York: Dodd, Mead, 1970). Paul Starr has recently argued that corporate medicine threatens to challenge the

authority and autonomy of doctors in *The Social Transformation of American Medicine* (New York: Basic Books, 1982), 379–449.

9. Rose Laub Coser and Gerald Rokoff, "Women in the Occupational World: Social Disruption and Conflict," *Social Problems* 18 (Spring 1971): 548. See also Cynthia Fuchs Epstein, "Encountering the Male Establishment: Sex Status Limits on Women's Careers in the Professions," *American Journal of Sociology* 75 (May 1975): 965–82, and *Woman's Place: Options and Limits in Professional Careers* (Berkeley: University of California Press, 1970), 151–98; Arlie Russell Hochschild, "Emotion Work, Feeling Rules and Social Structure," *American Journal of Sociology* 85 (May 1979): 551–75.

10. "Women in Science, Why so Few?" *Science* 148 (April–June 1965): 1196–1202.

11. Dorothy Rosenthal Mandelbaum, *Work, Marriage and Motherhood: The Career Persistence of Female Physicians* (New York: Praeger, 1981), 6–7; H. Westling-Wikstrand, M. Monk, and C. B. Thomas, "Some Characteristics Related to the Career Status of Women Physicians," *Johns Hopkins Medical Journal* 127 (November 1970): 273–86; Lynne Davidson, "Choice by Constraint: The Selection and Function of Specialties among Women Physicians-in-Training," *Journal of Health Politics* 4 (Summer 1979): 200–219; "Symposium: Medical WomanPower—Can it be Used More Efficiently?" *JAMWA* 17 (December 1962): 973–85.

12. Mandelbaum, *Work, Marriage and Motherhood*, p. 32; Davidson, "Choice by Constraint," Marjorie Wilson and Amber Jones, "Career Patterns of Women in Medicine," in *Women in Medicine—1976:* Carolyn Speiler, ed., *Report of a Macy Conference* (New York: Josiah Macy, Jr., Foundation, 1977), 67–87.

13. Carol Gilligan, *In a Different Voice* (Cambridge: Harvard University Press, 1983), 174. For parallel or complementary arguments from other disciplines see Jean Bethke Elshtain, *Public Man, Private Woman: Women in Social and Political Thought* (Princeton: Princeton University Press, 1981); Nancy Chodorow, *The Reproduction of Mothering* (Berkeley: University of California Press, 1978); Lillian Rubin, *Intimate Strangers* (New York: Harper & Row, 1983); Carol McMillan, *Women, Reason and Nature* (Princeton: Princeton University Press, 1982).

14. For an interesting and perceptive feminist critique of what Anita Fellman has termed "maternal feminism" and Judith Stacey has labeled the "new conservative feminism," see Stacey, "The New Conservative Feminism," *Feminist Studies* 9 (Fall 1983): 559–84. See also Judith Lorber, "Minimalist and Maximalist Feminist Ideologies and Strategies for Change," *Quarterly Journal of Ideology* 5 (Fall 1981): 61–66.

15. "A Woman's Health School?" *Social Policy* 6 (September/October 1975): 50–53.

16. "Female Doctors Assess the Problems of Their Profession," *New York Times,* 12 October 1979; Carlotta M. Rinke, M.D., "The Professional Identities of Women Physicians," *JAMA* 245 (19 June 1981): 2419–21. See also Elizabeth Morgan, *The Making of a Woman Surgeon* (New York: Berkeley Books, 1981), 287 and *passim;* Michelle Harrison, *A Woman in Residence* (New York: Random House, 1982); Commentary, "Women in Medicine:

Two Points of View, I. The Future of Women Physicians, II. Medicine and Motherhood," *JAMA* 249 (14 January 1983): 207–10.

17. Commentary, "Women in Medicine: II. Medicine and Motherhood," 204–11; Marcia Angell, "Juggling the Personal and Professional Life," *JAMWA* 37 (March 1982): 64–68, and "Women in Medicine: Beyond Prejudice," *New England Journal of Medicine* 304 (7 May 1981): 1161–62; M. Heins et al., "Productivity of Women Physicians," *JAMA* 236 (October 1976): 1961–64, and "Medicine and Motherhood," *JAMA* 249 (14 January 1983): 209–10.

18. Adele N. Brodkin et al., "Parenting and Professionalism—A Medical School Elective," *JAMWA* 37 (October 1982): 227–30. See also, for example, Robert M. Veatch and K. Danner Clouser, "New Mix in the Medical Curriculum," *Prism,* November 1973, 1–5; "The Hard Facts," *Second Century Radcliffe News,* April 1984, p. 19.

19. Josephine J. Williams, "The Woman Physician's Dilemma," *Journal of Social Issues* 6 (1950): 38–45; C. Nadelson and M. Notman, "The Woman Physician," *Journal of Medical Education* 47 (March 1972): 176–83; Editorials, "What Women Want in Medicine Most—Power," *Medical News,* 18 February 1980; "Female Doctors Assess the Problems of Their Profession," *New York Times,* 12 October 1971; Marilyn Heins, M.D., "Women Physicians," *Radcliffe Quarterly,* June 1979, 11–14; Mary Jane Gray and Judith Tyson, "Evolution of a Women's Clinic: An Alternate System of Medical Care," *American Journal of Obstetrics and Gynecology* 126 (1 December 1976): 760–68; Editorials—"Women in Surgery," *Archives in Surgery* 102 (March 1971): 234–35; Carol Nadelson and Malka Notman, "Success or Failure: Women as Medical School Applicants," *JAMWA* 29 (April 1974): 167–72; Esther Haar, M.D., et al., "Factors Related to the Preference for a Female Gynecologist," *Medical Care* 13 (September 1975): 782–90; "An Interview with Dr. Estelle Ramey," *Perspectives in Biology and Medicine* 14 (Spring 1971): 424–31; Kathleen Farrell et al., "Women Physicians in Medical Academia," *JAMA* 241 (29 June 1979): 2808–12.

20. Brodkin, "Parenting and Professionalism," 227.

21. "The Hard Facts," *Second Century Radcliffe News,* April 1984, p. 19.

22. Editorial, "What Women Want in Medicine Most—Power," *Medical News* 18 February 1980; "Female Doctors Assess the Problems of Their Profession," *New York Times* 12 October 1979.

Index